Innovation and Tradition

at the University of Pennsylvania School of Medicine

DAVID Y. COOPER III
MARSHALL A. LEDGER

UNIVERSITY OF PENNSYLVANIA PRESS   Philadelphia

upp

Innovation

AND Tradition

AT THE UNIVERSITY
OF PENNSYLVANIA
SCHOOL OF MEDICINE

An Anecdotal Journey

Library of Congress Cataloging-in-Publication Data

Cooper, David Y., 1924–
   Innovation and tradition at the University of Pennsylvania School
of Medicine: an anecdotal journey/David Y. Cooper III, Marshall
A. Ledger.
     p.   cm.
   Includes bibliographical references.
   ISBN 0-8122-8242-6
   1. University of Pennsylvania. School of Medicine—History.
2. Medical colleges—Pennsylvania—Philadelphia—History.
I. Ledger, Marshall A. II. Title.
   [DNLM: 1. University of Pennsylvania. School of Medicine.
2. Schools, Medical—history—Philadelphia. W 19 C776i]
R747.U6837C66 1990
610'.71'174811—dc20
DNLM/DLC
for Library of Congress   90-12050
                                                                CIP

Design: Adrianne Onderdonk Dudden

This history is dedicated to
Cynthia, Lucy, and Allison
all gifts to me from the School of Medicine
of the University of Pennsylvania

and

To Martha, Kate, and Gabe Ledger

Be not dispirited at the difficulties which present, or obstacles you are to encounter. Let them serve rather as a spur to your industry. They will not stand in the way of men who are determined to surmount all opposition to their course. Regard them as left by others for you to master. Was there no difficulty remaining, you would have less scope for a genius of investigation; less honor in being barely followers of others. Both science and honor offer one fate to their votaries. They reward the courage of the brave and of the steady, and repel the fainthearted and irresolute. You have an ample field before you to cultivate. Inspired by a love of science, your diligent inquiry into natural causes and effects must produce discoveries and these discoveries prompt you with fresh alacrity to new researches; an employment as delightful and honorable as it is advantageous.

John Morgan, Charge to the Students. A Discourse Upon the Institution of Medical Schools in America

CONTENTS

FOREWORD   *Arthur K. Asbury*   ix

FOREWORD   *Jonathan E. Rhoads*   xi

PREFACE   *David Y. Cooper III*   xiii

PREFACE   *Marshall A. Ledger*   xv

ACKNOWLEDGMENTS   xvii

Introduction: History Rounds   1

1   Stirrings of Organized Medical Education   5

2   Early Teachers and Scientists   11

3   Conditions of Learning   29

4   The First Wave of Nineteenth-Century Luminaries   45

5   Creating a Change or Reacting to It   67

6   The Start of Several Modern Departments   87

7   A Chair for Surgery   115

8   Specialized Institutes   123

9   Reform, Gentlemanly and Otherwise   137

10   A New Building and New Research Groups in Surgery and Dermatology   145

11   Mergers and Graduate Education   167

12   Establishing Twentieth-Century Practice of Science   175

13   Science and Practice: The Next Phase   191

14   The Maloney Constellation and a Severe
      Self-Examination   211

15   Medical Physics   229

16   Discoveries That Turned into Household Names   243

17   Research During World War II and Afterwards   261

18   Advances in Pennsylvania's Pediatric Service at the Children's
      Hospital of Philadelphia   277

19   Introduction to the Modern Era   289

      APPENDIX I   *Leaders of the University of Pennsylvania School
                        of Medicine*   305
      APPENDIX II   *Buildings of the School of Medicine*   329
      APPENDIX III   *Buildings of the Hospital of the University of
                        Pennsylvania*   331
      INDEX   337

FOREWORD

The University of Pennsylvania School of Medicine celebrates in 1990 the 225th anniversary of its 1765 origin. This date coincides, as it always must, with the anniversary of the founding of the parent University of Pennsylvania, in this instance 250 years ago in 1740. As most know, the School of Medicine at Penn is the oldest medical school in the United States.

It is fitting that the publication of this book on the history of the School of Medicine also falls in 1990. That it does so is no accident. Intensive planning for the occasion of the 225th anniversary began over two years ago and includes another book (a pictorial history of medicine in Philadelphia); ceremonial dedication of the new Clinical Research Building erected on the Old Blockley site; a large celebratory event for students, house staff, faculty, and alumni in October 1990 at the Philadelphia Zoo; and many lectures, symposia, and colloquia. Credit must be given to those who have worked so hard to make all these plans happen, particularly Dr. Alfred P. Fishman, William Maul Measey Professor Emeritus of Medicine, and Dr. Fredric C. Burg, professor of pediatrics and vice dean for medical education.

Innovation and Tradition at the University of Pennsylvania School of Medicine: An Anecdotal Journey has its own story. The seeds of the project took root a number of years ago in the mind of David Y. Cooper III, M.D. Dr. Cooper, professor of surgical research, has been interested in the history of the School of Medicine since he was a student here in the 1940s. He browsed endlessly over the historical material available, gathering anecdotes and historical tidbits and verifying each detail painstakingly. Reams of draft manuscript were produced. Marshall A. Ledger, Ph.D., editor of the highly regarded *Penn Medicine* alumni magazine, wove together the many threads of this tale into finished cloth. The emphasis is on the people who made the school important and had a major effect on the course and direction of American medicine and the sum of biomedical knowledge.

Each chapter highlights some of the heroes of our past, recounting their skills and contributions and their foibles and failings. Altogether the story of the school is told in compelling fashion. Doctors Cooper and Ledger are to be congratulated.

When I first came to the University of Pennsylvania nearly sixteen years ago as chair of the Department of Neurology, I was struck by two highly positive features of the School of Medicine. First, the ease of communication and collaboration across departmental and discipline lines was remarkable and, parenthetically, quite different from the institutions with which I had been previously connected. Second, there were virtually no constraints imposed by the past on day-to-day activities. I had expected to be nearly suffocated by tradition, but astonishingly the processes and procedures of the past were relics only, and the concepts of and methods by which we conducted our professional affairs frequently had to be invented anew. This fact suggests that our institutional memory is short. If so, and there is abundant evidence that institutions have short memories, it is doubly important that we preserve in formal ways the knowledge of our past. This book by Cooper and Ledger does just that.

ARTHUR K. ASBURY, M.D.
Van Meter Professor of Neurology
Acting Dean, School of Medicine
Acting Executive Vice President of the Medical Center
University of Pennsylvania

September 1989

FOREWORD

Since its origin in 1765, the School of Medicine of the University of Pennsylvania has grown from a tiny medical college with two professors teaching only the theory and practice of medicine, anatomy, midwifery, and surgery to a giant, multidisciplinary institution.

Over its long history, the school's faculty have accomplished a great deal. Not only have they excelled in medical teaching but they have also developed new institutions for medical research, for clinical teaching, and for care of patients, while making original contributions to medical science. In the following pages the "transactions and studies" of the medical professors from the school's founding until the first half of the twentieth century are told. The story is stopped here because the pace of scientific research has increased to such an extent that to describe these new discoveries adequately would require another volume equal in length to this one.

Although many important discoveries in medical science have been made at Pennsylvania, all too frequently, good ideas have originated but have not been followed through and implemented. A possible reason is limited financial support and facilities; however, it is also possible that some of the failures resulted from the lack of courage and conviction in the medical faculty.

Be that as it may, it has not been the policy of the School of Medicine throughout its history to buy talent from other institutions, but rather to develop its own. Thus one of the school's most important accomplishments has been developing the scientific and clinical talent that has entered the faculties of every medical school in the United States, to flower elsewhere than at Pennsylvania. An index of the success of this policy is that Pennsylvania-born-and-nurtured department chairmen are found in every medical school in the country.

The most important fact that one gains from this study of the School of Medicine is that accomplishments, all too frequently done in limited facilities, have been possible because the trustees and the medical professors have maintained an environment which is free—in which the faculty can interact with each other, think, and pursue their ideas.

JONATHAN E. RHOADS, M.D.
Professor of Surgery

PREFACE: HISTORICAL SURPRISES

This book was not commissioned, nor was the author assigned the task of writing a history of the School of Medicine of the University of Pennsylvania. The idea to write this history arose after I read the critique of a grant request to the National Institutes of Health, which gave my proposal an unfundable priority score. The reviewers' criticisms of the proposed experiments were so contrary to concepts that I thought lead to great discoveries that I wondered what factors are involved in making scientific advances. Realizing that a number of important advances in medical science had been made from time to time by my colleagues at the University of Pennsylvania School of Medicine, I decided to examine systematically how these scientists' ideas originated and their advances were made.

What I thought would be a relatively easy task soon became a complex one, for I soon found that, in addition to the many scientific contributions made by the faculty, the School of Medicine had a history that was richer and more distinguished than I or anyone I talked with realized. To my surprise, my investigations uncovered the fact that, even before the end of the eighteenth century, the faculty of the Medical "Department" had begun original experimentation and, within a short time, had made discoveries equaling those of their colleagues in Europe. As the new country developed, the Medical Department made every effort within its often meager means to improve its teaching, rebuild its facilities, and meet the medical challenges of a growing nation.

From the start, the University of Pennsylvania and its Medical Department had a faculty interested not only in the practice of clinical medicine and surgery but also in problems of basic medical science.

Many of the contributions made by the faculty have been simultaneously so fundamental and so early (for instance, bromine sensitization of the photographic plate, Muybridge's work on body motion, the birth-control pill) that, when they were incorporated into common or scientific use, the public or the benefiting scientist had long forgotten who made the indispensable discovery for the advance, or where and how it was done; typically credit for the advance was given not to the originator but to those making the most recent adjustment or revision.

Another thing I noticed as the history unfolded was that the important contributions have occurred randomly in the various medical disciplines. There is no set pattern determining who will make the next advance, or when or where. The only common denominator is the ingenuity of the scientist; and genius is an unpredictable phenomenon that silently invades our presence, making discoveries and originating ideas that others can confirm and perhaps even advance but could never conceive. Over the years the University has maintained an environment in which scientists are free to pursue their own ideas. It is an environment that allows for the random events required for discovery, along with stresses that stimulate but do not overwhelm.

Because scientific advances result from the function of minds working in environments influenced by random events, a historian can describe the making of discoveries, but should not force the process of discovery into a general concept. Following that principle, I have resorted to an anecdotal format rather than a conceptual one. What emerges, in addition to the accumulation of accomplishments, is the importance of the interaction of chance and originality in science.

DAVID Y. COOPER III

PREFACE: A WRITER/ EDITOR'S TALE

I came to the University of Pennsylvania Medical Center in 1987 to start a new alumni magazine, which became *Penn Medicine*. As part of my initiation, I read George W. Corner's *Two Centuries of Medicine*, a history of the University of Pennsylvania School of Medicine written in 1965. That book is a fine introduction to those who contributed to the growth of Penn's medical school, but (even in a new and exciting job!) I wished for myself the leisure to investigate in detail the achievements of the school's scientists and clinicians.

Luckily David Cooper walked into my office one day. I had heard that he had been writing a history of the medical school. He gave me a short, unpublished paper on the exact location of the amphitheater in the Thomas Eakins painting known as "The Agnew Clinic."

I enjoyed Cooper's sleuthing. He had compared photographs of surgical amphitheaters both in Medical Hall (sometimes identified as the site) and at the Hospital of the University of Pennsylvania. Agnew appears in the HUP photograph. Moreover, the newer HUP facility seemed more likely to be the setting, given Agnew's interest in the new aseptic approach to surgery. The biography of Agnew written by the surgeon's son-in-law also placed the surgical clinic at HUP.

But Cooper could not find evidence that HUP had an amphitheater of the dimensions that Eakins depicted, and no older members of the medical and nursing staff could recall any. He happened to see the 1981 annual report of The Philadelphia Contributionship for the Insurance of Houses from Loss by Fire, America's oldest insurance company, founded by Benjamin Franklin. That report mentioned that the company had insured HUP a century earlier. Cooper wondered whether it had insured the hospital in 1874 (when the original part was completed) and, if so, whether the Contributionship retained plans of the original building. The answer was yes to both questions, and architectural documents proved that HUP was the site of the Agnew Clinic.

I was happy to publish Cooper's article, which appeared during the one-hundredth anniversary of the painting. One lesson was clear: There is a poignant and unavoidable tug-of-war between the tragedy of destroying architectural treasures when they fall behind technologically and the continual requirement to build anew in order to meet the advancing needs of medical science.

I shortly discovered that Cooper was compiling a manuscript on the accomplishments in the University of Pennsylvania's medical history, the work that I longed to undertake. I was invited to help give shape to his draft. I jumped at the opportunity to contribute to the story that needed telling.

MARSHALL A. LEDGER

ACKNOWLEDGMENTS

What has been the greatest pleasure in assembling the information for this book has been meeting the curators, archivists, and librarians of the various institutions who possessed the required books, papers, and documents. I cannot adequately thank Hamilton Y. Elliott, Jr., Maryellen C. Kaminsky, and Mark F. Lloyd of the Archives of the University of Pennsylvania and Thomas Horrocks and June Carr of the Historical Collections of the College of Physicians of Philadelphia for their help. Thanks must also go to Christine A. Ruggere of the Rare Book Collection of the Van Pelt Library of the University of Pennsylvania, Beth Horrocks and Robert Goodman of the American Philosophical Society, Chris Wjtowicz (Smith) of the Philadelphia Contributionship and Mutual Assurance Company, who led me to important sources concerning the building of the University, as well as Gail Farr, and Jack Eckert for their help in leading me to important sources of information. Alice Kennedy, Elizabeth Berwick, Eleanor Goodchild, and Valerie A. Pena of the Biomedical Library of the School of Medicine of the University of Pennsylvania must also be thanked for their help in finding books and papers in the medical library. Nadine Landis has been very helpful in supplying old photographs of the Hospital of the University of Pennsylvania. Thanks must also be given to Linda Mills for her encouragement and editing of the early versions of this manuscript. Especial thanks must be given to Francis C. Wood, Jonathan E. Rhoads, Eliot Stellar, and George Koelle, who have read early versions of the manuscript and who have not only encouraged the completion of this work but also offered many helpful suggestions for its improvement. Thanks must also go to Terry Woodward of the College of Physicians of Philadelphia, Patricia Smith, Alison Anderson, and Carl Gross of the University of Pennsylvania Press for putting up with an amateur historian.

For the fact that this history is a part of the celebration of the 225th anniversary of the founding of the School of Medicine of the University of Pennsylvania the authors thank Frederic C. Burg, Arthur K. Asbury, and Alfred P. Fishman.

The authors are especially grateful to the Penn Medical Class of 1939, which generously applied its fiftieth anniversary gift to the publication of this book.

INTRODUCTION: HISTORY ROUNDS

No one walks alone through the halls of the University of Pennsylvania Medical Center. All those who travel through the School of Medicine and the Hospital of the University of Pennsylvania are accompanied by the many portraits on the walls, the busts on pedestals, and the memorabilia in display cases that tell in passing a history of an institution that extends 225 years—further than any other American medical school can claim. Portrait painting is a welcome tradition at the school. It has visually preserved the faces of former faculty (and some others) and continues to do so. But, in themselves, the art and artifacts are mute. They require words, the medium of stories, to flesh out what otherwise is only hinted at.

Words have not often told the full story. Dean Joseph Carson wrote a short history, apparently culled mostly from official school minutes, in 1869. George Corner, a physician with no official link to the University of Pennsylvania, wrote a substantial history for the school's 200th anniversary in 1965. Corner assiduously traced the founding and the growth of the school, then the hospital, chiefly through the augmentation of faculty and programs.

The book you are holding looks at the medical advances that faculty and associates (and sometimes students) made while at Penn. It covers the aspect of history that helps induce physicians to teach here and convinces students to attend school here. But such history is not easy to write. Done to the nth detail, it would be encyclopedic. Consequently this history is eclectic by design. It covers early Penn history, not to supplant Corner (its approach is too different from his) but to show that, early on, Penn was both first in date and preeminent in medical contributions. Then it moves on to show that medical advances never ceased coming from the school's laboratories and examining rooms.

This history is intended to arrest that individual who has walked the halls of the school and hospital but has been too pressed for time to examine the stories behind the portraits or statuary or artifacts. Today's students are certainly as harried as anyone and have little time to pause. Yet they probably have more reason to pause than anyone else. They are the ones in danger of graduating smart in medicine but ignorant of their own professional history. And how many have already graduated with less awareness of their surroundings than they ought to have had?

History Rounds, begun in the fall of 1988 for first-year medical students, was meant to prevent the worst. After hearing about the various buildings in Penn's medical history (accompanied by a poster-type display of drawings and photographs), the students took a tour of a few hallways and had the portraits explained. They heard about the first cordial then strained relationship between the school's major founders, John Morgan and William Shippen, Jr. They heard about the relationship between Robert Hare's oxygen-hydrogen blowpipe (the nineteenth-century device that first produced temperatures sufficient to melt metals with high melting points) and recent space ventures, which rely on such antecedents as Hare's work.

They heard about a host of Penn firsts: the first professors of chemistry, physiology (originally called "institutes of medicine"), pharmacology (originally "materia medica"), and surgery; the first endowed professorship; the first hospital built to teach students; a number of first institutes—one devoted solely to the study of anatomy, another to tuberculosis, another to public health, still another to the application of physics to biology and medicine; the first chemical laboratory to service a hospital.

The firsts continued: the first person to use daguerreotype to make portraits; the first head of the American Medical Association (twenty-three other Penn-affiliated presidents have served since). The students heard about firsts missed because, years back, the discoverer did not publish his results or died too soon or, too often, did not recognize the discovery for what it was (incredibly, the X ray and chemotherapy are two of these). And the students heard about the characters of the place. The physician who courted the wife of the hospital director, who, in turn, shot the philanderer in the back—commemorated by the bullet hole in the inkstand, which is on display. The renowned basic scientist who was so eager to avoid arguing with his colleagues that they dubbed him "the first invertebrate." The physician who (in unrelated activities) introduced urology to Penn, brought the Army-Navy football game to Philadelphia, and fought the last pistol duel.

The students also heard about the confused history of the staff-and-snake, both the staff and single snake of Aesculapius and the staff and twin snakes of Mercury. The material kept on coming, a lot for an hour—appropriate, certainly, for a book. And that is the rationale for this book: Penn medical history rounds for all.

In the seventeenth century Hermann Boerhaave summed up the arduous years of medical school and residency when he said:

> The person who can perform the several actions proper to the human body with pleasure and certain constancy is said to be well and that condition of the body is termed health. But if he either cannot perform those actions or if he performs them but with difficulty, pain, and sudden weariness, he is then said to be ill. And the state of the body is called disease.

Of course, physicians must know much more than that, just as they need much more than a stroll past the portraits to understand Penn's history. Medical study will resolve the former. This book is intended to resolve the latter.

1
STIRRINGS OF ORGANIZED MEDICAL EDUCATION

These are deeds which should not pass away and names that must not wither.

Edgar Fahs Smith

Settling new colonies was, as Benjamin Franklin called it, "drudgery." Only after a country passed that phase would a sufficient number of inhabitants have, again in his words, the "ease and . . . leisure to cultivate the fine arts and improve the common stock of knowledge."[1]

By the fourth decade of the eighteenth century, Franklin deemed, the American colonists had reached that stage. He, of course, was their premier example because of the wide variety of organizations he started and his scientific work, especially in electricity. His electrical experiments not only had scientific value but also represented the spread of Baconian science: the idea that knowledge is power, that it could free humankind from dogmas of any sort.[2] The success of Franklin's experiments suggested more: that it was one's duty to investigate the environment and that understanding how it functioned would itself be a means for attaining freedom. His clear description of the behavior of electrical fire dispelled the two-fluid theory of electricity and won the respect of scientists in France and England. It made the statement that American science had arrived.[3]

Medically, Franklin helped promote the first American hospital. He put forth the idea in *The Pennsylvania Gazette*, started the subscription for funds, and persuaded the Pennsylvania Assembly to grant matching funds to the £2,000 of private gifts. The result was the Pennsylvania

Hospital, which was granted its charter in 1751 and opened its door to patients the next year.[4]

Franklin expected that the new hospital would provide medical training, as European hospitals did. Hospitals were ideal sites for instruction, he pointed out, because they treated a "multitude and variety of cases" and because instruction could be "speedy and effective," especially for students from afar who intended to return home.

Shortly after the Pennsylvania Hospital opened, students began visiting the wards. Most were apprentices to members of the hospital staff or to consultants of the hospital. After they finished their clinical service, they were given a certificate drawn up by Thomas Bond to acknowledge this training.

Such an enlightened environment inspired apprentices in many fields. One of the most apt pupils of the era, in activity, ambition, and breadth, was John Morgan, the son of a Philadelphia shopkeeper.[5] At the age of fifteen, he began a six-year apprenticeship with Dr. John Redman, one of the founders of the Pennsylvania Hospital. While he was learning, Morgan served as the hospital's apothecary, and in his spare time, cataloged a gift of fifty books presented to the hospital by the sister of Dr. Benjamin Morris. Morgan's bibliographic effort was eight years before the Pennsylvania Hospital's library was officially founded by the Managers in 1763.[6]

During his apprenticeship he responded to an advertisement for students to the Academy of Philadelphia—the institution that would become the University of Pennsylvania. Morgan finished his college studies in 1756 and graduated in the first class of the new college in 1757.[7]

Armed in both medicine and liberal arts, Morgan left Pennsylvania Hospital to become regimental surgeon of the Pennsylvania provincial troop.[8] Here he had the opportunity to watch English surgeons operate. They repeatedly told him that if he wanted to reach the top of his profession he must have a European medical degree—an opinion corroborated by the Philadelphia physicians he esteemed, who had studied abroad. His decision to study in Europe was hastened when the Pennsylvania troop was disbanded.[9]

Another ambitious pupil of the times was William Shippen, Jr. A great-grandson of a Philadelphia mayor and a nephew of the Chief Justice of Pennsylvania, he had graduated from the College of New Jersey (later Princeton University) and spent a four-year apprenticeship with his father, a physician.[10] Shippen's father packed him off to Europe "to gain all the knowledge he can in anatomy, physic, and surgery," especially to observe dissections and a wider variety of operations than were available at home.

Shippen indeed had a grand tour. In addition to pursuing an active social life, he enrolled in John and William Hunter's famous school of anatomy and lived at their home for eight months. He studied midwifery with Colin Mackenzie, the leading teacher of the discipline, and attended deliveries at Mackenzie's lying-in home. Shippen visited the major hospitals and observed operations by the noted surgeon Percival Potts. He traveled to Scotland, where he heard lectures of William Cullen, the country's most distinguished physician, and Alexander Monro, the anatomist. Shippen received his medical degree from the University of Edinburgh in 1761; two years later, Morgan received his medical degree from the school.

Although no documents exist to prove who first proposed a medical school in Philadelphia, discussions of establishing one evidently took place at the home of Dr. John Fothergill, a busy London practitioner who welcomed every American medical visitor warmly. Fothergill's father and brother were eminent Quaker preachers who had traveled through most of the American colonies. Although he never visited America, Fothergill, better than almost any other Englishman, understood the colonists' needs. He had recognized the importance of Franklin's electricity experiments and ushered Franklin's small book describing them through the press.[11]

Shippen breakfasted with Fothergill frequently and informed his host about the Pennsylvania Hospital, the practice of every notable practitioner in the city, and the training of medical apprentices—pointing out, finally, the crying need for more formal medical teaching in the colonies.

The first recorded mention of any such plan appears in a letter from Fothergill to Dr. James Pemberton, a Philadelphian. Fothergill wrote that he "recommended . . . to Dr. Shippen to give a course to such as may attend." He also mentioned that Shippen "will soon be followed by an amiable assistant Dr. Morgan." Both of them, with the aid of the legislature, might "erect a school for physic" to furnish students "with a better idea of the rudiments of their profession than they have at present on your side of the water."[12]

In the early part of 1761 Morgan and Shippen were in London

together, so they had ample time to discuss with Fothergill and each other their plans to found a medical school in America. They reached an agreement to start classes with Shippen as professor of anatomy and midwifery and Morgan as professor of physic.

Their plans were hardly private. Samuel Bard, a New Yorker studying in Edinburgh, wrote to his father in 1762 about Shippen's anatomical class in Philadelphia and Morgan's plans to lecture on the theory and practice of physic when he graduated. Admitting his own ambition to start a school at the College of New York (later Columbia University), Bard wrote, "I own I feel a little jealous of the Philadelphians."[13]

The course Bard referred to was opened in the autumn of 1762, just after Shippen returned to Philadelphia. Shippen initiated it with an introductory lecture in the State House on November 16, an impressive occasion attended by many laymen as well as medical students.

Shippen clearly intended his anatomy class to expand into something larger.[14] Described by an unknown student, Shippen, in the introductory lecture,

> inform'd his audience with the method he intended to pursue in his instruc-
> tion of his pupils. He would begin with that great & material part the
> Blood, then the bones, &c: afterwards with Dissection and Bandages, and
> between whiles would introduce a small Part of Physiology, but upon the
> arrival of his friend & fellow citizen John Morgan, he would readily resign
> that Branch & refer his pupils to his further instruction.

Meanwhile, Fothergill had hoped that the new school would have institutional connections. He assembled a collection of anatomical material for illustrating lectures and had it sent, along with a cash gift, to the Pennsylvania Hospital. The material included a human skeleton, a fetus, three cases of anatomical models in plaster, and a set of 18 crayon drawings by Jan van Rymsdyk, the celebrated medical artist who had illustrated the dissections of the London anatomist Charles Nicholas Jentry.[15]

Pennsylvania Hospital's board of managers, strapped for funds despite Fothergill's donation, did not start a school but offered the instructional material to Shippen, who used it in special sessions and charged a separate fee to benefit the hospital.

Shippen's courses in anatomy and midwifery were the first systematic teaching of medical subjects approaching an academic level in the American colonies. In January of 1765 he advertised in *The Pennsylvania Gazette* a course of twenty lectures on midwifery open to both sexes, to train physicians as well as midwives. To provide his students with patients, Shippen arranged lodging for a few poor women who were ready to deliver; he also employed a matron acquainted with the problems of lying-in.[16]

For his regular course Shippen charged each student five pistoles (about $20) and that sum again for seeing subjects prepared for lectures or for learning the "art of displaying blood vessels by colored injections."

The school gained more pupils each year, despite increasing opposition from a public which abhorred dissection and accused Shippen of grave-robbing. One jingle declared,

Don't go and weep upon my grave
And think that there I be;
They haven't left an atom there
Of my anatomie![17]

Shippen was not always let off so lightly. On one occasion, the windows of his dissecting room were smashed. On another, he had to run for his life through an alley while his carriage was pelted with bricks and stones and perforated by a musket ball. Shippen finally settled the disturbance by assuring the public that he was not raiding cemeteries but using bodies of executed criminals and suicides given to him by municipal authorities.

It is not known whether Shippen ever intended to affiliate his private enterprise with Pennsylvania Hospital or with the College of Philadelphia. In either case, he could have enlisted the help of his father, who served on the boards of both. Perhaps those institutions, young and cautious, discouraged close ties, noting the public's objection to anatomical teaching and feeling that training male physicians in obstetrical practice was too risky.

Later, Shippen said that he delayed because he was waiting for John Morgan to return from Europe. But he may not have been up to the rigors of putting together an entire school. Despite being an excellent teacher and physician, he showed himself to be a poor organizer in his subsequent career; and he apparently dissipated time by indulging in the good things of life. In any case, he left the field to the far more aggressive Morgan.[18]

NOTES

1. J. Bigelow, *The Life of Franklin Written by Himself*, vol. 1 (Philadelphia: Lippincott, 1900), pp. 274–75.

2. I. B. Cohen, "Franklin and Newton," *Memoirs of the American Philosophical Society* 43 (1956):438–41; B. Franklin (1769), *Experiments and observations on electricity, made at Philadelphia in America. To which are added letters and papers on philosophical subjects* (London: printed for David Henry; and sold by Francis Newbery); B. Franklin (1774), *Experiments and observations on electricity, made at Philadelphia in America. To which are added letters and papers on philosophical subjects*, 5th ed. (London: printed for F. Newbery).

3. F. H. Anderson, *Francis Bacon—Baron of Verulam, Viscount St. Albans—The New Organum and Related Writings* (New York: The Liberal Arts Press, 1960).

4. Bigelow, *Life of Franklin*, pp. 295–98; G. W. Corner, *Two Centuries of Medicine* (Philadelphia: Lippincott, 1965) p. 4.

5. W. J. Bell, Jr., *John Morgan—Continental Doctor* (Philadelphia: University of Pennsylvania Press, 1965).

6. *Ibid.*, p. 27; Pennsylvania Hospital Minutes, 3 mo. 29, 12 mo. 29, 1755.

7. Bell, *John Morgan*, pp. 26, 27.

8. *Ibid.*, p. 30.

9. *Ibid.*, p. 43.

10. H. A. Kelley and W. L. Burrage, *A Dictionary of American Medical Biography* (Boston: Milford Press, 1928), pp. 1104–5; B. C. Corner, *William Shippen, Jr.—Pioneer in American Education* (Philadelphia: American Philosophical Society, 1951); J. Carson, *A History of the Medical Department of the University of Pennsylvania, From its Founding in 1765.* (Philadelphia: Lindsay and Blakiston, 1869), p. 105.

11. Corner, *Two Centuries of Medicine*, pp. 9–10.

12. *Ibid.*, p. 9.

13. *Ibid.*, p. 10.

14. W. J. Bell, Jr., "William Shippen, Jr.'s Introductory Lecture, 1762," in *The Colonial Physician and Other Essays*, pp. 215–16.

15. Corner, *Two Centuries of Medicine*, pp. 11–13, 15.

16. *Ibid.*, p. 13.

17. J. F. Watson, *Annals of Philadelphia* (Philadelphia: Cary and Hart, 1830), pp. 607–8; W. L. Turner "The Charity School, the Academy, and the College Fourth and Arch Streets," in *Historic Philadelphia*, ed. Luther P. Eisenhardt, issued as vol. 43, part 1 of *The Transactions of the American Philosophical Society*, 1952, and reprinted 1980, pp. 179–86. Turner gives a description of early buildings of the University of Pennsylvania. The colored map included shows the location of William Shippen Sr.'s property at Fourth above High Street. William Shippen, Jr., lived at the southwest corner of Fourth and Prune Streets (now the Shippen Wistar House, sold to Caspar Wistar in 1798—an early location of the famous Wistar Parties). There is some confusion in various accounts that state Shippen's Anatomical School was at the Prune Street location. Watson's annals and a map prepared by the American Philosophical Society both show that Shippen's school and his later anatomical lectures in the Medical Department were given at Fourth above High Street, a little over a block from the Philadelphia College.

Thomas Morris wrote in his diary that Shippen, accused by a mob of exhuming a body for dissection, was pelted by bricks and stones on December 20, 1787 in the alley near his father's home on Second Street. Thomas Morris's diary is in the document collection of the Hagley Museum, Greenville, Delaware.

18. Corner, p. 14.

2
EARLY TEACHERS AND SCIENTISTS

It is often said the master word of medicine is work. Of course this is true in one sense of the word work. *But I don't like masters and I don't like work—in the other sense. The best that I can wish—is that you will find in medicine not a master, but a mistress: charming, intelligent, amusing, arousing love, passion, and a desire to serve.*

O.H. Perry Pepper, M.D.
Address to the Senior Class, University of Pennsylvania School of Medicine,
Spring 1955

Commencement, 1765, at the College of Philadelphia. John Morgan, M.D., was the speaker, but his talk was too long to fit within the ceremony's allotted time; the audience adjourned and returned the next day for the conclusion.[1]

In his speech, Morgan drew a shocking picture of his medical colleagues and the state of medical knowledge in the colonies. The physician, he argued, usually has a contracted view of medicine that "limits him to a few partial indications in the cure of disease—he repeats over and over again his round of prescriptions." Physic has arrived at a certain "degree of perfection," he continued, but it would be too much to expect any one "untutored in this art" to learn it by himself. Thus his plan "for transplanting Medical Science into this seminary and for the improvement of every branch of the healing art."

Morgan tugged at the heart. As for the physician, who ought to welcome deeper education: "If not past all feelings of humanity, what compunctions of conscience, what remorse would not fill his breast from practicing at random and in the dark; not knowing whether his prescription might prove a wholesome remedy, or a destructive poison."

Morgan encouraged special training for surgery, pharmacy, and midwifery. He suggested that Philadelphia was an ideal location for formal medical training because of the city's financial wealth and critical mass of physicians and natural philosophers. In addition, he recommended that Philadelphia physicians follow the London and Edinburgh model of separating the practices of apothecary and medicine, rather than charging one fee for their advice and their drugs. To offset popular misunderstanding, Morgan explained his ideas in a 26-page Apology included as the preface to his Discourse when it was published later in 1765.[2]

Morgan had instigated the Commencement address on his own. Within a few days of his return from his European studies, he approached the College of Philadelphia trustees and disclosed his plan to found a medical school under their guidance and patronage. He also asked them to elect him professor of the theory and practice of physic. Impressed by his presentation and the honors he had gathered in Europe, the trustees acceded to his requests, approving the plan for the medical course of study on May 3, 1765.[3]

During the summer Morgan alone made plans for his course, which would begin in the fall. He did not approach, nor was he approached by, his former colleague and co-strategist Shippen.[4]

Shippen, for his part, was irritated at Morgan's initiative and the trustees' actions. A bitter feud developed between Morgan and Shippen and continued throughout their lifetimes. Nonetheless, on September 17, Shippen applied successfully to the trustees for an appointment as professor of anatomy, surgery, and midwifery in the college. The *Pennsylvania Gazette* carried the announcement, signed by both Morgan and Shippen, that their medical lectures would begin on September 26.[5]

On November 14, Shippen delivered his first lecture in his anatomical rooms near the college buildings. Four days later, Morgan began his course in materia medica in the college's lecture hall. Over the next four months, Morgan gave about forty-eight lectures, Shippen sixty. Morgan's fee was four pistoles, about $16; Shippen's six pistoles. Students also paid the college a dollar each to purchase books for a medical library. Morgan attracted about twenty students; it is not known how many attended Shippen's course.[6]

No pretense was made that these two courses constituted a complete medical curriculum; as the *Gazette* announcement stated, the course would be helpful to those attending the practice at Pennsylvania Hospital. Other courses were added over the next few years.[7] Provost

William Smith lectured on natural and experimental philosophy. Ebenezer Kinnersly talked about electricity. Thomas Bond, a founder of Pennsylvania Hospital, reinforced the medical teaching by initiating a course of clinical lectures at the hospital.[8]

In 1767, after two years of medical courses, the medical members of the board—the medical professor and Provost Smith—formed a set of rules for the new offerings. They established a bachelor's degree in physic. Courses in anatomy, materia medica, chemistry, and the theory and practice of physic were required. So were a knowledge of Latin and "such branches of mathematics, natural and experimental philosophy as shall be judged requisite to a medical education." Also required were the clinical lectures, a year of practice at Pennsylvania Hospital, a knowledge of pharmacy, and an apprenticeship "to some reputable practitioner in physic."[9]

The bachelor's degree in medicine was apparently an English custom. Oxford and Cambridge Universities granted the M.D. only after the candidate had done further clinical or research work. On the other hand, the University of Edinburgh issued an M.D. without the M.B. prerequisite. Judging that the new Philadelphia school did not offer a medical education equivalent in quality to that of Edinburgh, the trustees of the College of Philadelphia initially adopted the English system.[10]

Still, they provided for the advanced doctor's degree in physic, stipulating that the candidate have earned a bachelor's degree at least three years previously, be at least twenty-four years old, and write and defend a thesis publicly.[11]

The first medical diplomas were awarded in 1768 to John Archer, David Cowell, Samuel Duffield, Jonathan Elmer, Humphrey Fullerton, David Jackson, John Lawrence, Jonathan Potts, James Tilton, and Nicholas Way. In 1771, Elmer, Potts, Tilton, and Way returned to their alma mater, defended their Latin theses, and received their M.D. degrees. But they were not the first in the American colonies to earn that distinction. Samuel Bard, who earlier had felt outdone by Morgan and Shippen, had started a medical school at King's College in New York (now Columbia University) in 1768. Its sole degree was an M.D., which it granted to two candidates in 1770.[12]

The medical faculty began to expand in 1768, when Adam Kuhn was appointed professor of botany and materia medica. Kuhn had picked up some medical training from his father, a Swabian doctor in Lancaster, Pennsylvania, then traveled to Sweden to study under the world-famous

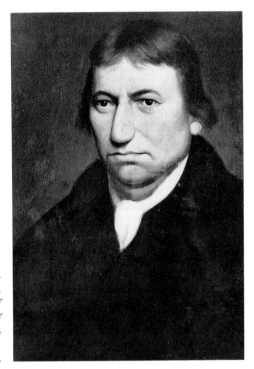

John Archer, from a painting in the portrait hall of the School of Medicine of the University of Pennsylvania. (Archives of the University of Pennsylvania.)

Carolus Linnaeus. Kuhn's work in Sweden was so well regarded that Linnaeus named an American variety of the thistle after him. Kuhn may not have been particularly imaginative—his lectures were said to have merely revised those he heard from Cullen in Scotland—but he had a profound talent for observation and systematization of details and was credited as a competent practitioner. Kuhn's subject matter represented an important advance in the curriculum, for students gained from him a better understanding of herbs and plants and the drugs that could be prepared from them.[13]

Chemistry was added in 1769, when Benjamin Rush was elected to the first chair of chemistry in America.[14] Rush was born in Philadelphia and raised by his mother, a greengrocer. He completed an apprenticeship with John Redman, attended the University of Edinburgh, and stayed a few months in London dissecting and observing anatomical procedures with the Hunters.

But his career started with more emotion and impetuousness than a bare description suggests. Rush was one of the ten students in Shippen's first anatomical course.

He was also a student in the first medical class of the College of Philadelphia when Morgan singled him out as a candidate for the chemistry chair. As Rush was planning to earn his M.D. from Edinburgh, Morgan suggested that Rush prepare himself instead for this subject by giving special attention to the lectures of Joseph Black, the famous chemist. Redman, wary of Morgan's taking too much into his own hands, advised Rush to be certain that the position promised by Morgan would be offered when he returned.

Rush went to Edinburgh, attended Black's lectures for two years in succession (in those days, students could repeat a course for cumulative credit), obtained his M.D. degree, and wrote a thesis on the chemistry of digestion; he dedicated the work to Black, Morgan, Shippen, and Benjamin Franklin. Furthermore, Rush persuaded John Fothergill to recommend him to Thomas Penn, the proprietor of Pennsylvania province, as "a very expert chemist" and to have Penn purchase a set of chemical apparatus and send it to the college in Rush's care. He was appointed to the chemistry chair three weeks after his return to America.

Morgan ceased active involvement in the medical school in 1775, when he was appointed director general and chief physician of the Continental Army. In 1777, he was dismissed from this office because of complaints of incompetence from troops under his care and because of vicious attacks by Shippen. He was replaced by Shippen, who was later court-martialed, charged with dishonesty and incompetence. By one vote the court dismissed the charges against Shippen for lack of proof. Subsequently, after being reappointed Director of Hospitals, Shippen was compelled to resign.[15]

Morgan never recovered from his dismissal from the Army. He spent his remaining years writing articles defending his Army service and attacking Shippen. His life ended in this sad scene described by Rush on October 15, 1789:

This afternoon I was called to visit Dr. Morgan, but found him dead in a small hovel surrounded with books and papers on a light dirty bed. He was attended by a washerwoman, one of his tenants. His niece Polly Gordon came in time enough to see him draw his last. His disorder was influenza but he had been previously debilitated by many disorders. What a change

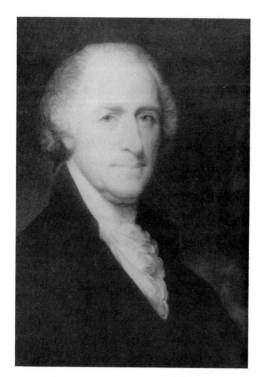

William Shippen, Jr. Portrait attributed to Gilbert Stuart. Original is in possession of the Wistar Institute. (Archives of the University of Pennsylvania.)

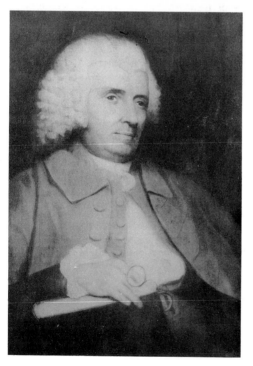

John Morgan, founder and Professor of the Theory and Practice of Physic. Painted about 1787 (two years before his death) by Thomas Spencer Duche. Original is in the possession of the Historical Society of Pennsylvania.

from his former rank and prospects! The man who once filled half the world with his name, had now scarcely friends enough to bury him.[16]

For good and ill, Benjamin Rush probably attracted the greatest attention among Pennsylvania's early physician-teachers.[17] By the time he died in 1813, he was considered one of the world's outstanding doctors, known chiefly for his studies of mental diseases.

When Rush joined the staff of the Pennsylvania Hospital in 1783, he was drawn to the two dozen insane patients there. Ever since the hospital opened, it had housed a section for the care of the insane, but Rush immediately found it inadequate. The cells, he complained to the hospital's managers, were damp in winter and too hot in summer and failed to circulate air; patients caught cold easily and several died of consumption. Rush also lobbied the legislature, which in 1792 appropriated $15,000 to construct an insane ward, a "mad house" in the parlance of the day. Patients moved into the new wing in 1796. Rush pleaded for even further improvements, and rooms with warm and cold baths were eventually added.[18]

Rush had advanced notions of treating the mentally ill, especially in assigning them definite tasks or occupations. He kept careful clinical records of his patients. (One of his patients was his son John, who was confined to the hospital for twenty-seven years after the turn of the century; John's constant pacing back and forth in a room on the ground floor wore grooves in the wooden flooring which became known as Rush's Walk.[19]

Rush used the occasion of his institutes of medicine lectures to teach his ideas on the psychology of the mind and the mechanism of its functions. Rush incorporated his long study and notes in his epoch-making *Medical Inquiries and Observations Upon Diseases of the Mind*, published in 1812.[20]

He evidently was an earnest if rigidly patterned instructor. During his lectures he seldom rose from his chair, reading slowly and distinctly what he had fully written out in little pamphlets.[21] He singled out students whom he thought receptive to his ideas and invited them to his home. He administered frequent quizzes in order to convince his classes to accept without question his speculations and medical theories.[22]

His inflexibility made him infamous during Philadelphia's yellow fever epidemic in 1793. Rush stubbornly held to a pet theory that all diseases were caused by "irregular convulsive or wrong action in the system affected." He also thought that the human body contained about 12 quarts of blood, twice the actual amount.[23] Together, these notions led him to a treatment of yellow fever through bloodletting and purging, in which he removed up to a quart of blood at intervals of forty-eight to seventy-two hours. His colleagues claimed that at least 40 percent of his patients died from his prescription.

Later in his life, Rush overcame the criticism and enjoyed fame. He served as the medical school dean and was known as a reformer for freedom and health on all fronts. He was a staunch republican[24] and abolitionist[25] and tried to relieve the tyranny of crime and poverty.[26] Much of his medical practice was devoted to care of the poor, and he helped establish the first public dispensary in the United States.[27] He was so vehemently opposed to the excessive use of alcohol that many regard him as the originator of the temperance movement. He opposed capital punishment. He favored education for women and proposed a series of colleges that would pyramid to a national university.[28]

Samuel Powell Griffiths, a 1781 graduate, was the first alumnus of the medical school to join the faculty, but he stayed for only six sessions, teaching materia medica and pharmacy. Although his lectures were praised for substance and organization, being a lecturer "was not all together congenial to his feelings." He founded the Philadelphia Dispensary and served it for forty years. He also encouraged the establishment of a national pharmacopoeia and, after a long dormant period, helped the College of Physicians of Philadelphia formulate it.[29]

Benjamin Smith Barton became professor of natural history and botany in 1789; previously botany had been taught as part of materia medica by Kuhn. The college created the chair in natural history—the first in America—in order to secure Barton's talents. His dissertation, *on Hyoscyamus Niger* of Linnaeus, written at the University of Edinburgh, had already earned him renown; and he was known as much for his capabilities in illustration as for his investigation of plants.[30]

He was an early collector of botanical specimens from various regions of the American continent. And in 1804 he founded *The Philadelphia Medical and Physical Journal*, one of the first periodicals in the city, which was chiefly devoted to natural history.

Although Barton's course was not required, his enthusiasm for the subject and his well-illustrated lectures drew students in sufficient numbers to support him. As a teacher he was described as "eloquent, instructive"; in temperament, he was called "irritable and even choleric, though in his gentle moods he was kind, tender, and intelligent."

As a Quaker, Caspar Wistar refused to enlist in the Revolution, instead offering his services for the care of the wounded in Germantown. That stint convinced him to enter medicine.[31]

During the institutional split that briefly created simultaneously a college and a university, Wistar joined the faculty of the college as professor of chemistry and of the institutes of medicine.[32] The latter name identified a subject new to the American medical curriculum, a subject recommended by Wistar to the trustees just prior to his appointment. The name derived from the book *Institutiones Medicae* by Hermann Boerhaave, published in Leyden in 1707. In it Boerhaave outlined the functions of the body, which he treated as a separate scientific discipline—as such, a forerunner of physiology. The lawyerly resonance of the name derived from *Institutiones Gaii* and *Institutiones Justiniani*, Roman legal treatises in which *institutiones* signifies "principles" or "elements."[33] In using the name, the college trustees followed the precedent of the University of Edinburgh. Thus Wistar was the first to hold a chair of physiology in America.[34]

When the college and university were reunited, he became adjunct professor of anatomy under Shippen. Upon Shippen's death, he moved into the chair, which included midwifery; midwifery was separated from anatomy in 1810, and Wistar thereafter focused on his specialty.

Despite his vast knowledge of his subject, Wistar felt insecure before audiences and came across as a poor teacher. But he studiously overcame his difficulties, eventually becoming one of the greatest speakers of his time.[35] He illustrated his lectures with actual dissections of the human body as well as with splendid wooden models of small anatomical parts, items carved for him by William Rush, a sculptor of ship figureheads.[36]

In 1811 Wistar published *A System of Anatomy*, the country's first textbook on this subject.[37] His most significant original contribution was a description of extensions of the roof of the nasal bone, called the "Wistar pyramids." He pointed out that the structures, though distinct in infancy and early childhood, later become cellular and grow into the sphenoid bone, forming the medial wall of the sphenoid sinus.[38]

His name is also associated with the "Wistar parties," Sunday soirees over tea, coffee, wine, and cake, although the menu gradually expanded. Usually the guests invited numbered about fifteen and included the faculty of the medical school, local "literati," members of the Board of Trustees, and distinguished visitors to Philadelphia—Baron Von Humboldt, James Madison, Abbé José Francisco Correa da Serra (a scientist and the first Portuguese ambassador to the United States), and others.[39] (In a substantially different form, these parties, under the name of the Wistar Association—made up of some members of the American Philosophical Society—have continued to this day.) He is also remembered by the flowering vine, *Wisteria sinensis* (*W. chinensis*), Chinese Wisteria, which his friend Thomas Nuttall brought back from China and named for him.[40]

Wistar became one of Philadelphia's most beloved and distinguished physicians. He was one of the few physicians who remained in the city during the yellow fever epidemic in 1793. His gentle personality, combined with caution and care of his patients, brought him a large practice. His medical fees were extremely low; and once when he was very ill, he asked his sister to destroy his records so that no one would owe his estate any money after he died. His patients took to sending him gifts anonymously so that he could not return them. In January 1818, he was seized with a high fever and died from malignant endocarditis.[41]

James Woodhouse became the most celebrated American chemist of his era, but not for his lectures.[42] They were called "dull and monotonous" and were considered too short because they rarely exceeded forty minutes in length. Brevity was a principle with him because, he said once when asked about it, "no man could dwell, in discussion, on a single topic more than five minutes without talking nonsense."[43]

He did much better in his small laboratory, which he set up in the first floor of Surgeon's Hall. He prepared demonstrations for his classes and conducted original chemical investigations. Although a close friend with Joseph Priestley, who discovered oxygen, he did not believe, as Priestley did, that burning material during combustion releases as flame a hypothetical substance called phlogiston. Rather, Woodhouse was a strong admirer of the French chemists, and was the first in America to support Antoine Laurent Lavoisier, who realized that during combustion (or oxidation) oxygen combines with the material being oxidized and increases its molecular weight.

In his 1919 book *Chemistry in Old Philadelphia*, Edgar Fahs Smith credits Woodhouse with being the first to isolate potassium. Smith says that Woodhouse purified it by heating potash with soot in an iron vessel as early as 1804, about the same time as Joseph Louis Gay-Lussac and Louis Jacque Thénard succeeded in purifying it. Yet Woodhouse received no acclaim for that important work.[44]

John Redman Coxe, professor of chemistry and later of materia medica, contributed to the reputation of the young medical school through his experiments and writings.[45]

His interest in using the static electric machine in chemistry led to his improving the apparatus. He conceived of a telegraph for conveying messages during emergencies, and he described this communication system in a paper published in the *Emporium of Arts and Sciences* in 1812.[46] He also designed an apparatus to mix gases efficiently with water in flow-through systems.[47]

Coxe helped introduce vaccination in Philadelphia. He obtained some smallpox vaccine from Thomas Jefferson, who had procured it from the Boston physician Benjamin Waterhouse to inoculate his slaves. On the day it arrived, Coxe vaccinated himself and four others. Subsequently he vaccinated many more, including his oldest child and the children of his friends Benjamin Rush and Charles Willson Peale. To test the "full efficacy of this procedure," he gave smallpox to his son, whom he had named Edward Jenner Coxe after the discoverer of the vaccine. The success of this experiment helped convince Coxe's medical colleagues of the vaccine's protective powers.[48]

Even when one of his projects fell through, Coxe made an important contribution. He tried to organize pharmacy education in Philadelphia, but his efforts were rebuffed; as a direct result, the Philadelphia College of Pharmacy, America's first such institution, was founded in 1821.[49]

Coxe wrote widely, producing, among much else, *The Importance and Respectability of the Science of Medicine* and the *Philadelphia Medical Dictionary*. He also edited the six-volume *Philadelphia Medical Museum* and the five-volume *Emporium of Arts and Sciences*.

He served as the medical school's dean, but his classroom days came to an untimely end. He was considered so pedantic that students, some armed with daggers, shouted him down in 1835. He was formally dismissed after that, but continued his scholarly work until he died in 1864 at the age of 91.[50]

Among other early contributors was Thomas Chalkley James. He held the chair of midwifery after it was separated from anatomy in 1810. About this time, he presented details of his most significant contribution—artificially inducing premature labor in a patient with a contracted pelvis. Both the mother and child survived, in what was called the first case in America of delivering a baby prematurely while it was still small enough to pass through the birth canal.[51]

One medical advance in this early period was credited to a student, John Richardson Young, whose thesis for the M.D. degree was completed just seven months after he entered medical school.[52] He demonstrated how the stomach digests food, a significant step in understanding the physiology and chemistry of digestion.

The digestive process supposedly worked (to mention a few theories) by concoction, by fermentation, by patrefaction, by material effervescence, or by a contracting force equivalent to 400,000 pounds of pressure. Young used frogs to prove the powerful action of gastric juices on ingested substances. Then he devised a "living principle" to explain why the process does not work on living material, including the frogs' own stomachs. Most important, he concluded that acid was required for gastric processes (but wrongly concluded that gastric juice contained phosphoric acid).

Young died in 1805 when he was twenty-two years old. His thesis was reprinted in *Medical Theses* of that year. Like much scientific work in those times, it escaped the attention of anyone qualified to appreciate its importance. Not until 1908 was his work rediscovered in the University of Pennsylvania library; then it received belated acclaim.

In addition to being the first medical school, Penn's was the only one of America's eighteenth-century medical schools whose founding was motivated chiefly by its academic connection. Columbia's medical school, founded in 1768, and Harvard's, founded in 1782, originated from medical societies concerned with regulating and controlling medicine in their respective cities. Pennsylvania can rightly claim a more intellectual foundation, traceable to the influence of Benjamin Franklin. It was this tradition that contributed to its being a center of medical learning for most of the nineteenth century.

Even so, there was much settling of the sands. Professorships were allotted and reallotted ingeniously. The curriculum fluctuated; botany was discontinued as a degree requirement. The bachelor of medicine degree was dropped and the M.D. alone conferred, according to the practice of the University of Edinburgh.

Some appointments were abruptly cut off, exemplified by James H. Hutchinson's short term of two years. At the time of the Revolution, he had hastened home from his studies in Europe. The ship carrying him was captured by the British. He escaped in an open boat but lost a fine library that he had assembled in France and England. Serving as a university trustee during the institutional split, he worked to lessen the hard feelings between the separate faculties; in fact he refused two professorships until the rights of the college were restored. When Hutchinson died in the yellow fever epidemic of 1793, the chemistry professorship remained unfilled until James Woodhouse accepted it in 1795; but he died suddenly in 1809.

In one sense there had been continuity in the chair. All incumbents after Rush had been his students. But Rush had always tried in his lectures to relate chemistry to medical problems. Woodhouse had not followed this tradition faithfully. His death raised a problem that would plague the University of Pennsylvania until the 1850s: who should teach chemistry, already a distinct discipline, to medical classes—a chemist without a medical background or a physician with inclinations toward the field?

Many practicing physicians questioned whether the chair of chemistry belonged to the medical faculty at all. But Rush and other medical professors had no doubts; furthermore, they demanded that appointments to the medical department be filled exclusively by men of the medical profession. Rush successfully promoted the election of his own student, John Redman Coxe.

When Coxe moved from chemistry to materia medica in 1818, the controversy over the need for chemistry in the medical curriculum arose again. Rush and Wistar were no longer alive to defend the old, cultivated, scientifically oriented physician from the new medical instructor who wanted to teach only practical medicine. Nevertheless, the trustees declined the pressure to abolish or transfer the chair of chemistry and elected Robert Hare to the post. The appointment signified the solidity of the basic departmental divisions in the medical curriculum. These divisions have not changed substantially since then, although they have evolved, some of their names have changed, and their scope of knowledge has expanded exponentially.

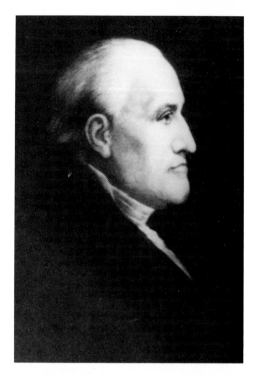

Adam Kuhn, Professor of Material Medica and Pharmacy. From a painting that hangs in the Portrait Hall of the School of Medicine of the University of Pennsylvania. (Archives of the University of Pennsylvania.)

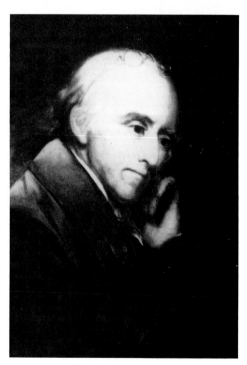

Benjamin Rush, first Professor of Chemistry in America. Painting by Thomas Sully that hangs at the American Philosophical Society. (Copied from a photograph in the Archives of the University of Pennsylvania.)

By 1818 the infancy of the Penn medical school had ended. All of the original faculty were dead. The school weathered the difficult period of starting up and even the jealousies and arguments inevitable among its faculty. Significantly it was an established source of new and competent physicians and of original investigations that deserved worldwide recognition.

NOTES

1. W. J. Bell, Jr., *John Morgan—Continental Doctor* (Philadelphia: University of Pennsylvania Press, 1965).

2. J. Morgan, *A Discourse Upon the Institution of Medical Schools in America* (Philadelphia, 1765). A fascimile was published by the Johns Hopkins University Press in 1937 (introduction by Simon Flexner) and by the University of Pennsylvania in 1965.

3. G. W. Corner, *Two Centuries of Medicine* (Philadelphia: Lippincott, 1965); T. H. Montgomery, *A History of the University of Pennsylvania, 1749–1770* (Philadelphia: G. W. Jacobs, 1900); E. P. Cheyney, *History of the University of Pennsylvania 1740–1940* (Philadelphia: University of Pennsylvania Press, 1940); J. Carson, *A History of the Medical Department of the University of Pennsylvania, from its Founding in 1765* (Philadelphia: Lindsay and Blakiston, 1869); Bell, *John Morgan*, pp. 120–28; J. T. Scharf and T. Wescott, *History of Philadelphia—1609–1884* (Philadelphia: L. H. Everts, 1884).

4. Bell, *John Morgan*, pp. 124–25.

5. *Ibid.*, pp. 132–33.

6. *Ibid.*, p. 134; Corner, *Two Centuries of Medicine*, pp. 23–24; Carson, *History of the Medical Department*, pp. 56–57.

7. Corner, *Two Centuries of Medicine*, p. 23.

8. Bell, *John Morgan*, pp. 146–47.

9. Minutes of the Faculty of the Medical College, Philadelphia College, May 1768; Carson, *History of the Medical Department*, pp. 65–66.

10. Carson, *History of the Medical Department*, pp. 69–72; Corner, *Two Centuries of Medicine*, pp. 27–28.

11. Carson, pp. 75–76.

12. Corner, *Two Centuries of Medicine*, p. 31. Benjamin Cowell's name is listed in the hall of the Medical Laboratories as David Cowell and the name on the photostat of his diploma in the Archives of the University is also given as David Cowell.

13. *Ibid.* pp. 64–65; C. Caldwell, *An Autobiography of Charles Caldwell, M.D.*, with a preface, notes and appendix by Harriot W. Warner (New York: Da Capo Press, 1968), pp. 123–25.

14. N. G. Goodman, *Benjamin Rush—Physician and Citizen* (Philadelphia: University of Pennsylvania Press, 1934); C. Binger, *Revolutionary Doctor, Benjamin Rush (1746–1813)* (New York: W. W. Norton, 1866); J. T. Flexner, *Doctors on Horseback* (New York: Viking, 1937).

15. Flexner, pp. 83–85; L. Butterworth, *Letters of Benjamin Rush*, vol. 1 (Princeton, N.J.: Princeton University Press, 1951), Letter to Nathaniel Green, February 1, 1778, p. 194; to William Shippen, February 1, 1778, pp. 196–97; to George Wash-

ington, February 25, 1778, pp. 200–4; to Daniel Roberdeau, March 9, 1778, pp. 204–8; to William Henry Drayton, Samuel Huntington, and John Banister, April 20, 1778; to John Morgan, June? 1779, pp. 225–29; to William Shippen, November 18, 1780, pp. 256–60; Bell, *John Morgan*, pp. 229–36, 238.

16. Bell, *John Morgan*, pp. 263–64.

17. Goodman, *Benjamin Rush*, pp. 179–95; Binger, *Revolutionary Doctor*, pp. 217, 223; J. H. Powell, *Bring Out Your Dead: The Great Yellow Fever Epidemic in Philadelphia, 1793* (Philadelphia: University of Pennsylvania Press, 1949), pp. 64–89; W. J. Bell, Jr., *The College of Physicians, A Bicentennial History* (Canton, Mass.: Science History Publications, 1987), pp. 26–33, 32.

18. Binger, *Revolutionary Doctor*, pp. 255–56.

19. *Ibid.*, pp. 282–83.

20. B. Rush, *Medical Inquiries and Observations upon the Diseases of the Mind*, with an introduction by Dr. S. Bernard Wortis (New York: New York Academy of Medicine [The History of Medicine Series, vol. 3, no. 15] 1962).

21. E. T. Carlson, J. L. Wollock, and P. S. Noel, "Benjamin Rush's Lectures on the Mind," *Memoirs of the American Philosophical Society* 144(1981):15–17.

22. *Ibid.*, pp. 15–17: Caldwell, *Autobiography*, pp. 146–47.

23. Powell, *Bring Out Your Dead*, pp. 162–63; Binger, *Revolutionary Doctor*, p. 229.

24. Goodman, *Benjamin Rush*, pp. 283–84.

25. *Ibid.*, pp. 48–49.

26. *Ibid.*, pp. 272–73, 298; Binger, *Revolutionary Doctor*, pp. 197–98.

27. Goodman, pp. 274–79.

28. *Ibid.*, pp. 321–22, 307–11.

29. Carson, *History of the Medical Department*, pp. 102–3.

30. *Ibid.*, pp. 126–30.

31. H. A. Kelley and W. L. Burrage, *Dictionary of American Medical Biography* (Boston: Milford Press, 1928), pp. 1318–19.

32. Carson, *History of the Medical Department*, pp. 93–94.

33. Corner, *Two Centuries of Medicine*, p. 40; Carlson, Wollock, and Noel, *Benjamin Rush's Lectures on the Mind*, pp. 17–18.

34. Carson, *History of the Medical Department*, p. 97; Corner, *Two Centuries of Medicine*, pp. 41–44.

35. Carson, pp. 137–40; Caldwell, *Autobiography*, pp. 129–30.

36. Carson, pp. 139–41.

37. C. Wistar, *A System of Anatomy for Use of Students of Medicine*, 2 vols. (Philadelphia: T. Dorland, 1811–1814).

38. C. Wistar, *System of Anatomy for Use of Medical Students*, with notes and additions by W. E. Horner, entirely remodeled by J. Pancoast (Philadelphia: Thomas Cowperthwait, 1846), pp. 78–81, plate opposite p. 80.

39. Caldwell, *Autobiography*, pp. 135–36; I. J. Wistar, *Autobiography*, p. 504; I. Richman, *The Brightest Ornament* (Bellefont, Pa.: Pennsylvania Heritage, 1967), pp. 165–67; W. B. McDaniel II, "The Wistar Party and the College of Physicians of Philadelphia," *Transactions and Studies of the College of Physicians of Philadelphia* 4th ser., 39(1972):164–67.

40. W. J. Bell, Jr., "Caspar Wistar," in *Dictionary of Scientific Biography*, ed. C. C. Gillispie, A. E. Verrill, and J. Zwelfer, vol. XIV, pp. 456–57.(Bell states that although Nuttall named the plant for Caspar Wistar, he spelled it Wister, the name of the other branch of the family in Philadelphia, therefore the name of this plant should

be spelled wistaria); M. Meyerson and D. P. Winegrad, *Gladly Learn and Gladly Teach* (Philadelphia: University of Pennsylvania Press, 1978), p. 43. A portrait of Abbé José Francisco Correa da Serra, the first Portuguese ambassador to the United States, that previously hung in the front hall of the Wistar Institute bears the inscription stating he classified the vine *glicinea*. He was a guest at many Wistar parties, and named the plant for his friend Caspar Wistar.

42. E. F. Smith, *James Woodhouse, A Pioneer in Chemistry* (Philadelphia: James Winston and Co., 1918); Carson, *History of the Medical Department*, pp. 107–10; H. S. Klickstein, "A Short History of the Professorship of Chemistry of the University of Pennsylvania School of Medicine," *Bulletin of the History of Medicine* 27(1953):43–68.

43. C. Caldwell, *Autobiography*, pp. 173–76.

44. E. F. Smith, *Chemistry in Old Philadelphia* (Philadelphia: Lippincott, 1919), p. 23.

45. Carson, *History of the Medical Department*, pp. 157–59; Smith, *Chemistry in Old Philadelphia*, pp. 52–61; Kelley and Burrage, pp. 262–63.

46. J. R. Coxe, "Description of a Revolving Telegraph, for conveying Intelligence by Figures, Letters, Words, or Sentences," in *The Emporium of Arts and Sciences*, ed. John Redman Coxe (Philadelphia: Joseph Delaplain, 1812), pp. 99–109.

47. Smith, *Chemistry in Old Philadelphia*, p. 57.

48. J. R. Coxe, *Practical Observations on Vaccination, or Inoculation for the Cow-pock* (Philadelphia: Humphry, 1802); Kelley and Burrage, pp. 262–63.

49. Corner, *Two Centuries of Medicine*, pp. 72–73.

50. Corner, pp. 80–85.

51. Kelley and Burrage, pp. 646–47.

52. J. R. Young, *An Experimental Inquiry into the Principles of Nutrition and the Digestive Process*, with an introduction by W. C. Rose (Urbana: University of Illinois Press, 1959).

3
CONDITIONS OF LEARNING

The business of a professor is to place before students in full light, at their first entrance upon any study, the true object of that study and to ascertain their proper pursuit. . . . He thus points out the road that leads to science. . . . He confirms [the student's] steps, smooths the rugged path he has to tread, assists him in climbing the steep ascent, and before dismission informs him how to conduct himself in order to reach at length the summit of his profession.

John Morgan
A Discourse

The turmoil associated with the outbreak of the American Revolution brought the College of Philadelphia and its medical curriculum to the brink of disaster. In 1777, the school was closed for a period because British troops were billeted in its buildings. Worse, the school was perceived as Anglican, aristocratic, and Tory by the radical Constitutional Party that had seized power in the state; the upshot was that the legislature suspended the powers of the trustees. Power was restored in 1779, but not to the old trustees. They and the college faculty were dismissed in favor of a new board with its own faculty, and the college's name was changed to the University of the State of Pennsylvania.[1]

The new board appointed Shippen to evaluate the medical curriculum and present a plan "for establishing the school on the most respectable footing."[2] This resolution is the first time the group of medical courses was referred to as a "school."[3]

The board also appointed the medical professors of the old college to the new university, but at first Shippen was the only one to accept. By 1783 Rush, Kuhn, and Bond had returned to the faculty. Courses were shortened from four to three months to accommodate students from surrounding states who could not afford longer stays away from home.

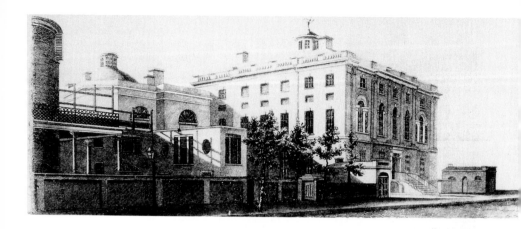

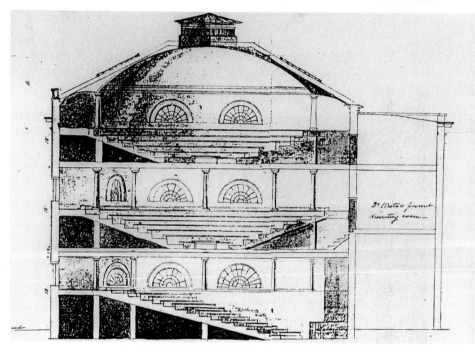

TOP: *University of Pennsylvania at 9th Street between Market and Chestnut Streets. The large house was built as a residence for the President of the United States. The addition, designed by Benjamin Latrobe, containing a lecture room and the anatomical amphitheater was built in 1807. Drawing by William Strickland. (Archives of the University of Pennsylvania.)* Bottom: *William Strickland's proposed renovation of Medical Hall showing the original lecture hall and the anatomical amphitheater. Strickland proposed to build a new anatomical amphitheater on the third floor and convert the existing one to a second lecture hall. (Archives of the University of Pennsylvania.)*

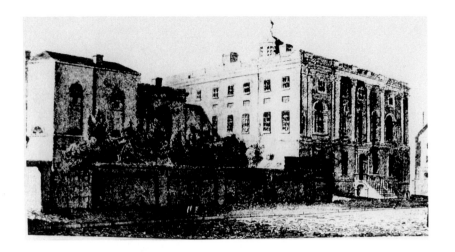

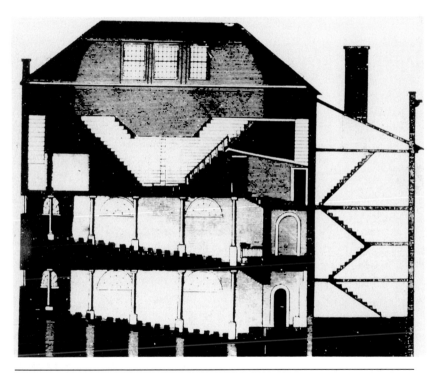

TOP: *Medical Hall after renovation in 1817. (Archives of the University of Pennsylvania.)* Bottom: *Interior of Medical Hall reconstructed in 1817. From an engraving in the* American Medical Recorder, *frontispiece, vol. 1, 1818. (Historical Collections of the College of Physicians of Philadelphia.)*

Even in the best light, medical lectures during this period of reorganization were irregular, as was the awarding of degrees: in 1781, two students received M.B. s; in 1782, eight.[4]

In 1788 conservatives returned to power in the Pennsylvania legislature, promptly restoring the privileges and property of the College of Philadelphia.[5] From 1789 to 1791, the school existed as two institutions. Since the college regained its buildings, the university moved to Philosophical Hall, the new building of the American Philosophical Society.[6] In 1889 Rush was elected to the chair of Theory and Practice of Medicine in the College and Kuhn resigned his professorship and took the medical chair in the University. Naturally rivalry developed between the two faculties, which was "singular from the fact of an inosculation existing in the person of Dr. Shippen, who held professorships in both."[7]

In 1791, the legislature united the college and university under the university's name.[8] Rush was so ecstatic over the reunion that he prefaced his introductory lecture in the fall with his rapturous approval.

When the college and university were reunited, the lease of the rooms at Philosophical Hall was dropped, and the medical classes were held in the academy and in Anatomical, or Surgeon's, Hall.[9]

The name Surgeon's Hall no doubt stems from the famous medical building of the same name at the University of Edinburgh. Its American namesake was the first building in the new country used exclusively for medical teaching. The anatomy and chemistry lectures of both college and university were held there during the institutional division. It was located on Fifth Street north of Walnut Street.[10]

Most of Surgeon's Hall's history prior to 1792 is obscure. Classes were first held in it sometime between 1775 and 1779, and the university referred to it as "the laboratory." By the time the schools rejoined in 1791, the structure sorely needed repairs, which Shippen and Wistar funded from their own estates. Among the renovations were the installation of a stove in the anatomical amphitheater and the building of a second story. A winding stair led to a cupola, an octagonal structure with glazed windows that served to illuminate the anatomical dissecting room. One of William Birch's famous lithographs of Philadelphia, executed in the 1790s, shows it as a narrow structure with its distinctive cupola.

In 1800, the university bought the mansion at Ninth and Market Streets that the Commonwealth of Pennsylvania had built for President

John Adams.[11] The medical faculty applied for accommodations there. In 1802 the committee on the "new Building" offered them the West Bow room on the second floor and space for a chemistry laboratory on the first floor. Facilities for dissection and anatomy classes were not offered.[12] These arrangements were not satisfactory, so the medical faculty stayed in "the laboratory." In 1804 they asked to use the old academy buildings on Fourth Street, but the trustees refused.[13] In 1806 the physicians had a new proposal: to build an addition to the mansion and to accept responsibility for the interest on the cost. The trustees approved. A new Medical Hall was designed by Benjamin Latrobe and completed in time for classes in 1807.[14]

Within a decade, these facilities, too, were insufficient. They were renovated and enlarged by Latrobe's student William Strickland.[15] But by 1828 even these quarters were outgrown. The trustees decided to demolish all of the structures on this site and build two new buildings, one for the medical school and one for the University. William Strickland was hired as the architect for this project as well.[16]

The result for Medical Hall was described in an 1844 report.[17] The central location was praised, since students could live nearby. In addition, "the large space around it allows of the free circulation of air which is especially necessary, in an establishment of this kind, to comfort and preservation of health." There were three 600-seat lecture rooms, one dedicated to chemistry, "in its extent and arrangement as a laboratory nowhere surpassed."

Another was reserved for "other demonstrative branches" and built under the supervision of the anatomy professor, who provided for both maximum light and proximity of the students. William Horner wrote about the innovative seating in his report from the surgical service at the Philadelphia Hospital:

> The seats are elevated on the plane of an inverted cone (not like a funnel, as is common in amphitheaters), whereby every row of students has the same angle of demonstration over the row in front (an idea first carried into execution by myself so far as I know).[18]

Sports arenas and theaters today employ this principle of amphitheater construction.

The medical course was taught over a four-month period and lengthened by two weeks in the early 1840s. The faculty favored demonstra-

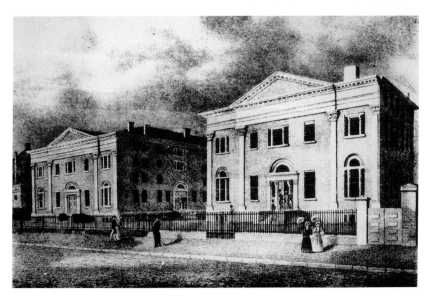

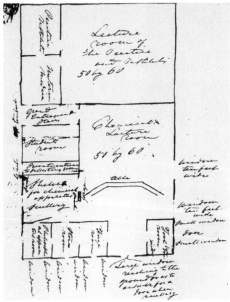

TOP: *Medical Hall of the University of Pennsylvania, designed by William Strickland, erected in 1829. (Archives of the University of Pennsylvania.)* Bottom: *William Strickland's original sketch for the new Medical Hall. The diagram was glued in the Minutes of the Medical Faculty when the proposed new building was planned. (Archives of the University of Pennsylvania.)*

tions whenever possible, illustrating their lectures with carefully made anatomical dissections and representative pathological specimens of disease removed during surgery or at autopsy. Teachers of institutes of medicine and materia medica—disciplines which did not lend themselves to biological material—used, instead, accurate models, oil paintings, dried plants, and diagrams obtained from Europe.[19]

EXAMINATION OF THE MEDICAL STUDENTS IN THE "GREEN BOX"

As other medical schools opened, competition for students grew—not only among schools but among professors, who wanted to attract large classes to sell more tickets and thereby increase their income and prestige. Some students, and professors as well, accused the university examiners of favoring their own students by asking them easy questions while directing hard questions at rival students.

To make the examinations fair, the faculty decided in 1810 to examine candidates behind a screen.[20] And so the "rules governing examinations" declared that the candidate be placed behind a screen and the examination be so conducted that no professor but the dean of the faculty should know the candidate. For nine years, a green baize frame enclosed all students sitting for examination. In 1819, some students petitioned that the so-called Green Box be discontinued; they felt it was demeaning and stressful. Others wished to continue the procedure, however; thus for the next two years, students were given an option of sitting directly before the faculty or behind the screen. In 1821 the faculty finally agreed that the Green Box should be "altogether abolished."

CLINICAL TEACHING

There is no doubt that a thorough medical training requires direct contact of students with patients. Apprenticeship traditionally provided that contact, but the advent of medical schools demanded a new relationship. Although schools, as Morgan anticipated, easily eclipsed the amount of knowledge that previously could be passed on to new gen-

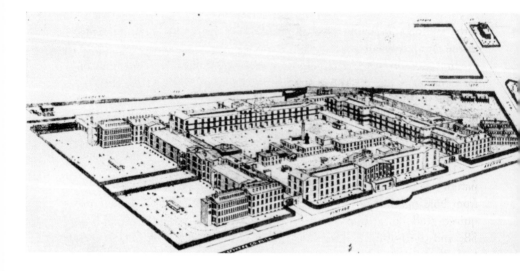

The Philadelphia Hospital, designed by William Strickland and erected in 1834. Drawing shows the hospital as it existed in 1890. (Philadelphia General Hospital picture collection, Historical Collections of the College of Physicians of Philadelphia.)

erations of physicians, they tended to distance students from actual disease cases.

A new arrangement was quick in coming. In 1766, Thomas Bond initiated clinical instruction for the medical students by taking them to the wards of Pennsylvania Hospital.[21] A few years later, Bond and an associate began clinical obstetrics by allowing students of "good character" to attend cases of labor at the Philadelphia Almshouse.[22]

As the numbers of medical students attracted to Philadelphia increased, the professors solicited the almshouse's Board of Guardians "to extend the convenience of the house for accommodating the students." The first step was to increase the number of medical officers there; Gerardus Clarkson, Adam Kuhn, and Benjamin Rush were among the initial additions.[23]

In 1803 Thomas C. James and John Church offered their services to the lying-in wards if they could be accompanied by a pupil from their private obstetrics school for each case. Their request was granted, as was that of Charles Caldwell, who instructed a class of twenty, and later forty, students on the medical wards. By 1806 lectures were being given in the dead house, too.

In 1811 the almshouse surgeons asked the board for room suitable for conducting operations on patients in front of the medical classes, arguing that the separate space would "remove from the wards a source of mischief to the other sick." The board had a second floor added to the dye-and-wash house and installed a lecture room with adjoining wards.[24]

The board had its own restrictions on access to the almshouse patients.[25] It disqualified members of the Pennsylvania Hospital staff from holding staff positions in the almshouse. After 1805, it also required students to purchase tickets to attend the clinics; a ticket was $8, and the purchase of two tickets gave "perpetual attendance privileges."

In 1812, Pennsylvania Hospital instituted a ticket policy. To compete, the almshouse board allowed students with the hospital's ticket to attend a case of labor. When this proposal was advertised in the newspaper, a protest arose over the indiscriminate opening of the lying-in ward. Protestors also complained about the board's exclusion of the Pennsylvania Hospital staff. The board was forced to rescind both policies.[26] (When the Jefferson Medical College petitioned the board in 1827 for equal status with Penn in the almshouse, however, Penn objected—successfully.)[27]

The almshouse moved to new buildings in Blockley Township in 1834.[28] For the students, "transportation was no inconsiderable item," wrote D. Hayes Agnew years later as he looked back on his medical-school days. But he recalled the rewards: "more invigorating air," for one; for another, "the most capacious and finely arranged amphitheater in the country, and capable of seating seven to 800 persons"; and most of all, the hospital itself, "the great clinic school of the country, annually opening its exhaustless treasures of disease to crowds of educated, zealous inquirers of medical knowledge."[29]

But tensions arose periodically between the almshouse's stewards and the resident physicians and their students. The stewards complained about the students' inexperience in treating the patients, the constant staff changes, and the lack of student supervision. In 1845, in particular, the board learned that some of the bodies of dead patients had been disposed of improperly after autopsy. In June of that year, a complete split occurred. The precipitating event, according to Agnew, centered on a cockroach "which had rashly taken a near cut across the table instead of going around."[30] The table in question was the steward's, at which the resident physicians boarded. The insect was squashed, but the physicians demanded to board at the matron's table. Rebuffed, they resigned and took the students with them.

The Board of Guardians submitted a different account.[31] It determined that the physicians were angry at the steward for allowing a resident physician whose term had recently expired to remain at the table. The board decided that the steward's permissiveness was improper but ordered the physicians to resume boarding at his table.

In September, the board established four specific positions for physicians. The almshouse stayed closed to the medical students until 1854, however, when Henry Hollingsworth Smith and John Livingston Ludlow visited every member of the board, which was persuaded to reinstall the students.

The next few years were unstable. In 1856 the chief medical officer was accused of improper management and dismissed (and his position abrogated). The new position was that of chief resident. The first incumbent resigned in June of 1857 when the board arbitrarily decided to discontinue student instruction. It might have reversed itself before the new academic year began, but the new chief resident created a new problem. He had formulated some "family medicines," whose ingredients he kept secret. When he failed to disclose them, his staff accused him of quackery and resigned, closing off clinical education for a year. In October 1858 the students petitioned the board, "praying" for it to reestablish instruction at the almshouse. The board listened and consented. From then until the mid-1970s, when the hospital (by then called Philadelphia General Hospital) was permanently closed and demolished, it remained open for medical students.[32]

SAINT JOSEPH'S HOSPITAL

Penn students also received training at Saint Joseph's Hospital, founded in 1849 for the care of poor Irish immigrants.[33] Many physicians on the Penn faculty had appointments on its staff, and they brought their students there until the 1870s, when the Hospital of the University of

Pennsylvania was founded and the medical department moved to West Philadelphia.

THE ANATOMICAL SCHOOLS AND CHAPMAN'S ACADEMY

Students had additional ways of obtaining information, even back in the days when Morgan, Shippen, Kuhn, and Rush dominated medical training. In pre-Revolution Philadelphia, Abraham Chevat (Chovet), not a member of the faculty, taught anatomy in his house, where he became known for wax anatomical models. Many students no doubt attended his lectures and visited his museum. His collection later became part of the collection at the Wistar Institute and was used by Penn professors well into the 19th century.[34]

Subsequently students could learn in proprietary institutions run by their own instructors. When the medical school moved out of "the laboratory," the building was rented to faculty members Thomas Chalkley James and Nathaniel Chapman, who taught extra medical courses there privately as Chapman's Medical Academy.[35]

Far from usurping the functions of such schools, formal medical education stimulated them. For most of the nineteenth century, medical classes were large, containing between four hundred and five hundred students—numbers necessary to maintain the faculty's income and support the medical department. Classes of this size, however, could be taught only by lectures illustrated by demonstrations, preserved specimens, wax models, and table experiments. Medical Hall had no student laboratories and limited space for anatomical dissection.

For practical dissecting experience, then, students enrolled in a proprietary school, much like their European counterparts, who filled such establishments as William Hunter's Great Windmill Street School of London. One of the more enduring in Philadelphia was the Philadelphia School of Anatomy, opened in 1820 by James Valentine O'Brion Lawrence. It had no charter, granted no degrees, and operated "without a well-known faculty." Still, it stood for fifty-five years, outlasting many larger and more prestigious competitors, partly because of its ideal location near both Penn and Jefferson.

In 1838 James McClintock started a dissecting room on the corner of Eighth and Walnut Streets, but his neighbors complained bitterly about both the odors that emanated from it and the nature of the work. He then moved the school to the building next to the Philadelphia Dissecting Rooms. After several changes of hands over time, Agnew bought it for $600 in 1852.

Agnew was an enthusiastic teacher of anatomy. His rooms were open twelve to eighteen hours each day, and he lectured five evenings a week during the school year, three evenings a week during summers. James Edmund Garretson, Samuel David Gross, Richard J. Levis, and William Williams Keen were among his many demonstrators. His enrollment grew from 9 to 250 students, culled from Penn, Jefferson, and the Pennsylvania Dental College; students from Hahnemann and Women's Medical College were not accepted. In 1854 he opened a floor to demonstrate current operative procedures on cadavers. Agnew sold the school in 1862 to Garretson for the same amount he paid for it.[36]

FOUNDING OF THE AMERICAN MEDICAL ASSOCIATION

Because the level of quality (not to mention the prejudices) of private schools was so haphazard and student involvement was voluntary, the quality of a young person's medical education depended largely upon the individual's own ambition.

Because the new medical schools were successful, a large number of new schools were founded between 1820 and 1845. Faculties of the established institutions worried that students would flock to the least expensive schools and those with the lowest admission requirements.

In response, talk circulated about the "failure" of the American system of medical education, and reform was bruited as early as 1839. An attempt at a national convention in 1840, sponsored by the New York State Medical Society, failed because no medical society or faculty accepted the invitation.[37]

Medical societies replied more positively to a meeting held in New York in 1846, but only about one-third of the schools sent delegates; Penn was not among them. Among the reforms proposed was improvement of the preliminary preparation and office training of apprentices; lengthening of lecture courses from four to six months; and the creation of state licensing boards to control those who practice.

At that meeting, a convention was set for Philadelphia in 1847 to found the American Medical Association. It met at the Academy of Science in May; Penn was one of twenty-eight schools (out of some thirty-six) to send delegates. It came away with the chief officers: Chapman as president, Alfred Stillé as one of two secretaries, and Isaac Hayes as treasurer. As one reformer noted, Chapman's election "was not based on any of his services to organizing the movement but on his personal standing as one of the oldest and most eminent teachers in the Union, he stood appropriately at the head of the whole profession."[38]

The Penn faculty moved to alter its curriculum along the lines recommended at the convention, despite the fact that its courses, five and a half months long, were already longer than those at most schools. Two weeks of preliminary lectures began in October; then the regular courses began, ending on the last day of March. Course fees were reduced from $20 each to $15 and the graduation fee from $40 to $30. No other medical school in the city responded to the advice of the convention, however; by 1853 Penn's faculty reverted to a term of nineteen weeks.[39]

As for other proposed reforms, control of licensing was left to the state legislature. The Penn professors noted that the preliminary training of students depended on the cooperation of physicians who chose them. That, of course, was only part of the educational problem. More stringent solutions remained elusive as long as the competence of the practitioners who gave hands-on experience could not be monitored, and as long as professorial salaries were set by the number of students in each medical class. Another twenty years would pass before reform reached these areas.

NOTES

1. E. P. Cheyney, *History of The University of Pennsylvania 1740–1940* (Philadelphia: University of Pennsylvania Press, 1940), pp. 112–25; G. W. Corner, *Two Centuries of Medicine* (Philadelphia: Lippincott, 1965), pp. 32–37; J. Carson, *A History of the Medical Department* (Philadelphia: Lindsay and Blakiston, 1869), pp. 86–90.

2. Corner, *Two Centuries of Medicine*, p. 36; Carson, *History of the Medical Department*, pp. 89–90.

3. Cheyney, *History of the University of Pennsylvania*, p. 136.

4. Carson, *History of the Medical Department*, p. 91; Corner, *Two Centuries of Medicine*, p. 37.

5. Carson, pp. 92–93.

6. Cheyney, pp. 152–53.

7. Carson, p. 93.

8. Carson, p. 97; Corner, *Two Centuries of Medicine*, pp. 41–44.

9. Carson, p. 206.

10. L. C. Parish and T. N. Haviland, "Surgeon's Hall—The Story of the First Medical-School Building in the United States," *New England Journal of Medicine* 273(1965):1021–24: C. E. Peterson "Library Hall: Home of the Library Company of Philadelphia—1790–1880, in *Historic Philadelphia*, ed. Luther P. Eisenhardt, issued as vol. 43, part 1 of the *Transactions of the American Philosophical Society*, 1952, and reprinted 1980, p. 131.

11. Cheyney, *History of the University of Pennsylvania*, pp. 180–81.

12. Carson, *History of the Medical Department*, p. 207.

13. Carson, p. 208; Corner, *Two Centuries of Medicine*, p. 50.

14. Corner, p. 50.

15. Corner, p. 68; Carson, p. 209.

16. Corner, p. 79; Carson, p. 209; Minutes of the Faculty of the Medical Department, Archives of the University of Pennsylvania.

17. *Medical Department of the University of Pennsylvania* (Philadelphia, 1844). (A history of the Medical Department authorized by the medical professors of the University of Pennsylvania.)

18. W. E. Horner, Art. 5, "Clinical Report on the Surgical Department of the Philadelphia Hospital, Blockley, for the Months, May, June, and July, 1837" *American Journal of Medical Sciences*, 21, 99–112 (1845): 100–101.

19. G. B. Wood, M.D. professor of the theory and practice of medicine, in *Descriptive Sketches of Medical Professors of Philadelphia*, No. 1, *The University of Pennsylvania, by a graduate in medicine, published by the author, 1857. For sale only at George A. Wentz's Segar Store, No. 8, South 9th Street, first door north of the university.*

20. Corner, *Two Centuries of Medicine*, pp. 61–62; Minutes of the Faculty of the Medical Department, Archives of the University of Pennsylvania.

21. Corner, p. 24.

22. W. S. Middleton, "Clinical Teaching in the Philadelphia Alms House Hospital," in *Old Blockley: Proceedings of the Bi-Centenary Celebration of the Building of the Philadelphia Alms House* (New York: Froeben Press, 1933), p. 95.

23. *Ibid.*, p. 96.

24. *Ibid.*, pp. 100–101.

25. *Ibid.*, pp. 101–2.

26. *Ibid.*, p. 102.

27. D. H. Agnew, "The Medical History of the Philadelphia Almshouse," in J. W. Crosky, *History of Blockley—A History of the Philadelphia General Hospital* (Philadelphia: F. A. Davis Co., 1929), p. 38.

28. Crosky, p. 37; R. G. Curtin, "The Philadelphia General Hospital," in *Founders Week Memorial Volume* (Philadelphia: City of Philadelphia, 1909); R. J. Hunt *The Origin of the Philadelphia Hospital, Blockley Division* (Philadelphia: Rittenhouse Press); *Old Blockley.*

29. Crosky, p. 39.

30. *Ibid.*, pp. 31–32.

31. Minutes of the Board of Guardians of the Poor of the City of Philadelphia, Archives of the City of Philadelphia, 1845.

32. Crosky, pp. 40–42.

and Incidents of the City and its Inhabitants from the Days of the Pilgrim Founders (Philadelphia, 1830), p. 609.

35. I. Richman, *The Brightest Ornament* (Bellefont, Pa.: Pennsylvania Heritage, 1967), p. 76.

36. J. H. Adams, *History of the Life of D. Hayes Agnew M.D., LL.D.* (Philadelphia: F. A. Davis, 1892), pp. 76–105.

37. N. S. Davis, *History of the American Medical Association from its Organization to January, 1855* (Philadelphia, 1855).

38. Richman, *The Brightest Ornament*, pp. 182–83.

39. G. B. Wood, *Introductory Lecture to the Course of Materia Medica in the University of Pennsylvania, Delivered October 21, 1847* (Philadelphia: John Young, 1847), pp. 13–19.

4

THE FIRST WAVE OF NINETEENTH-CENTURY LUMINARIES

*It is true that the history of science is very different from the science of history—
we are not—attempting to study the working of blind forces—operating on
crowds of obscure people—The men whose names are found in the history of
science are not hypothetical constituents of a crowd—We recognize them as men
like ourselves and their actions and thoughts, being more free from the influence
of passion and recorded more accurately than those of other men are better
material for the study of the calmer parts of human nature.*

James Clerk Maxwell

PHILIP SYNG PHYSICK

Throughout the nineteenth century, the medical school was distinguished by its professors of anatomy and surgery. At about the time the University was beginning its move to Ninth and Market Streets, one member of its faculty, Philip Syng Physick, was becoming a world-prominent surgeon.[1] Retiring and soft-spoken, a relentless experimenter and inventor, he joined Benjamin Rush as one of the first of the New World physicians to gain a reputation among his European counterparts.

Born in Philadelphia in the year of the medical school's first graduation, Physick, in his youth, appeared unlikely to become known as the father of American surgery.[2] After graduating from the College of Philadelphia, under his father's advice, he began a preceptorship with Adam Kuhn and attended lectures at the medical school. Without obtaining his medical degree, however, he embarked for London with his father to further his medical training.

Shortly after arriving, the elder Physick not only obtained a position for his son with John Hunter but also persuaded the famous surgeon and anatomist to let Philip live at his home.[3] When the father asked what books his son would need for his studies, Hunter took him to the dissecting room, pointed to the cadavers, and said, "These are the textbooks. The printed ones are fit for very little."[4]

Philip availed himself of the opportunities in the dissecting room. He also studied surgery at Saint George's Hospital and attended lectures on midwifery by John Clark and William Osborne. He eventually took a medical degree at the University of Edinburgh.[5]

In September 1792, Physick returned to the United States and opened a surgical practice. Few patients came, and he fell into debt, becoming disillusioned with surgery.[6] His financial distress was relieved during the yellow fever epidemic of 1793 when he was one of four young physicians appointed to attend the sick at Bush Hill Hospital, which had been opened for care of the stricken poor.[7]

Physick allied himself with Rush in the arguments on treating yellow fever, and Rush helped him gain appointment to Pennsylvania Hospital.[8] For the remainder of his career, Physick was loyal to Rush's ideas. He remained an ardent believer in bleeding and refrained from joining the College of Physicians of Philadelphia, from which Rush had resigned in the controversy over that form of treatment.

With his staff position secure, Physick applied his ingenuity to a host of surgical problems.[9] He designed and made novel instruments to treat the urinary tract. He developed a procedure for making bougies with "bees wax and fine new linen," which he attached to the end of catheters to serve as a filiform guide.[10] For more difficult urethral strictures, he invented a device that contained a lancet in a tube, with which he could cut the constriction.[11] He improved the gorget used to enter the bladder in lithotomy.[12] (One of his patients was Chief Justice John Marshall, from whom Physick successfully removed more than a thousand stones.)[13]

While performing his first lithotomy, Physick accidentally divided the internal pudendal artery. He controlled the profuse bleeding by compressing the artery with his left hand while passing a hooked instrument under the artery. Then he cast a ligature around it and tied it off. He stopped the bleeding, but too much of the surrounding tissue was damaged by the tie. To reduce the amount of tissue included, he designed his celebrated forceps for carrying ligatures under deep-seated vessels.[14]

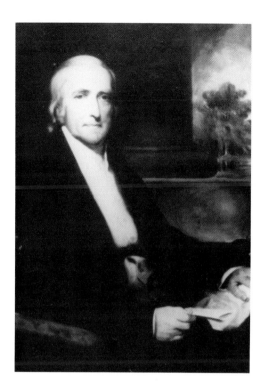

Philip Syng Physick, Professor of Surgery, 1805–1818; Professor of Anatomy, 1818–1832. From a portrait by Henry Inman that hangs in the Portrait Hall of the School of Medicine of the University of Pennsylvania. (Archives of the University of Pennsylvania.)

For some prostatic obstructions, he used a catheter to which he tied a pouch made from sheep intestines. After he inserted the instrument into the bladder, he filled it with tepid water, plugged it, and then retracted it. The effect repressed the enlarged prostate and gave patients months of relief by making it easier for them to urinate.[15]

One of Physick's most impressive accomplishments was the closure of an artificial anus (abdominal fistula). In 1809, nearly twenty years before a similar operation was described in France, he fused the two ends of the bowel to each other like the two barrels of a shotgun. When he was satisfied that the ends of the colon adhered to each other, he passed a needle with a ligature from one part of the intestine into the other, "through the sides which were in contact." In three weeks the septum between the two ends of bowel had broken down. Now feces passed through the intestine and the patient had normal bowel movements. He covered the abdominal opening with a lint bandage held in place with a truss.[16]

With Dr. Alexander Monroe (secundus) of Edinburgh, Physick shares the honor of being the first to wash out the stomach and actively lavage it using a large flexible tube and pewter syringe. Physick was called to treat three-year-old twins whose mother had mistakenly given them an overdose of laudanum. The children had convulsed after the dose and become comatose with a pulse that had almost ceased when Physick arrived. The children could not swallow, so Physick introduced his gum elastic tube into their stomachs and injected ipecac mixed with water. He repeated the procedure until he had emptied their stomachs. By this time, "all signs of animation in both children had ceased." Determined to save them, Physick injected some spirits mixed with water and vinegar into their stomachs through the tube while administering external stimuli. In a few moments the pulse and respiration returned to each child. Through this procedure he managed to save one of the twins.[17]

Physick developed a double-wire snare passed through a tube or cannula for removing scirrhous tonsils and for removing hemorrhoids.[18] And he improved methods of treating fractures and developed new ones to treat fractures. He stimulated bone growth in nonunited fractures by passing a seton through the fracture line.[19]

Probably his greatest and most lasting contribution to surgery was his work on absorbable sutures. He noticed that ordinary ligatures of silk or flax prevented wounds from healing; they were customarily left in wounds for weeks or even months, causing painful inflammation and drainage and pain. Physick proposed the use of animal ligatures to secure an artery long enough to cause the obliteration of the vessel. In 1816 he described how the idea occurred to him and how it worked:

> Several years ago, recollecting how completely leather straps spread with adhesive plaster and applied over wounds for the purpose of keeping the sides in contact were dissolved by the fluids discharged from the wound, it appeared to me that ligatures might be made of leather or some animal substance [he used thin leather strips cut from kid gloves] with which the sides of blood vessels could be compressed for a sufficient time to prevent hemorrhage; that such ligatures would be dissolved in a few days and would be evacuated with the discharge from the cavity of the wound.[20]

From this point, Physick used animal ligatures, even though other surgeons did not pick up the technique rapidly—perhaps because they did not take the time to prepare the animal tissue in advance.

Until 1800 surgery had been taught by the professor of anatomy. At this time the students petitioned Physick by letter, asking him to lecture to them on surgery. His initial lecture, given at Pennsylvania Hospital and attended by his supporter Rush, was judged a huge success.[21] From this time, Physick's reputation as a teacher of surgery grew among his colleagues to such an extent that a separate chair of surgery was created for him in 1805. He held it until 1818, when John Syng Dorsey, the anatomy professor, died. Then Physick shifted to the anatomy professorship, which he held until his retirement in 1831.[22]

WILLIAM E. HORNER

As professor of anatomy, Physick was assisted by William E. Horner, a polite, retiring, deeply religious Virginian. Although considered by some colleagues to be a mediocre scholar,[23] through "sheer force of will and indomitable purpose " Horner exceeded the accomplishments of his critics as a teacher, scientist, and administrator.[24]

Horner was best known for his anatomical observations of the eye.[25] He first described the function of the tensor tarsi muscle, whose structure had been described some 75 years earlier.[26] The tensor tarsi keeps the edges of the eyelids properly adjusted to the ball and helps the gathering of tears; it is called "Horner's muscle." Horner wrote that he had been primed for the discovery, in part, by observing how the lower eyelids of Caspar Wistar fell from his eyeballs in a fainting spell during his last illness.

Horner also devised the Z-plasty, an operation still used today, to revise wound scars. He used this procedure to correct the ectropion of the eye of a patient at the Philadelphia Hospital.[27] Previously V-shaped and Y-shaped incisions had been used. Horner's simpler operation became the more useful procedure when the plastic surgeon J. Stage Davis reintroduced it in the early 1900s.[28]

Horner made two other significant contributions to surgery. In one, he, along with Physick, suggested the extraperitoneal approach for a Caesarean section.[29] In the other, he described the first successful repair of a ruptured Achilles tendon.[30] He passed a thin ribbon through the

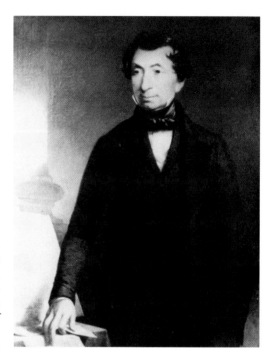

William E. Horner, from a painting by John Nagle. School of Medicine of the University of Pennsylvania. (Archives of the University of Pennsylvania.)

torn ends of the tendon, and removed the ribbon when the wound began to suppurate. (This principle of stimulating growth with a seton was the same as that used by Physick to heal nonunited fractures.)

It was in the wards of Philadelphia Hospital, where he practiced surgery, that Horner and his colleagues William Gibson and Joseph Pancoast were among the first in Philadelphia to use ether anesthesia successfully, about a year after the 1847 demonstration of the technique at Massachusetts General Hospital.[31]

Because of his expertise in anatomy as well as surgery, Horner was frequently called upon to perform autopsies on the patients of his colleagues in addition to those he did on his own. He summarized the knowledge accumulated in these cases in his 1829 *Treatise of Pathological Anatomy*, the first textbook of pathology published in the United States.[32]

Horner also made original clinical contributions in pathology. During the city's cholera epidemic of 1832, he made microscopic studies of the colons of cholera patients. He concluded that the intestinal tract had an area greater than that of a large dining-room table filled with glandular structures. He reasoned that large volumes of fluid could readily be lost from this large intestinal surface. He explained correctly that the rice-water stools of cholera were formed when this huge fluid volume washed the mucus secreted by the irritated intestinal glands from the surface of the intestinal lumen as it rushed from the colon as a diarrheal stool.[33]

He also wrote *Lessons in Practical Anatomy for the Use of Dissectors* (1823), which went into five editions.[34] And he published his lecture notes as *Treatise on Special and General Anatomy* (1826), a textbook that went through eight editions; the final three revisions reflect his appreciation of the importance of the achromatic and astigmatic microscope, introduced about 1830.[35]

Among his other anatomical discoveries, Horner described the membrane that lined the larynx, which he called the vocal membrane. He also clarified how the epiglottis defends the trachae from fluids and food particles. He showed that the larynx is closed by being pulled up into the base of the epiglottis rather than by pulling the epiglottis down over it.[36] He was especially pleased at this discovery, because it explained a famous French case at the time—why Baron Larrey's patient who had had the upper part of his epiglottis destroyed by a musket ball could swallow food without aspirating it.

Horner was appointed dean in 1822 and stayed in that post for thirty years. He required students to take 704 hours of instruction, the highest standard of medical education at the time. Lengthy study tended to reduce enrollment, which in turn reduced the income of the faculty and the school, but the trustees supported his policies: three years of study, a course in clinical instruction, and a faculty-approved thesis free of bad spelling and grammar. He was also praised for able handling of the school's finances.[37]

Horner was also active in the city's medical community, helping to found Saint Joseph's Hospital in 1849, and he was made the first president of its medical board.[38] He left his books and surgical instruments to Saint Joseph's. He left his dissecting instruments and anatomical collection to the Wistar Museum, to which his name was added until the Wistar Institute was established at the end of the century.[39]

JOSEPH LEIDY

Joseph Leidy, who dominated the chair of anatomy for most of the second half of the century, differed from the earlier Penn anatomists because he was a naturalist, not a surgeon.[40] He received his M.D. degree from Penn in 1844 after presenting his thesis on "The Comparative Anatomy of the Eye of Vertebrate Animals." He abandoned a short-lived private practice to travel with Horner to Europe in 1848, then became professor of anatomy upon Horner's death in 1852. He was lively, expressive, and animated in lectures, unceremonious, and good-natured to the point of avoiding controversy of all kinds; his friends even mocked him as being an "invertebrate."

Leidy made advances and discoveries in botany, comparative anatomy, mineralogy, paleontology, and many areas of medicine that affected public health. It was Leidy who first determined that America was the ancestral home of the horse.[41] In addition, his profound knowledge of osteology enabled him to identify a fragment of a fossilized tooth found in Nebraska as that of a rhinoceros. Skeptical contemporary naturalists dropped their doubts about his theory when, coincidentally, a skull, unmistakably that of a rhinoceros, was found in the same region of Nebraska. Embedded in its jaw were the remains of the very tooth Leidy had identified.[42]

Years ahead of Louis Pasteur and Charles Darwin, Leidy discussed the questions of spontaneous generation and the origins of life. In a paper with the interesting title "Monas, Vibrio, Euglena, Volvox, Leucophys, Paramecium, Valecella, etc.," he asserted his belief in evolution:

An attentive study of geology proves that there was a time when no living bodies existed on the earth. Living beings, characterized by a peculiar structure and series of phenomena, appeared upon the earth at a definite though very remote period. Composed of the same ultimate elements which constitute the earth, they originated in the pre-existing materials of their structure. . . . The study of the earth's crust teaches us that very many species of plants and animals became extinct at successive periods, while other races originated to occupy their places. This probably was the result in many cases of a change in exterior conditions incompatible with life of a certain species and favorable to the primitive production of others. Living beings did not live on earth prior to their indispensable conditions of action but wherever these have been brought into operation concomitantly, the former originated. Of the life present everywhere, with its indispensable conditions and coeval in its origin with them, what was the eminent cause? It could not have existed upon earth prior to its essential conditions, and is it therefore the result of these? There appear to be but trifling steps from the oscillating particle of organic matter to a Bacterium; from this to a Vibrio, thence to a Monad, and so gradually up to the highest orders of life. The most ancient rocks containing remains of living beings indicate the contemporaneous existence of the more complex as well as the simplest organic forms; but nevertheless, life may have been ushered upon earth through oceans of the lowest type long previously to the deposits of the oldest Palaeozoic rocks known to us. . . . Probably every species has a definite course to run in consequence of a general law, an origin, an increase, a decline, and an extinction.[43]

Joseph Leidy lecturing in the Anatomical Amphitheater of Medical Hall. (Archives of the University of Pennsylvania.)

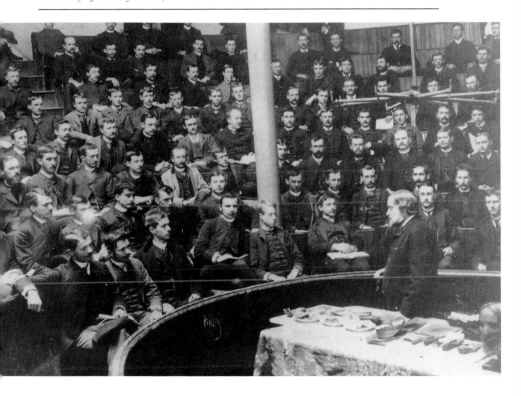

This paper was published six years before Darwin published *The Origin of Species* but produced no significant response in the scientific world.

One of Leidy's most practical contributions to medical science came early in his career, in 1846, when he reported that he had found *Trichina spiralis* in the superficial thigh muscle of pigs. In keeping with his keen sense of observation and curiosity, he had noted minute white specks in a piece of ham served to him at his breakfast table. Under the microscope they proved to be *Trichina spiralis*.[44] Leidy knew such parasites occurred in human muscle, for they had been discovered previously by Sir James Paget and studied in detail by Richard Owen, who gave them their name. Prior to Leidy's discovery, however, no one had suspected that pork was the source of this dangerous infestation in humans. Fourteen years later, the epidemiological significance of Leidy's discovery was provided by Friedrich Albert Zenker in Dresden. Zenker related the muscular and intestinal forms in humans to a single organism in whose life cycle the pig played an intrinsic part.

Leidy also advanced ideas on hookworms before their time. In 1886 he reported an autochthonous infestation of hookworm in cats. Although now the cat is considered only an experimental host for this parasite, his early finding raised interest in Europe and the United States in the distribution of hookworm.[45] Leidy's reports reinforced the growing suspicion that hookworms are a cause of anemia. Early on, Leidy investigated flies as transmitters of disease at a time when cleanliness was only beginning to seem important in medicine. Some time elapsed before his understanding of bacterial parasites in disease was fully appreciated.

WILLIAM GIBSON

William Gibson, born in Baltimore, studied medicine there, in Scotland, and at Pennsylvania. He boasted to his Penn classmates that he would replace the "old man"—Physick —in the chair of surgery. He did, indeed, in 1819, after Physick took the chair of anatomy.[46]

Gibson helped care for casualties at the Battle of Waterloo, where he, too, was wounded. He had already made a mark as the first surgeon to tie off a common iliac artery when he tried to stop the bleeding caused by a gunshot wound. The patient died, nonetheless, from loss of blood. Evidently he was a graphic teacher, according to this description by a student:

> In teaching gunshot wounds, he illustrates all that is said by showing us the character of such injuries by shooting the different parts of a subject, tracing the ball, and exhibiting the peculiarities of the wound to the class. The superiority of this method over that of simply talking on a subject is at once evident to all. He does not content himself with giving abstract notions of dislocations by merely showing dry bones displaced; but by having the joints opened and dividing the ligaments, he displaces the bones in the various ways that we know to result from accident. Thus it has very nearly the exact appearance that the real injury would present.[47]

ROBERT HARE

While Physick and Horner were advancing anatomy and surgery, Robert Hare was assuring Penn first rank in chemistry.[48] He had a significant hand in planning the facilities. Having taught in the renovated Medical Hall of 1819, he knew its limitations for teaching and experimentation. When the faculty decided to build a new facility, Hare consulted with Strickland, the architect; the result was one of the most modern and best-equipped chemical laboratories of its time.

It was an all-purpose structure that could be used for lecture demonstrations, original experimentation, and student benches. Hare provided for high-temperature furnaces, electrical apparati, a sand-and-water bath to heat and distill flammable chemicals, as well as for storage of expensive glass and other devices. The design incorporated proper heating and ventilation and allowed for the safe use of highly combustible materials.[49] He insisted that one side of the lab have a southern exposure to ensure adequate light in winter for demonstrating the development of precipitates and the colors of solutions.

Hare was a student of James Woodhouse, but for the most part he taught himself chemistry.[50] A fellow student at the same boarding house was Benjamin Silliman. They persuaded their landlady to let them convert a small cellar kitchen into a laboratory. Here the two worked together, extending their education far beyond what they learned from Woodhouse, whom Silliman thought a poor teacher. Silliman went on to a distinguished career at Yale University. He and Hare remained close friends and exchanged their scientific ideas in long letters until they died.

Hare never received his M.D. degree and so was deemed less than ideal to teach medicinal chemistry.[51] The faculty delayed his election to the chemistry chair until 1818. By this date, Rush and others were no longer present to block the appointment of a nonmedical instructor.

Still, the prejudice against his education persisted, and Hare was looked on as a second-class member of the faculty. When he was first appointed, he was not permitted to examine students, sign diplomas, or participate in faculty decisions involving medical affairs. He did not fret, however, over his restricted authority; it freed him from routine administrative duties and allowed him to get on with his chemistry.

He did get on with it. He was considered America's foremost chemist, the equal of America's foremost physicist, Joseph Henry, at Princeton.[52] Both these early American scientists were interested in the

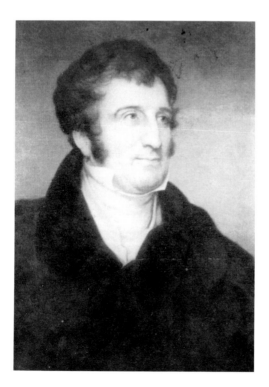

Robert Hare. (Archives of the University of Pennsylvania.)

same problem: finding a means to generate large electrical currents. Since one was a physicist and the other a chemist they employed different methods to attain their goal. Henry generated electricity by induction with electromagnets while Hare produced large currents with chemical reactions, using batteries.

Hare was only twenty years old when the Chemical Society of Philadelphia appointed him to a committee to discover how a "greater concentration of heat might be obtained from chemical processes." Much more oxygen, the committee determined, would have to be introduced into any combustion procedure. Hare wrote that he had already made a machine to do it. It was his oxygen-hydrogen blowpipe, and he was invited to demonstrate it before the society.

He reported that he had been readily able to fuse heavy spar, alumina, silica, lime, and magnesia, while platinum, gold, and silver "were thrown into a state of ebullition." He repeated the demonstration for the American Philosophical Society, which was so impressed that it elected him to membership. The blowpipe was the forerunner of oxygen acetylene welding as well as the basis for the fuel system of rocket motors in space exploration.[53]

Hare extended his experiments to the use of electricity to generate intense heat. In 1818 he revealed a calorimotor, in which he wired, in parallel, larger copper and zinc plates than had been used previously. When they were dipped into sulfuric acid, they generated currents sufficient to burn iron rods and even to fuse them.[54]

He also invented the "deflagrator," another galvanic instrument that generated even stronger currents. When zinc and copper plates were immersed in acid solutions, Hare noted, the current generated was greatest instantly after immersion; a few seconds later, the current fell to low equilibrium levels. Accordingly, he constructed a rack that held a number of large copper and zinc plates. The rack could be immediately immersed into or removed from an acid bath. Just after the rack of plates was immersed, intense electrical currents arced between the tips of iron rods placed close to each other and fused them when they touched one another. Producing a heat capable of fusing metals was the origin of electric welding.[55]

Hare held the chemistry chair for twenty-nine years. Although he may not have been the best of teachers, there is ample testimony that he was a master demonstrator of chemical experiments and adequately explained their rationale.[56]

Still, he inspired discovery in others. In 1839 Paul B. Goddard, one of Hare's students, developed the bromine sensitizing method which made practical the photographic process invented by Daguerre.[57] Prior to Goddard's discovery, portraiture required exposure times of minutes. His method increased the sensitivity of Daguerre's iodine procedure and reduced the exposure time required for good photographs to seconds. (John Goddard—no relation—described the method independently in England in 1840.)

Paul Goddard was assisted in his experiments by Hare and Professor Martin Boye. He was also associated with Robert Cornelius, whose self-portrait, taken in November 1839, is probably the earliest photograph of a human being. Goddard's view of Philadelphia, also taken in 1839 and preserved at the Franklin Institute, is the earliest instantaneously exposed photograph. Goddard later joined Penn's anatomy department and became a prolific medical writer.

Upon Hare's retirement in 1855, Pennsylvania's trustees hoped that Henry would take the chemistry chair. Henry, however, had been invited to head the new Smithsonian Institution, and he went to Washington. Hare's treasured chemical apparatus followed; Hare donated it to the new museum, hoping that Henry would arrange to preserve it. For a time it was set up for display as well as used in a room across from Henry's office.[58] Subsequently it was dismantled and stored. It was destroyed in a fire early in the twentieth century.

The only piece of Hare's equipment that remained at Penn was the small cannon he used to demonstrate to students the forces created by combustion. Edgar Fahs Smith used the cannon for this purpose in his chemistry lectures until he retired.[59]

NATHANIEL CHAPMAN

Nathaniel Chapman held the chair of the theory and practice of physic from 1816 to 1850. He also held the chair of the institutes of medicine until 1835, when Samuel Jackson took over that responsibility.[60] Chapman was elegant and flamboyant, a persuasive teacher who eclipsed the precise teaching styles of Physick, Horner, and Hare, despite a nasal voice resulting from a defect in his palate produced by a childhood injury. His most important contribution may have been founding the *Philadelphia Journal of Medical and Physical Sciences* in 1820; later it was called the *American Journal of Medical Sciences* and was considered one of the country's foremost medical periodicals.[61] Chapman himself was ever embroiled in controversies yet always remained popular with his colleagues—as was indicated by his election as the first president of the American Medical Association when the organization was founded in Philadelphia in 1847.[62] He was called, variously, Philadelphia's "brightest ornament," "a man of irreversible mind," and an "intellectual bankrupt" who refused to accept scientific advances.[63] Chapman, a Virginian, studied medicine under Elisha Cullen Dick, who treated George Washington in his final illness.[64] He came to Philadelphia in 1797, worked in Rush's office, and attended Pennsylvania's medical lectures, graduating in 1800 after writing a thesis on hydrophobia.[65] After foreign training, he settled in Philadelphia and from the outset aimed to succeed Rush as professor of theory and practice of physic.[66] He joined the staff of the Philadelphia Almshouse when Charles Caldwell was forced to resign involuntarily following a violent dispute with Thomas C. James.[67] Chapman broke with Rush and jeopardized his chances to assume his chair. Although Rush signed the younger physician's application for membership in the Philadelphia Medical Society, he blocked his appointment to the staff of Pennsylvania Hospital.[68] Chapman, though, had many ways to cultivate the city's proper people. In 1808 he advanced his career by joining with James to teach a popular, independent course on midwifery. He managed after all to connect himself with the prestigious hospital despite Rush.[69] In 1807, the physicians of the hospital appointed two doctors to visit all poor patients with disease; they placed John Syng Dorsey in charge of the city's northern district and Chapman in charge of the southern. Those two became the first of many distinguished physicians to occupy these posts until 1818,[70] when the city opened two dispensaries.[71] When Rush died in 1813, Benjamin S. Barton succeeded him, but Chapman was not overlooked. He was given Barton's former post as professor of materia medica. When Barton died in 1815, Chapman gained the chair he wanted.[72]

In the 1820s he overcame an unpleasant association with an elixir named Swaim's Panacea, made by a New York harness maker or bookbinder. Its ingredient was essentially sarsaparilla syrup mixed with oil of wintergreen flavoring. Chapman and other physicians heartily endorsed the concoction, and Swaim prospered. As rumors began to circulate that some batches of the remedy contained mercuric chloride, a poisonous compound, the physicians worried about Swaim's use of their testimonials. The Philadelphia Medical Society investigated it and other specifics. It also asked the physicians who seemed to support it whether their endorsements were being used as they intended. Chapman was one of the first to recant. (Though Swaim was proclaimed a quack, the remedy continued to be used into the twentieth century.)[73]

WILLIAM WOOD GERHARD

The first doctor of physic to advance clinical medicine was William Wood Gerhard.[74] After earning his Penn medical degree, he traveled to Paris, then the medical center of the world. He was one of the so-called American Argonauts, who included George W. Norris, Caspar W. Pennock, and Alfred Stillé from Philadelphia, and Oliver Wendell Holmes, James Jackson, Jr., and George C. Shattuck from Boston.[75] He was still in France in 1832 when he joined Pennock in publishing an article on cholera. At that time typhus was prevalent in Paris. There was also a similar disease to which one of Gerhard's teachers, Pierre-Charles-Alexandre Louis, had given the name typhoid. Gerhard observed that French clinicians confused the two, and when he visited the British Isles in 1833, he noticed that physicians there also confused them. On his return to Philadelphia, Gerhard served as resident physician at the Pennsylvania Hospital and was elected to the staff of the Philadelphia Almshouse in 1835. While working on the almshouse wards, he, along with his colleagues Pennock and Stillé, established that the disease called "spotted fever" in Philadelphia was identical to the disease Louis had called typhoid. Gerhard widened his studies to include patients at the hospital. In more than fifty autopsies, he found many cases without the enlarged spleen and the ulcerations of the lymphoid follicles of the intestines characteristic of typhoid, although they had a skin rash similar to that caused by typhus. He proved that typhus was characterized by an absence of an enlarged spleen or intestinal lesions.[76] The honor of first distinguishing the two diseases has been given to many, including Gerhard and Pennock, Lemuel Shattuck of Boston, Robert Perry of Glasgow, and Lombard of Geneva. But Gerhard's 1837 papers in *The American Journal of Medical Sciences* are the first clear descriptions of the clinical and anatomical distinctions between the diseases. In *Principles and Practice of Medicine* (1892), William Osler awards the laurels to Gerhard.[77]

Gerhard contracted typhoid fever in 1837 at the age of 30. He recovered, but his health was permanently damaged. He subsequently withdrew from investigating infectious diseases and confined his practice to Pennsylvania Hospital and the almshouse and to teaching the institutes of medicine at Pennsylvania Hospital.

HENRY HOLLINGSWORTH SMITH

Henry Hollingsworth Smith succeeded William Gibson as professor of surgery.[78] Smith had worked in the department of anatomy and aided his father-in-law, William E. Horner, in his duties as dean; Horner paid Smith $150.00, half the dean's salary.

As a surgeon, Smith became interested in methods to treat false

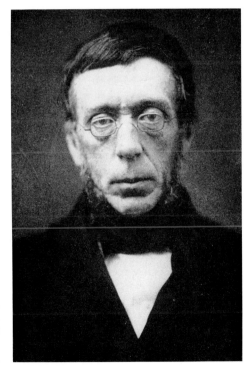

William Wood Gerhard. (Historical Collections of the College of Physicians of Philadelphia.)

joints (pseudarthrosis or nonunited fractures).[79] In 1855 he wrote that he urged

> the advantage of pressure and motion as obtained by means of a soft artificial limb, and experience has hence shown no case of failure even when the union of the bone did not ensue.[80]

Smith displayed his organizational capabilities during the Civil War. He devised the plan for removing the wounded from the battlefield after the Battle of Winchester to major hospitals in Reading, Philadelphia, Harrisburg, and other large cities in the region. As an administrator-surgeon in the Union Army, he established the practice of embalming the dead on the battlefield, facilitating their removal and return to their families. He organized and directed a corps of surgeons and used a steamer as a floating hospital to treat the wounded at the siege of Yorktown and managed the treatment of wounded in the Seven Day Battles around Richmond.[81]

During his productive career Smith wrote a textbook of surgery, an atlas of anatomy with Horner, and numerous works on the treatment of fractures.[82]

NOTES

1. J. Randolph, *A Memoir of the Life and Character of Philip Syng Physick, M.D.* (Philadelphia: Collins, 1839); W. E. Horner, "Necrological Notice of Philip Syng Physick," *Proceedings of the American Philosophical Society* (Philadelphia: Barrington and Haswell, 1838).

2. Randolph, pp. 14, 15.

3. *Ibid.*, pp. 12, 16, 17, 18.

4. J. Kobler, *The Reluctant Surgeon* (Garden City, N.Y.: Doubleday and Co., 1960), p. 194.

5. Randolph, pp. 18, 19, 21, 22, 28, 29.

6. *Ibid.*, pp. 31, 32, 33.

7. *Ibid.*, pp. 33, 34; J. H. Powell, *Bring Out Your Dead: The Great Yellow Fever Epidemic in Philadelphia, 1793* (Philadelphia: University of Pennsylvania Press, 1949), pp. 154–57.

8. Randolph, pp. 33, 36, 38.

9. J. S. Dorsey, *Elements of Surgery for Use of Students* (Philadelphia: Kimber and Conrad, 1813); Horner, "Necrological Notice."

10. Dorsey, pp. 136–38, plate opposite p. 138.

11. *Ibid*, pp. 138–40, plate opposite p. 140.

12. Description of Dr. Physick's improved gorget, in a letter from R. B. Bishop, Surgeon's Instrument Maker to Dr. Coxe (with plate), *Coxe's Medical Museum* 1(November 1, 1804):186–87. Dorsey, *Elements of Surgery*, pp. 149–59, plate opposite p. 150.

13. Randolph, pp. 97, 98; Horner "Necrological Notice," p. 21.

14. Dorsey, *Elements of Surgery*, pp. 156–57, plate opposite p. 157.

15. Randolph, pp. 103, 104, 105.

16. B. H. Coates, "Extracts from an account of a case in which a new and particular operation for artificial anus was performed in 1809 by Philip Syng Physick, M.D., Professor of Surgery in the University of Pennsylvania, etc., drawn up for publication by B. H. Coates," *Philadelphia Journal of Medical and Physical Sciences* 13(1826):199–202.

17. P. S. Physick, "Account of a new mode of extracting poisons from the stomach," *Eclectic Repository* 3 (1813): 111–13.

18. P. S. Physick, "Art. II: Use of the Double Catheter and a wire recommended in the operation of extirpation of scirrhous tonsils and hemorrhoidal tumors," *Philadelphia Journal of Medical and Physical Sciences 1*(Philadelphia: Cary and Sons, 1820): 17–21.

19. Dorsey, *Elements of Surgery*. vol. I, pp. 96–283; P. S. Physick, "Case of Luxation of the Thigh Bone forward, and mode of reduction," *Coxe's Medical Museum* 1(12 April, 1805):428–30.

20. P. S. Physick, Letter to the editor, *Medical and Philosophical Intelligence for The Eclectic Repertory*. "The Editors are pleased to have it in the interesting communications from Dr. Physick, which has just been handed to them. Had it been sooner received it would have occupied a more appropriate place in the number." *Eclectic Repertory* 6 (1816): 389–90.

21. Randolph, pp. 68, 69, 70, 71.

22. *Ibid.*, p. 88: Horner, "Necrological Notice," p. 12.

23. S. Jackson, *A Discourse Commemorative of the Late William E. Horner, Professor of Anatomy, October 10, 1853*, published by the class (Philadelphia: T. K. and P. G. Collins Printers, 1853), p. 7.

24. W. S. Middleton, "William Edmonds Horner (1793–1853)," *Annals of Medical History* 5(1923):33–44; C. R. Bardeen, *William E. Horner* (Baltimore: American Medical Biographies, 1920), pp. 595–97; S. Jackson, *Discourse Commemorative*; W. Horner, "William E. Horner," in S. D. Gross, ed., *Lives of Eminent American Physicians* (Philadelphia, 1861), pp. 627–21; J. Walsh and C. H. Goudiss, "Notes on the Life of William Edmonds Horner," *Records of the American Catholic Historical Society of Philadelphia* 14 (1903):275–98, 423–38; A. R. Shands, "William E. Horner (1793–1853)," *Transactions and Studies of the College of Physicians of Philadelphia* 4th ser., 22 (February 1955): 105–11; D. Y. Cooper "William E. Horner (1793–1853), America's First Clinical Investigator," *Transactions and Studies of the College of Physicians of Philadelphia* 5th ser., 8 (1986):183–200; D. W. Albert and H. G. Scheie, *A History of Ophthalmology at the University of Pennsylvania* (Springfield, Ill.: Charles C. Thomas, 1965), pp. 24–33.

25. W. E. Horner, "A Description of a Muscle Connected with the Eye, Lately Discovered by W. E. Horner, M.D.," *London Medical Repository* 18(1822):32–33; W. E. Horner, "Description of a Small Muscle at the Internal Commissure of the Eyelids," *Philadelphia Journal of Medical and Physical Sciences* 8(1824):70–80.

26. Jacques Fabian Gautier D'Agoty, *Essai d'Anatomie, en tableaux imprimés, qui représentent au natural tous les muscles de la face, col, de la tête, de la langue et du larinx, d'après les partes dissequées et preparées par J. G. Duverney* (Paris, 1745).

27. W. E. Horner, "Method for Correcting Ectropion of the Lower Eyelid," *American Journal of Medical Sciences* 21(1837):99–112

28. R. Ivy, "Who Originated the Z-Plasty?" *Plastic and Reconstructive Surgery* 47(1971):67–72; A. F. Borges and T. Gibson, "The Original Z-Plasty," *British Journal of Plastic Surgery* 26(1973):237–46.

29. W. P. Dewees, *A Compendious System of Midwifery* (Philadelphia, 1824), p. 580.

30. W. E. Horner, "Observations on a Case of Ruptured Tendo Achillis and the Method Adopted for its Cure," *Philadelphia Journal of Medical and Physical Sciences* 12(1826):407–9.

31. *American Medical Association, Transactions* 1(1848):188–89, 220–21; report (by H. H. Smith) of cases in which ether and chloroform were used in the surgical clinic of the University of Pennsylvania in the session of 1847–1848. I. Parrish, "Annual Report on Surgery," *Transactions of the College of Physicians of Philadelphia, Summary* 2 (1846–49):156; describes William Gibson's amputating a medical student's finger successfully under ether anesthesia; in the case of Horner, amputation of a breast had to be discontinued and was considered unsuccessful; both cases occurred May 1847. Horner later that year successfully used ether anesthesia to operate on anal fistula.

32. W. E. Horner, *Treatise on Pathological Anatomy* (Philadelphia, 1829).

33. W. E. Horner, "On the Anatomical Character of Asiatic Cholera with Remarks on the Structure of the Mucous Coat of the Alimentary Canal," extracted from the *American Journal of Medical Sciences* 1835 (Philadelphia: Joseph R. A. Skerrett, 1835); W. E. Horner "On the Anatomical Characters of Asiatic Cholera with remarks on the Structure of the Mucous Coat, Parts I and II," *American Journal of Medical Sciences* 16(1835) 58–81, 277–95.

34. W. E. Horner, *Lessons in Practical Anatomy for Dissectors* (Philadelphia, 1823).

35. W. E. Horner, *Treatise on Special and General Anatomy* (Philadelphia, 1826); W. E. Horner, *Special Anatomy and Histology* (Philadelphia, 1843).

36. W. E. Horner, *Lessons in Practical Anatomy for Use of Dissectors* (Philadelphia: Carey and Thomas, 1827), p. 161.

37. W. S. Middleton, "William E. Horner (1793–1853)," *Annals of Medical History* 5(1923):33–44; A. R. Shands, "William E. Horner (1793–1853)," *Transactions and Studies of the College of Physicians of Philadelphia* 4th ser., 22(1955): 105–11.

38. John Mulchinock Crucie (1873-1956) papers, Historical Collections of the College of Physicians of Philadelphia.

39. Jackson, *Discourse Commemorative*, p. 45.

40. H. F. Osborne, "Biographical Memoirs of Joseph Leidy, 1823–1891," *Biographical Memoirs of the National Academy of Sciences* 7(1913):335–96; *The Joseph Leidy Commemorative Meeting, Held in Philadelphia, December 26, 1923, a pamphlet containing estimates of his work and personal characteristics by several eminent scientists* (Philadelphia: College of Physicians of Philadelphia, 1923); W. S. W. Ruschenberger, "A Sketch of the Life of Joseph Leidy, M.D., L.L.D.," *Proceedings of The American Philosophical Society* (Philadelphia: MacCalla, 1892).

41. Osborne, p. 337.

42. *Ibid.*, pp. 338–39.

43. *Ibid.*, pp. 367–68.

44. *Ibid.*, p. 356; J. Leidy, "On the Existence of an Entozoon (*Trichina Spiralis*) in the Superficial Part of the Extensor Muscles of the Thigh of a Hog," *Proceedings of the Academy of Natural Sciences, Philadelphia* 3(1846):102–8.

45. J. Leidy, "Remarks on parasites and scorpions," *Transactions and Studies of the College of Physicians of Philadelphia* 3d ser., 8(1886):441–43.

46. H. A. Kelley and W. L. Burrage, *A Dictionary of American Medical Biography* (Boston: Milford Press, 1928), pp. 465–466.

47. H. J. Abrahams and W. D. Miles, "William Gibson, M.D., Anatomist, Surgeon, and Student in 1823," *Transactions and Studies of the College of Physicians of Philadelphia* 4th. ser., 38(1970–71):184–88.

48. E. F. Smith, *The Life of Robert Hare. An American Chemist, 1781–1858* (Philadelphia: J. B. Lippincott, 1917); H. S. Klickstein, "A Short History of the Professorship of Chemistry of the University of Pennsylvania, 1765–1847," *Bulletin of the History of Medicine* 27(1953):46–68.

49. R. Hare, "Description of the Laboratory and Lecture Room in the Medical Department of the University of Pennsylvania" (with a plate), *American Journal of Science* 19(1831):26–28; E. F. Smith, *Chemistry in America* (New York, D. Appleton and Co.), plate opposite p. 158; Smith, *Robert Hare*, pp. 172–75.

50. Smith, *Robert Hare*, pp. 7–8.

51. *Ibid.*, pp. 493–503.

52. T. Coulson, *Joseph Henry—His Life and Work* (Princeton, N.J.: Princeton University Press, 1950), pp. 65–95.

53. R. Hare, *Memoir on the Supply and Application of the Blow Pipe* (Philadelphia: H. Maxwell, Columbia-House, 1802).

54. R. Hare, *A Compendium of the Course of Chemical Instruction in the Medical Department of the University of Pennsylvania* (Philadelphia: J. G. Auner, 1827); Smith; *Chemistry in America*, p. 189.

55. R. Hare, "A memoir on some new modification of galvanic apparatus with observations in support of his new theory of galvanism," *Philadelphia Journal of Medical and Physical Sciences* 1(1820):270–85; Smith, *Chemistry in America*, p. 188.

56. Smith, *Robert Hare*, pp. 55–57.

57. S. B. Burns, *Early Medical Photography in America (1839–1883)* (New York: The Beacon Archive, 1983), pp. 944–45; J. S. Berkowitz, *College of Physicians of Philadelphia Portrait Catalogue* (Philadelphia: College of Physicians of Philadelphia, 1984), pp. 56–57; Kelley and Burrage, p. 474.

58. Smith, *Robert Hare*, p. 214.

59. Corner, *Two Centuries of Medicine*, p. 102.

60. I. Richman, *The Brightest Ornament* (Bellefonte. Pa.: Pennsylvania Heritage, 1967).

61. *Ibid.*, pp. 119–23.

62. *Ibid.*, pp. 21–22.

63. *Ibid.*, pp. 1–8, 105.

64. *Ibid.*, pp. 21–22.

65. *Ibid.*, pp. 24–25.

66. *Ibid.*, pp. 64–65.

67. *Ibid.*, pp. 45–46.

68. *Ibid.*, pp. 64, 62–63.

69. *Ibid.*, pp. 64–65.

70. *Ibid.*

71. *Ibid.*, p. 64.

72. *Ibid.*, pp. 69–70.

73. *Ibid.*, pp. 134–38.

74. T. Stewardson, "Biographical Memoir of William W. Gerhard," *Transactions and Studies of the College of Physicians of Philadelphia* 3d. ser., 132 (1864): 473–81; Kelley and Burrage, pp. 465–66; J. F. Fulton, *William Wood Gerhard* in *Dictionary of American Biography*, vol. 7 (New York: Charles Scribner's Sons, 1931) pp. 218–19; E. B. Krumbhaar, "The History of Pathology at the Philadelphia General Hospital," *Medical Life* 40 (April 1933):162–77; W. S. Middleton, "William Wood Gerhard," *Annals of Medical History* 7 (January 1938):1–18; F. B. Rogers, "William Wood Gerhard: Pioneer in Nosography," in *Early Dickinsoniana, The Boyd Lee Spahr Lectures in Americana, 1957–1961* (Carlisle, Pa.: Library of Dickinson College, 1961), pp. 237–51.

75. W. R. Steiner, "Some Distinguished American Medical Students of Pierre-Charles-Alexandre Louis of Paris," *Bulletin of the History of Medicine* 7(1939):783–85; G. Hinsdale, "American Medical Argonauts: Pupils of Pierre-Charles-Alexandre Louis," *Transactions and Studies of the College of Physicians of Philadelphia* 3rd ser., 132(1945):37–43; W. Osler, "The Influence of Louis on American Medicine," *Johns Hopkins Hospital Bulletin* 8 (August-September 1897):161–67.

76. W. W. Gerhard, "On Typhus Fever, which occurred in Philadelphia in the spring and summer of 1836; illustrated by clinical observations at the Philadelphia Hospital; showing the distinction between this form of disease and Dothinenteritis or the Typhoid Fever with alteration of the follicles of the small intestine," *American Journal of Medical Sciences* 19 (1836):289–322; W. W. Gerhard, "On the Typhus Fever Which Occurred in Philadelphia in Spring and Summer of 1836," *American Journal of Medical Sciences* 20(1837):289–322.

77. W. Osler, *The Principles and Practice of Medicine* (New York: D. Appleton and Co., 1892), p. 2.

78. Kelley and Burrage, p. 1127.

79. Account Book of the Department of Anatomy by W. E. Horner, unpublished, Historical Collections of the College of Physicians of Philadelphia.

80. H. H. Smith, *On the treatment of ununited fractures by means of artificial limbs, which combine the principle of pressure and motion at the seat of pressure, and lead to the formation of an ensheathing callus* (Philadelphia: Collins, 1855).

81. Kelley and Burrage, p. 1127.

82. H. H. Smith, *Minor Surgery: or Hints on the Everyday Duties of the Surgeon* (Philadelphia: Barrington, 1843), 4 editions, the last published in 1859; H. H. Smith, *System of Operative Surgery; Based Upon the Practice of Surgeons in the United States: and Comprising a Bibliographical Index and Historical Record of Many of their Operations During the Period of Two Hundred Years* (Philadelphia: Lippincott, 1852); H. H. Smith, *Treatise on the Practice of Surgery* (Philadelphia: Lippincott, 1856); H. H. Smith, *Civale on the medical and prophylactic treatment of stone and gravel* (1841); H. H. Smith, *Anatomical Atlas Illustrative of the Human Body* (under the supervision of W. E. Horner) (Philadelphia: Lea, 1844) [8 editions of this work were published, the last in 1867]; Thomson Spencer, fl.1848–1883, "A Dictionary of Domestic Medicine and Household Surgery." 1st American ed. from the last London ed., rev. with additions by Henry H. Smith (Philadelphia: Lippincott, 1868); H. H. Smith, *United States Dissector* (1846) 5th ed. of W. E. Horner's *Lessons in Practical Anatomy for the Use of Dissectors*, 1st ed. (Philadelphia: Cary, 1823); H. H. Smith, *Principles and Practice of Surgery Embracing Minor Operative Surgery. With a Bibliographical Index of American Surgical Writers from the Year 1783 to 1860 Arranged for the Use of Students* (Philadelphia: Lippincott, 1863).

5
CREATING A CHANGE OR REACTING TO IT

Enough if something from the hands have power
To live and serve the future hour.

William Wordsworth

Except for the loss of the Southern students, the Civil War did not significantly impinge on the activities of the medical department as it ended its first century. Nor did it bring forth major advances in medical science. It did, however, lead indirectly to improvements in medicine.

Joseph Leidy, colleague Robert Rogers, and future trustee S. Weir Mitchell joined Smith in the local military hospitals. Treating the wounded soldiers taught them and other medical officers much about the management of fractures, use of anesthesia, and hospital design. And they learned the value of specialized hospitals. In *Gunshot Wounds and Other Injuries of Nerves*, Mitchell, George R. Morehouse, and W. W. Keens described the advantages at the United States Hospital for Diseases of the Nervous System, organized in May 1863. At first, the authors stated, they encountered many "difficulties and embarrassments" but eventually gained by focusing on "a limited class of cases":

> No sooner did the class of patients begin to fill our wards than we perceived that a new and interesting field of observation was opened to view. . . . Among them were representatives of every conceivable form of nerve injury—from shot and shell, from saber cuts, contusions and dislocations.[1]

Physicians at such hospitals learned the importance of obtaining special knowledge of diseases of the various organ systems; such lessons eventually contributed to medical specialization.

Other lessons from the war would modify medical education. Maintaining the health of masses of soldiers boosted the importance of public health, leading to new hygiene courses in Pennsylvania's post-war curriculum. Medical teachers observed how the sick and wounded were improperly managed both on the battlefield and in military hospitals and led a drive to improve instruction in patient management.[2]

Surgical inexperience added to the battlefield tragedies, as William S. Forbes, a Philadelphia anatomy teacher, observed, "because of a want of practical anatomy on the part of many surgeons." Schools could not give their students proper experience, he felt, because they lacked an adequate supply of human cadavers for dissection. In response to this need, Forbes drew up an anatomical bill that provided a legal mechanism for medical schools to use unclaimed bodies. Although initially defeated, the bill passed in 1867, after lobbying by a committee appointed by the College of Physicians of Philadelphia.[3]

At Penn, the ever-lasting struggle between a curriculum too oriented to practical medicine and one well-rounded in sciences auxiliary to medicine emerged again in 1865. One of the reformers was George B. Wood, a trustee, who felt that the curriculum had become stagnant in practicality. Wood persuaded his fellow members of the board to bring back the study of such natural sciences as botany, comparative anatomy, and zoology and to introduce a course in hygiene. Wood backed his proposals by donating $50,000 to the University for establishing the Auxiliary School of Medicine.[4]

The school was a step toward eliminating the archaic method of obtaining academic salaries through the sale of lecture tickets. Lecturers teaching the basic sciences in the new school could not be supported by the lecture fees, so they were paid fixed salaries for their part-time work.[5] The first faculty consisted of Harrison Allen as professor of comparative anatomy and zoology, Henry Hartshorn as professor of hygiene, Ferdinand V. Hayden as professor of geology and mineralogy, John J. Reese as professor of medical jurisprudence, and Horatio C. Wood (nephew of George B. Wood) as professor of botany. Only Hayden was not a Penn graduate.[6]

Hartshorn was Penn's first hygiene professor, but neither he nor his successor for one year, Horace Binney Hare, had special training in the discipline. In 1877 Joseph G. Richardson, a microscopist and pathologist, took over the course until 1887, when the chair was given to Samuel G. Dixon, who organized the first hygiene laboratory in America.[7]

Beginning in 1866 the five teachers of the auxiliary school each delivered thirty-four lectures during April, May, and June, after the regular medical course was completed. Wood's endowment allowed any student or graduate of the medical department to attend free; others were charged $10 for one course or $35 for all five. In the first year the school enrolled one hundred students, expanding to more than 400 within a decade.[8]

The teaching was by didactic lectures with no opportunity for laboratory work. Unfortunately, most of the students had already finished much of their medical work, so knowing the basic sciences could not help them study medicine. But it did broaden their education; later, these courses would be offered first in the regular curriculum.[9]

At first, no degree was awarded for this extra work, but in 1872 the faculty petitioned the trustees to give a second degree when two courses and proper examinations were completed. They suggested the German title of doctor of philosophy, Ph.D., a degree practically unknown in

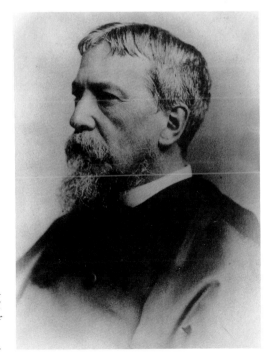

S. Weir Mitchell. (Historical Collections of the College of Physicians of Philadelphia.)

England and the United States. They argued that attending the auxiliary courses taught some general culture to add to the technical skills of the medical courses—analogous to the practice that students studying for degrees in history and philosophy were required to take courses in natural science.[10]

The trustees agreed, making these Ph.D.s the first awarded by the University of Pennsylvania. (Mary Alice Bennett, a graduate of Women's Medical College, was the first woman to earn the degree, in 1880.) But later in the decade, the trustees had second thoughts. The new Johns Hopkins University began granting the Ph.D. for advanced study in 1876.[11] Its course of study was closer to the German model, considerably more rigorous than Penn's. So the Penn trustees reduced their degree to bachelor of science, although they permitted those already enrolled for the higher degree to receive it.

The faculty made further attempts to improve the curriculum by lengthening it. In 1868 it instituted an "autumn" course to be given by lecturers not on the faculty.[12] The first teachers were James Tyson in microscopy, Edward Rhodes in physical diagnosis, D. Hayes Agnew in regional anatomy, H. Lenox Hodge, Jr., in skin diseases, and William Pepper, Jr., in morbid anatomy. In 1872, the Summer Medical Association of the University was organized; its teachers, faculty and non-faculty alike, represented almost all of the disciplines. This summer course replaced the "autumn" course.[13] Later the "Summer Association" course was replaced by the spring course which was given in April, May, and June, and what previously had been called the autumn course was renamed the "preliminary" course.[14]

In the 1893–94 school year, the regular curriculum was lengthened to four years, and the spring and preliminary courses were discontinued. Two of the auxiliary courses were dropped in 1895 and the school was disbanded in 1898.[15]

FOUNDING OF THE HOSPITAL OF THE UNIVERSITY OF PENNSYLVANIA

The weakest link in medical education was the recurring shortage of patients for clinical instruction. Penn's connections to the Philadelphia Almshouse and Pennsylvania Hospital were unofficial, maintained by the faculty who were members of those hospitals' staffs. Lay boards of prominent Philadelphians governed both hospitals, and access of Penn students to the wards was periodically restricted, making Saint Joseph's Hospital a major location for clinical teaching.[16] The fragile ties led to the organization of a University hospital whose staff and faculty could be controlled by the medical faculty and the Penn trustees.

Leadership came from William Pepper, Jr.[17] He was a tall, handsome man with a pleasant voice and a persuasive manner with which he convinced his many friends to contribute to the building of Penn's medical school. He generously gave monies from his personal estate when matching funds were required for public or private grants. Under Pepper's leadership the medical school moved to West Philadelphia, where it organized and built the first university hospital and clinical pathology laboratory in the United States.

The University began discussing moving to West Philadelphia in the late 1860s. Older medical faculty objected; the prospective location was inconvenient, distant from hospitals. Younger faculty were enthusiastic, especially young Pepper, recently appointed a lecturer in clinical medicine, who realized that existing facilities were antiquated and cramped, with no room for expansion at the Ninth and Market Streets location.

Most important, Pepper reasoned that the most serious objections to the move could be overcome by building a new hospital west of the Schuylkill River near the proposed medical department. The idea of a hospital available exclusively to medical students and faculty, linked directly to the University, was new for its time, and it required the proper presentation for acceptance.[18]

Pepper dropped a hint of his intended project at the annual dinner of the alumni society in 1870. In response to a toast to the medical department, Pepper praised the medical school for having "the best and most complete system of dispensary clinical teaching" in the country; but he went on to regret that American medical students, unlike their European counterparts, lacked thorough clinical instruction in specialized branches of medicine. He declared that a change was due.[19]

Change was at work within months, when construction of a University hospital was openly discussed. The trustees appointed a feasibility committee chaired by Morton McMichael, owner and editor of the *North American*, the oldest newspaper in the country; his endorsement of a new hospital was strong assurance that the idea would succeed. Indeed,

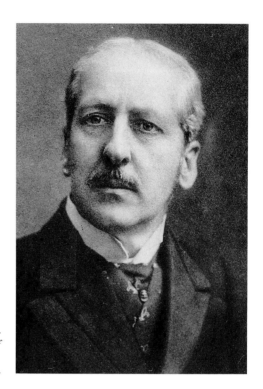

William Pepper, Jr. (Archives of the University of Pennsylvania.)

the committee urged that a new hospital be built. It was joined by a committee of the medical faculty, and the groups campaigned together for public funds.[20]

Pepper wrote an appeal for the enterprise and collected endorsements from 109 prominent citizens of the city. Pepper argued that the hospital would improve medical education, serve the city with more beds, and provide material advantage to the community. He also collected data showing that Philadelphia's hospital facilities were inadequate compared to those of other cities, including New York.[21]

University alumni were exhorted to urge their legislative representatives for support, and in April 1872 the legislature granted $100,000 for the project, on condition that the University match it with $250,000.[22]

A month later, the trustees designated, as a site for the hospital, newly acquired property north of Spruce Street, near the plot where

Houston Hall would later be built. If a more desirable location could be found, they added, it could be used. Pepper concluded that the ten acres granted for the new campus was inadequate, so he petitioned the city to grant to the trustees the ground between Spruce Street on the north, Pine Street on the south, 34th Street on the east, and 36th Street on the west. After considerable negotiation, on May 18, 1872, the city sold the land to Penn for $500 with the following stipulations: The hospital building must be completed within five years; the hospital must perpetually maintain no fewer than fifty free beds for use by the city, and the trustees must report annually to the city on the condition of the institution.[23] Pepper solicited his influential friends. He urged lawyers to suggest to clients drawing up wills and arranging to dispose of their property that they consider a gift to the hospital: $5,000 endowed a free bed in the donor's name and would give relief to an average of twelve persons a year. "In no way," he stated simply, "can the same amount of good be done by the same money." The success of Pepper's tactic may be measured by the many memorial plaques on the walls of the hospital.[24]

By November 1872 the $250,000 required by the state had been secured. But more was needed, and Pepper worked zealously to obtain another matching grant—$100,000 if private subscription could raise $100,000. The legislature approved, and that money was soon in hand.[25]

The hospital was designed by T. W. Richards, drawing instructor at the University. The style of "university Gothic" matched his design of College Hall, completed in 1872. Funds, however, could cover only the central and western wings of Richards's original plans.[26] Shortly after the hospital opened on June 4, 1874, Pepper again appealed to the legislature for a grant to erect the eastern wing of the plan. But he soon discovered that he had taught other institutions how to obtain state monies. The legislature was so deluged by similar petitions that his request was denied. The eastern wing was never completed, and seventeen years passed before the University again applied for funds from the state.

Once founded, the Hospital of the University of Pennsylvania prospered and grew.[27] In 1883 the Gibson Pavilion, funded by a gift from Henry Gibson of Baltimore, was opened. Through the efforts of Mrs. Richard D. Wood, the nurses' home was opened in 1886. A maternity ward was opened in 1889, followed by a maternity wing in 1894.[28] The

T. W. Richards's plan for the Hospital of the University of Pennsylvania. Only the central building (Administration) and west ward wing of this plan were erected. Opening Exercises of the Hospital of the University of Pennsylvania. The pamphlet containing the Hospital's plan is bound in the Annual Reports of the Hospital of the University of Pennsylvania *(*Annual Reports of the Hospital of the University of Pennsylvania.*)*

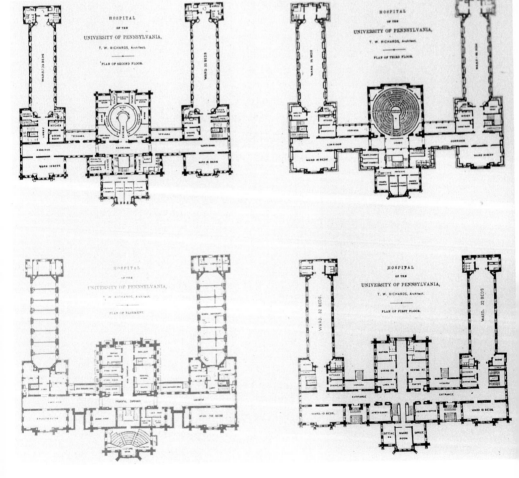

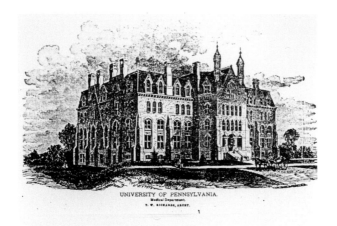

UNIVERSITY OF PENNSYLVANIA.
Medical Department.
T. W. RICHARDS, ARCHT.

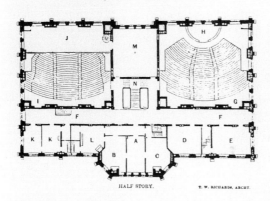

HALF STORY.   T. W. RICHARDS, ARCHT.

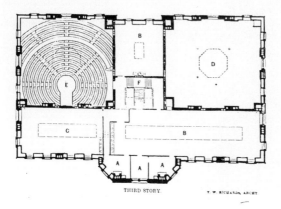

THIRD STORY.   T. W. RICHARDS, ARCHT.

Medical Hall. TOP: *T. W. Richards drawing of the Exterior.* BOTTOM: *Plan of the interior of Medical Hall showing the lecture hall and anatomical ampitheater. (Archives of the University of Pennsylvania.)*

William Pepper Laboratory, which Pepper Jr. erected in memory of his father, was completed in 1894.[29] The last structure added in the nineteenth century was the Agnew wing, which opened in 1897. It contained four operating amphitheaters, wards for surgical patients (men, women, and children), and gynecological patients, and a children's orthopedic ward. In the basement was a shop for making artificial limbs and other orthopedic appliances as well as a gymnasium fitted with equipment for strengthening limbs weakened by surgery or disease.[30]

RELATIONSHIP BETWEEN THE MEDICAL FACULTY AND THE CLINICAL (HOSPITAL) FACULTY

From the moment a University hospital was suggested, the medical faculty questioned the relationship between itself and the hospital staff, particularly about control of hospital policies.[31] It rejected an initial proposal, made by George B. Wood, that the hospital be staffed by clinical professors alone.[32] It agreed to a revised plan that placed the medical faculty in senior chairs over the clinical professorships.[33]

The first staff, as of February 1874, consisted of Alfred Stillé as professor of the theory and practice of medicine and clinical medicine, and William Pepper, Jr., as clinical professor of medicine; D. Hayes Agnew as professor and clinical professor of surgery and John Neil as associate clinical professor of surgery; R.A.F. Penrose as professor of obstetrics and the diseases of women and children and William Goodell as clinical professor of the diseases of women and children; William F. Norris as clinical professor of diseases of the eye; and George Strawbridge as clinical professor of diseases of the ear.[34]

REFORM OF THE CURRICULUM

These changes stemmed from forty years earlier when the American Medical Association was founded, partly, on the program of raising standards of medical education. Pennsylvania was one of the few institutions that responded by lengthening its medical course, but the reform failed when student enrollment declined; in the mid-1850s the faculty voted to return to the shorter course.

Reform became a serious topic again at the urging of Alfred Stillé.[35] An 1836 M.D. graduate, Stillé worked with Gerhard and Pennock on distinguishing typhoid fever from typhus and wrote independent papers on his observations of the symptoms of the two diseases. He also wrote important papers on cerebral meningitis and cholera as well as on dysentery and erysipelas. He became revered as an excellent clinician and teacher and served as president of the American Medical Association.[36]

At the alumni society meeting in 1873, Stillé spoke on the need to base a school on its merits, not the number of students. Competition for students, he charged, forced professors "to keep down the value of their wares and furnish them at a price as their rivals charged." Schools had to be independent "so that the earnest and true shall not be held back by the apathetic and incompetent." He favored an endowment to remove payment-by-lecture, a lengthened term, and a graded curriculum.[37]

Another major struggle between the medical faculty and the hospital staff erupted over the issue of improving the medical curriculum. In 1875, the medical faculty wrote to the trustees that

> the vast acquisition of medical and surgical knowledge which have been gained within the last quarter of a century . . . so enlarged the domain of the profession that the brief period allotted to medical instruction . . . is entirely inadequate. . . .[38]

A meeting was arranged among the medical faculty, a committee from the hospital staff, and the trustees—the implication being that the presence of the trustees made any decisions final.[39] The medical faculty were infuriated, feeling that the clinical professors had overstepped their bounds. Informal conciliatory meetings followed, but no changes were made in medical education.[40]

In 1876 the trustees appointed four new professors to the medical faculty. The medical faculty then moved to delay this action by writing a "communication" to the entire board of trustees, which was printed to be certain that it reached each member. One of the new professors appointed was William Pepper Jr.—evidence that the old guard in the medical faculty had lost its fight to retain control of the department.[41]

Four days later, long-sought administrative changes were made. Among the changes was installation of the three-year course, grading of the courses, and the guarantee of annual professorial salaries of $3,000.[42] Such sums were met mostly by tuition fees and aided by a gift of $50,000 from Mrs. John Rhea Barton, who endowed a chair of surgery in her husband's name.[43] In addition, the names of some chairs were altered: institutes of medicine became physiology, diseases of women and children became gynecology, and general therapeutics was added to materia medica and pharmacy.[44]

Since there was still some misunderstanding in 1877 about the status of the new professors, the trustees spelled it out: the clinical professors of medicine, surgery, pathology and morbid anatomy, and obstetrics and diseases of women and children would be full professors with the right to examine students, sign diplomas, share in the award of prizes, and deliver introductory and valedictory addresses.[45]

This action of the trustees was too much for Robert Rogers, who resigned the deanship on May 7, 1877.[46]

EXPLOITATION OF THE NEW ACADEMIC REQUIREMENTS

Some students found and exploited a loophole in the new requirements. They left school before second-year examinations, took summer (and easier) courses at another institution, then returned for their Penn degree in the third year.[47] The abuse surfaced publicly in an editorial in the *Philadelphia Evening Bulletin* in 1883, and the medical faculty responded by requiring readmission exams of returning students.[48]

THE FOUR-YEAR COURSE

When John Marshall became dean in 1892, the first problem he faced was the extension of the medical course to four years. Provost Pepper had begun to press for a four-year course in 1877. At first the medical faculty resisted adding an additional year by proposing that the curriculum be rearranged by placing the basic science courses in the first and second years and the clinical courses in the second and third. In 1891 Pepper proposed raising a guarantee to support the four-year curriculum. In 1892 he was able to announce that finally through a personal subscription of $10,000 from his estate and generous gifts from D. Hayes Agnew, J. William White, and Horatio C. Wood that the sum required for the guarantee—$20,000 a year for five years—had been raised.[49]

The four-year course which began in the school year of 1893–95 was essentially the same as the voluntary four-year course that had been available but little used since 1883. What was most important was that the four-year course provided additional time for studies in the clinical specialties.

Shortly after this announcement, through the efforts of S. Weir Mitchell and others of the medical faculty the school year was lengthened by beginning in October and ending in June, yielding an academic year of about eight months.[50] When the school year was lengthened in 1894 the autumn (preliminary) and spring courses were discontinued.

ENTRANCE EXAMINATIONS

Inauguration of the four-year course on October 2, 1893 was distinguished by the inaugural address of Dr. William Pepper dealing with the same subject he had addressed sixteen years earlier: *Higher Medical Education the True Interest of the Public and the Profession.* In this famous address he began by stating that in 1877 he had urged the faculty to institute these reforms: preparatory examinations for entrance to medical school, the lengthening of the annual term of studies; the grading of the course, clinical and laboratory instruction for the student; and the establishment of fixed salaries for professors rather than the old system of selling lecture tickets. The inauguration of the four-year course accomplished all of these high goals except the introduction of an entrance examination. Pepper started this drive for he knew as well as the faculty that the entrance requirements were still those of 1880, which permitted enrollment of a large number of ill prepared students to the study of medicine.[51]

The requirement of entrance examinations was inaugurated in 1896 when the faculty announced the minimal entrance requirement would be a high school diploma or its equivalent, proven by written test. As the faculty feared, enrollment plummeted, from a high of 926 students in 1896–97 to 472 in 1902–1903.[52]

THE WILLIAM PEPPER, SR. LABORATORY

As the academic changes developed, Pepper began the movement to establish a laboratory of pathology that would be a department of the medical school and the hospital. He combined a legislative grant of $100,000, $50,000 of his own money, and $30,000 of other subscriptions; and in 1895 the William Pepper Laboratory of Clinical Medicine was formally dedicated. The laboratory aimed to help the hospital's patients "by prosecution of minute clinical studies and original research, and to advance the interest of science by publication of the results of such work."[53]

R. A. F. PENROSE

In 1872 the professorship of midwifery and the diseases of women and children was divided into two services. R.A.F. Penrose continued as the professor of midwifery.[54] He was rated as a superb teacher; as one of his students put it,

> Who can forget the account of the essential scientific facts then known in regard to fertilization of the ovum in the guise of a charming fairy tale in which the spermatozoa figures as the prince and the ovum as his captive lady love awaiting liberation from the enchanted cell, the Graffian follicle. A Psyche to be awakened by Cupid's kiss?[55]

One of Penrose's most dramatic demonstrations was his "delivery" of a baby from the manikin dubbed Mrs. O'Flaherty, which he performed with all of the skill of a pantomime artist. Although Penrose died in 1908, Mrs. O'Flaherty was alive many decades later, memorialized by I. S. Ravdin when he reminded his residents to deal with their private and ward patients equally, stating "Treat them all like Mrs. O'Flaherty."

WILLIAM GOODELL

When the chair was divided, William Goodell was chosen as professor of the diseases of women and children. He had gained a distinguished reputation as the director of the Preston Retreat, a unique hospital that revolutionized midwifery, or obstetrics, in the United States.[56] He also developed the Goodell dilator for the cervix, which is still in use. Goodell identified infection as the cause of childbirth fever (puerperal sepsis) and developed effective methods to prevent it. He was the first

American obstetrician to apply the doctrine of antisepsis and asepsis in institutional practice. His work proved that large numbers of patients could be treated safely in a public institution, a feat which altered obstetrical practice in the United States. His methods were based on those set forth originally by the Philadelphia College of Physicians in 1836, some seven years before Oliver W. Holmes published his famous paper accusing physicians of spreading childbirth fever and, in effect, murdering patients. In 1860, the Hungarian obstetrician Ignaz Semmelweiss published his famous paper on "The Etiology, Concept, and Prophylaxis of Childbirth Fever" and was still trying to get his ideas

William Goodell's clinic in the large amphitheater in the second and third floors of the Administration Building of the Hospital of the University of Pennsylvania. (Archives of the University of Pennsylvania.)

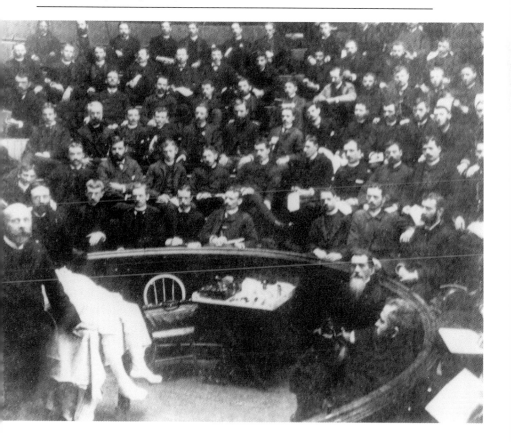

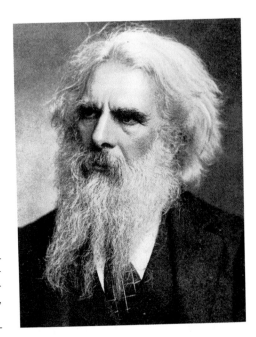

Eadweard Muybridge. (E. Muybridge, The Human Figure in Motion *[London: Chapman and Hall, 1901].)*

accepted in Europe when the Preston Retreat opened in 1866, using the hygienic precautions he recommended.[57]

EADWEARD MUYBRIDGE—STUDIES OF ANIMAL MOTION

One of the more unusual research activities in the medical department was conducted by the experimental photographer Eadweard Muybridge, who devised methods to show animal motion, an important step in the development of motion pictures.[58] Muybridge had immigrated from England in 1851, when he was twenty-two years old. He went West and in 1872 was commissioned to photograph the horse of Leland Stanford to settle an argument: did a running horse have all four feet off the ground at any single instant? Muybridge produced a photograph that stopped the horse's motion, but he did not have the equipment to take sequential photographs of the horse's strides. In 1877 he managed to arrange a series of cameras, trip wires, electromagnets, and a white screen that reflected sunlight correctly; and he proved that a running or trotting horse always has one foot on the ground.

In 1883 Muybridge came to Philadelphia to lecture. Pepper heard him. He and others contributed to establishing a studio for Muybridge in space behind the Hospital of the University of Pennsylvania and the Philadelphia Hospital, just east of the newly opened veterinary school.[59]

Muybridge began using his new studio in the spring of 1884 and

Muybridge's photographs of human motion. (E. Muybridge, The Human Figure in Motion *[London: Chapman and Hall, 1901].)*

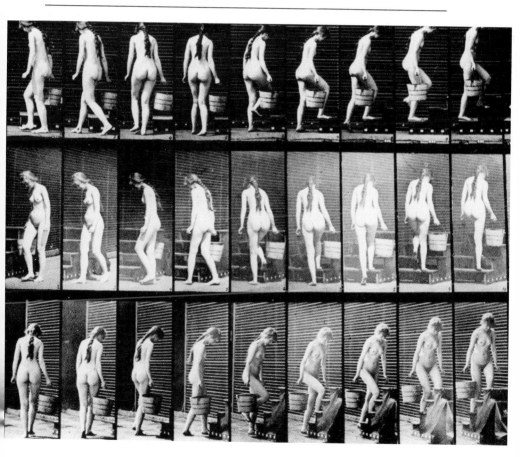

worked there into 1886. Three members of the medical faculty became involved in his work. Harrison Allen, from physiology, studied the motion of normal male and female subjects and wrote on it in Muybridge's book *Animal Locomotion*. His departmental colleague Edward Tyson Reichert had his own photographic facilities; he had Muybridge photograph the movements of an animal heart and make pictures of normal subjects, but most of this work was never published.[60]

Neurologist Francis X. Dercum asked Muybridge to photograph patients from the neurology clinics of the University hospital and Philadelphia Hospital. Dercum had devised a method to produce convulsions by muscle constraint using the patient's outstretched arm; he also studied hypnotism. He helped Muybridge assemble, classify, and describe his plates; Muybridge's studies, with comments by Dercum and Allen, were published in 1888 as *The Muybridge Work at the University of Pennsylvania: The Method and the Result*.[61]

NOTES

1. S. W. Mitchell, G. R. Morehouse, and W. W. Keen, *Gunshot Wounds and Other Injuries of Nerves* (Philadelphia, Lippincott, 1864), pp. 2–11.

2. G. W. Corner, *Two Centuries of Medicine* (Philadelphia: Lippincott, 1965), p. 128.

3. W. J. Bell, Jr., *The College of Physicians of Philadelphia: A Bicentennial History* (Canton, Mass.: Science History Publications, 1987), pp. 141–42.

4. Corner, *Two Centuries of Medicine*, pp. 126–27.

5. *Ibid.*, p. 128.

6. Minutes of the Medical Faculty, April 25, 1865, Archives of the University of Pennsylvania.

7. Corner, p. 128.

8. *Ibid.*

9. *Ibid.*, p. 127.

10. *Ibid.*, p. 126.

11. M. Meyerson and D. P. Winegrad, *Gladly Learn and Gladly Teach* (Philadelphia: University of Pennsylvania Press. 1978), p. 122.

12. Minutes of the Medical Faculty, Archives of the University of Pennsylvania.

13. *Ibid.*

14. *Ibid.*

15. *Ibid.*

16. Corner, p. 134; D. Hayes Agnew, *Lecture on the Medical History of the Philadelphia Alms House* (Philadelphia, 1862); Minutes of the Board of Guardians of Philadelphia.

17. F. N. Thorpe, *William Pepper, M.D., LL.D.* (Philadelphia: Lippincott, 1904).

18. *Ibid.*, p. 42.

19. *Ibid.*, pp. 42–43.

20. *Ibid.*, pp. 43–44.

21. *Ibid.*, pp. 44–45.

22. *Ibid.*, p. 49.

23. *Ibid.*, p. 51.

24. *Ibid.*, pp. 53–54.

25. *Ibid.*, pp. 55–58.

26. *Ibid.*, p. 167.

27. *Ibid.*, p. 29.

28. Annual Report of the Hospital Board of the Hospital of the University of Pennsylvania.

29. Thorpe, *William Pepper*, p. 134.

30. Program of the Opening Exercises of the D. Hayes Agnew Wing of the Hospital of the University of Pennsylvania.

31. Minutes of the Medical Faculty Meeting [hereafter abbreviated as "MFM"], June, 1873, Archives of the University of Pennsylvania.

32. MFM, January, 1874

33. MFM, February, 1874.

34. MFM, February, 1874.

35. H. A. Kelley and W. L. Burrage, *A Dictionary of American Medical Biography* (Boston: Milford Press, 1928), pp. 1169–70.

36. W. Osler, "Memoir of Alfred Stillé," *Transactions and Studies of the College of Physicians of Philadelphia* 3d. ser., 24(1902):xliii–lxxi

37. A. Stillé, M.D., Annual Address, *Proceedings of the Alumni Society given at the Anniversary Meeting 1873* (Philadelphia, Collins, 1873); MFM, June 18, 1875.

38. MFM, June 18,1875.

39. MFM, November 4, 1875.

40. MFM, November 11, 1875; November 18, 1875.

41. MFM, March 25, 1876

42. Report of the Special Committee on the Medical Department, presented March 28, 1876. [Printed for the use of the Board of Trustees, Guarantee of the Trustees, MFM, 1896].

43. W. A. Damon, "A Brief History of the John Rhea Barton Chair of Surgery," *Transactions and Studies of the College of Physicians of Philadelphia* 4th ser., 23(1955): 94–104.

44. MFM, May 28, 1887.

45. MFM, April 4, 1877.

46. MFM, May 7, 1877.

47. MFM, 1883.

48. MFM, 1892.

49. MFM, book 9, 1893, p. 127.

50. MFM, book 9, p. 193.

51. William Pepper, Jr., "Higher Medical Education the True Interest of the Public and Profession," Inaugural Address at the Opening of the Four Year Course of Medical Study in the University of Pennsylvania, October 2, 1893.

52. MFM, book 10, p. 15.

53. Thorpe, *William Pepper*, pp. 131–42.

54. Kelley and Burrage, pp. 957–58.

55. B. C. Hirst, "Memoir of Richard Alexander Fullerton Penrose, M.D.," *Transactions and Studies of the College of Physicians of Philadelphia* 3d ser., 32 (1910): lxviii–lxxii.

56. W. R. Penman and E. J. Penman, *Dr. William Goodell and Camp Paoli* (Paoli, Pa.: Serpentine Press, 1987).

57. W. R. Penman, "Charles Delucina Meigs, M.D.: An Assessment of His Role

in Philadelphia Obstetrics," *Transactions and Studies of the College of Physicians of Philadelphia* 4th ser., 43 (1975–76):121–24; J. W. Meigs, "Puerperal Fever and Nineteenth-Century Contagion," *Transactions and Studies of the College of Physicians of Philadelphia* 4th ser. 42 (1974–75):273–80.

58. R. B. Haas, *Muybridge: Man in Motion* (Berkeley and Los Angeles: University of California Press, 1976).

59. G. Nitzsche, Muybridge's Method and Apparatus, unpublished manuscript, Archives of the University of Pennsylvania; G. Nitzsche, Muybridge Moving Picture Experiments at the University of Pennsylvania, unpublished manuscript, Archives of the University of Pennsylvania; Francis X. Dercum, Letter to G. Nitzsche, May 10, 1929, describing his collaboration with Eadweard Muybridge. Archives of the University of Pennsylvania.

60. E. T. Reichert, no address, letter describing his collaboration with Eadweard Muybridge, Archives of the University of Pennsylvania.

61. E. Muybridge, *The Human Figure in Motion* (London: Chapman and Hall, 1901) [the results of Eaedweard Muybridge's investigations consisting of 781 photos, mezzo-tint engravings, with examples of more than twenty thousand acts of motion by animals, birds, and human beings were published in 1887 in eleven folio volumes, under the title of *Animal Locomotion*]; F. X. Dercum, "The Walk and Some of its Phases in Disease," *Transactions and Studies of the College of Physicians of Philadelphia* 3d ser., 10 (1888):308–38: M. R. McVaugh, *Francis X. Dercum and Animal Locomotion*; C. W. Burr, M.D., "Memoir of Francis Dercum," *Transactions and Studies of the College of Physicians of Philadelphia* 3d ser., 54(1932):lxv–lxxi: A. Brubaker, "Francis X. Dercum" [obituary], *Proceedings of the American Philosophical Society* 71(1932):39–41.

6

THE START OF SEVERAL MODERN DEPARTMENTS

Inveniemus viam aut faciemus [*Find a way or make one*]
Inscription over the gate between Williams Hall and Houston Hall on Spruce Street, University of Pennsylvania

After the move to West Philadelphia, the medical department began a transition into what we recognize as a modern medical school. Scientific medicine took hold. Specialties in medicine and surgery were introduced, and clinical laboratories established. The lecture halls, the hospital wards, the surgical amphitheaters, and new laboratories were populated by some remarkable people.

WILLIAM OSLER

Scarcely anyone enhanced the reputation of American medicine more than the Canadian-born William Osler.[1] He was chosen to fill the chair of clinical medicine, vacated when William Pepper succeeded Alfred Stillé in the senior medical chair. Osler revolutionized clinical teaching: he popularized bringing medical students to the patients' bedsides and teaching them there.

Penn considered Osler for the post only as an afterthought. According to Harvey Cushing, the medical members of Penn's board of trustees had drawn up a list of internal candidates; but the editorial staff of the *Medical News* was chagrined that a "wider view" had not been taken, especially mentioning Osler, then practicing in Montreal. Dean Tyson, one of the editors, felt that it was too late, but was convinced to move on it nonetheless.[2]

Horatio C Wood traveled to Montreal to learn more about Osler. As Cushing put it, "He went first . . . to the French hospitals and found that, among the French physicians, everyone spoke of him in highest terms; he then went to the Montreal General Hospital where he encountered such a degree of enthusiasm . . . he became himself a convert and returned home without interviewing any of Osler's colleagues on the faculty."[3]

Wood's report convinced the search committee to recommend Osler. Osler was visiting in Europe when the crucial next steps, including the famous examination by cherry-pit, occurred. They are described by Osler:

> On June 17 a coin was flipped at 14c Terch Street, Leipzig, which fell heads [deciding for Philadelphia]. . . . Dr. [Weir] Mitchell cabled me to meet him in London, as he and his good wife were commissioned to "look me over," particularly with regard to my personal habits. Dr. Mitchell had said there was only one way in which the breeding of a man for such a position, in such a city as Philadelphia, could be tested: give him cherry pie and see how he disposes of the stones. I had read of this trick before and disposed of them genteelly in my spoon and got the chair.[4]

Osler came to Philadelphia in October 1884.[5] He was an immediate contrast to his predecessor Pepper, who arrived in the amphitheater with great dignity and, still in the process of removing his gloves, might begin a brilliant dissertation on a topic, not always the one prescribed. Osler could be dignified and serious, but his mischievous, playful nature would break through the solemn mask of the medical teacher. His formal lectures required careful, extensive preparation, and he clearly was more at home on the wards. It was there, as he used patients to describe the history of their disease and pointed out changes in the physical signs of the disease, that he conveyed to students a relaxed feeling of confidence, a sense of a professor who wanted to teach them something useful.[6]

Within a short time students flocked to the wards where Osler was found every morning. They knew nothing about clinical research, and even if they had an interest in it, there were no facilities for laboratory studies on patients at the University hospital. Osler changed that, too. He outfitted a primitive laboratory under the hospital's amphitheater. In surroundings resembling a cloakroom, he stimulated the students to conduct laboratory studies on their assigned patients.[7]

Osler's lack of interest in building a large private practice mystified his Penn colleagues. He limited his outside work to consultations; and instead of devoting his afternoons to office hours or house calls, he went over to Philadelphia Hospital, affectionately called Old Blockley, where he gathered a group of students in the "dead house" and conducted postmortem examinations. "A breath of fresh air," one student observed, referring to Osler's teaching. Osler left Penn for Johns Hopkins in 1888 and concluded his career at Oxford. He left his mark on every institution at which he served.[8]

LOUIS DUHRING

What Osler did for clinical medicine, Louis Duhring did for dermatology. He established this new specialty in America.[9] A native Philadelphian and a Penn medical graduate, Duhring was drawn to skin diseases after hearing Francis Fontaine Maury lecture on managing skin lesions at the Jefferson Medical College in the 1860s. As a resident at Philadelphia Hospital, young Duhring showed such interest in the dermatological cases he saw that the hospital authorities granted him a room to study and care for the patients. This room soon became known as "the diseases of the skin ward," and from this modest start American dermatology began.

Duhring extended his knowledge by studying in Europe, mostly in the Vienna clinic of Ferdinand Hans von Hebra. On his return he opened the Dispensary for Skin Diseases on 11th Street; he eventually turned it over to one of his associates.

His success in treating skin diseases led the medical school to form a dermatology department, which he headed from 1875 to 1910, a period the specialty still refers to as the "era of Duhring."

Duhring's great *Atlas of Dermatology* first appeared in 1876; additional sections appeared at six- to seven-month intervals until it included nine sections containing 36 color plates. His worldwide fame, however, stemmed from 18 papers published between 1884 and 1891 on the disease or group of diseases he called *dermatitis herpetiformis*, subsequently known as "Duhring's disease." He showed that various cutaneous conditions previously described as different diseases were actually manifestations of one disease. He demonstrated that the

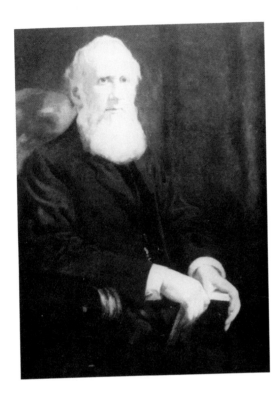

Louis   Duhring.   (Historical Collections of the College of Physicians of Philadelphia.)

symptoms, though variable, are generally chronic with occasional re-missions, They are also characterized by pruritis which is often intense, herpetiformity, and a symmetrical distribution of lesions. It usually follows profound psychological shock or nervous exhaustion.

Duhring was a bachelor and inherited considerable wealth from his family. These circumstances, plus a self-denying lifestyle, a remunerative practice, and judicious stock investments, led him to accumulate an estate worth over $1.5 million at the time of his death; he left the bulk of it to Penn and the College of Physicians of Philadelphia.[10]

HORATIO C WOOD

Penn also spurred the work of several basic scientists who fostered experimental biological research in the United States. Horatio C Wood was one of these.[11] He succeeded Joseph Carson as professor of materia medica. In addition to therapeutics, he was interested in neurology, and he held that chair as well. He also served the United States Pharmacopoeia for more than three decades.

Wood represented the ninth generation of an old English Quaker family who had come to Pennsylvania with William Penn. At an early age, he was attracted to natural science and was encouraged in it by Joseph Leidy, whom he met at the Philadelphia Academy of Natural Sciences. He graduated from Penn's medical school and served in a unit of the Army medical corps headed by Harrison Allen. His first position at Penn, in 1866, was as quizmaster and private teacher in the medical department.

Wood's early writings on myripoda attracted the attention of Louis Agassiz. Agassiz, who had recently acquired a collection of Brazilian myripods, put it at Wood's disposal for classification. Wood made two expeditions for specimens on behalf of the Smithsonian Institution; on the second trip, he became one of the first white men on record to see the Grand Canyon. In 1877 the Smithsonian published his 270-page work on fresh water algae; the book contained nineteen colored and two uncolored plates of 360 drawings Wood had made from microscopic slides.

Eventually Wood published more than three hundred papers on topics as varied as the action of atropine, veratrum, amyl nitrite, the oxytocic action of quinine, the vasomotor action of ergot, the action of alcohol on the circulation, and the biological action and behavior of ethyl bromide, strontium, chloramine, the volatile oils, and the anesthetics. His most important papers—on American hemp and hyoscine—were the first to appear on these subjects.

His monumental work was his book *A Treatise on Therapeutics.* In it, he revolted against empiricism, or as he harshly put it, against "clinical experience." In his introduction he wrote, "Empiricism is said to be the mother of wisdom. Verily she has been in medicine rather a blind leader of the blind." Instead, he aimed "to make the physiological action of remedies the principal point in discussion, not secondary, as had been the custom in preceding works on therapeutics."

HARRISON ALLEN

Harrison Allen, also descended from a Quaker Philadelphia family, studied dentistry after high school before entering medicine.[12] After army service during the Civil War, he practiced surgery at Saint Joseph's Hospital and at Philadelphia Hospital. He was considered technically skilled, but failed as a clinical surgeon because of his extraordinary fondness for detail; his power of intellectual perspective was lost in his study of the details. Yet this mental trait helped his research.

Although Allen regarded his time spent on dentistry as wasted, his familiarity with the anatomy of the mouth, as well as the head and neck, led to his studies on this part of the body. His papers describe the anatomy of the teeth, deformities of the face, and the importance of alveolar bone in preventing the loss of teeth.

He became an authority on diseases of the mouth. In one experiment he devised a method to measure the motions of the soft palate during speech. In a dramatic surgical success, he cured a case of epilepsy by extracting a tooth that remained over an impacted tooth. Allen extended his interest to include the nose, leading to his reputation as the father of rhinology. In 1874 he published his *Analysis of Life Forms in Art.*

In 1878 the medical faculty offered Allen the chair in physiology, although it knew that his interest was largely in anatomy. Allen accepted because there were no prospects of a position in his field of expertise. Later, he collaborated with Eadweard Muybridge in the photographer's experiments on animal motion. His career was short; he retired in 1885 because of failing health.

EDWIN TYSON REICHERT

Allen's successor was Edward Tyson Reichert, who devoted much of a long career to validating chemically Darwin's theory of the origin of species.[13] He carried out extensive projects, first on hemoglobin and later on plant starches, to devise a chemical classification of animals and plants. At this time physiologists believed that the active substance of all living things was the same. Reichert disagreed. He showed that different species of animals and plants could be distinguished positively by tracing their protoplasmic-chemical composition, which varied widely.[14]

In 1911 he published the results of his systematic work on the properties of hemoglobin crystals of 107 representative animals of various species. He pointed out that the hemoglobins of six species of baboons were similar in structure to man's—the nearest any scientist had come to offering chemical proof of Darwin's theory of evolution.[15]

Reichert had other research interests, too. He studied snake venom with S. Weir Mitchell. They crystallized a number of venoms and described their chemical nature. They showed that snake venoms are proteins and demonstrated experimentally some of their poisonous effects on blood and nervous tissue. In physiology he studied the centers of the brain that control thermoregulation; and in pharmacology he studied the physiological action of such drugs as caffeine, amyl nitrite, brucine, and strychnine.

Reichert was known for his interest in instrumentation, and he equipped his laboratory with the most modern instruments available, using them effectively to teach students as well as to conduct original research. His contributions were significant, and his tenure as physiology professor stretched to thirty-four years. Yet he had a retiring character and left less imprint on the medical school than might be expected.[16]

THEODORE G. WORMLEY

Theodore G. Wormley, a Pennsylvanian who had migrated to Ohio, was elected in 1877 to fill the chair of chemistry vacated by Robert E. Rogers when he resigned. Wormley was an M.D. who received his medical degree from the Philadelphia Medical College in 1849. After practicing medicine for a year he finally settled in Columbus, Ohio and remained there for 27 years. Here he became interested in the use of the microscope to study the properties of chemicals and the products formed during chemical reactions. This work led to his becoming America's first microchemist, following in the footsteps of Louis Pasteur. The micro-analytical techniques he developed became particularly important in the identification of poisons, thus Wormley was one of America's first toxicologists. His precise chemical analysis defining the chemical reaction conditions, reactant and product concentrations, limits of accuracy, and solubilities of each alkaloid did much to establish the field of microchemistry as a quantitative science in America.[17]

His experience using the microscope in chemistry and the procedures he developed were summarized in his textbook, *The Microchemistry of Poisons.*[18] After he had completed his text and it had been accepted for publication the publisher informed him he could find no one with the skill required to make the steel engravings of his drawings of crystals. To insure that the publication of this work would not be delayed and that the crystals would be properly illustrated, his wife learned the art of steel engraving and made nearly one hundred plates to illustrate her husband's chemical classic.[19]

PATHOLOGY IN THE MEDICAL DEPARTMENT FROM THE 1870s TO THE TURN OF THE CENTURY

Until the William Pepper Laboratory was built in 1895, most of the studies in pathology—clinical morbid anatomy—were carried out at Pennsylvania and Philadelphia Hospitals. For most of the century, pathology had not achieved independence as a discipline; it was a stepping stone to clinical medicine. William Pepper, Jr. served as curator of the Pathological Museum at Pennsylvania Hospital and later became a distinguished clinician because of his wide knowledge of the morbid anatomy of diseases.[20] James Tyson was Penn's first professor of general pathology, but even he moved on to become clinical professor of medicine, succeeding William Osler.

A change in attitude occurred in 1889, when Juan Guiteras, a graduate of Penn's medical school, was chosen to succeed Tyson as professor of general pathology and morbid anatomy.[21] Guiteras organized a more systematic course in the subject. He delivered lectures himself and established laboratory work for which the class was broken into groups conducted by "demonstrators" to study gross and microscopic specimens of diseased organs. He also introduced lectures on bacteriology.

Guiteras resigned and returned to his native Cuba when the Spanish-American War broke out in 1898. The position was offered to William H. Welch of Johns Hopkins. He turned it down but recommended his assistant, Simon Flexner.[22]

SIMON FLEXNER

Flexner had just returned from the Philippines, then a United States protectorate.[23] While studying dysentery among the soldiers stationed there, he discovered the bacillus that bears his name, *Shigella flexneri*.

He came to Penn in 1899 as professor of pathology (a title shortened from general pathology and morbid anatomy) and proceeded to organize the first full-time Department of Pathology at Penn. He complained about "the discomfort and disadvantages of inadequate quarters for teaching and research in the old building"—that is, Medical Hall—and he looked forward to the completion of the Medical Laboratories in 1904. Little wonder, considering the activity he generated, as recollected by Eugene Opie:

> Flexner continued his studies of toxalbumin and the reactions of the immunized animal to them. He directed [Hideyo] Noguchi to a highly successful study of the nature of snake venoms. He made experimental studies of pancreatic disease, begun in Baltimore and later continued in New York. He demonstrated a fat-splitting enzyme in foci of fat necrosis. He undertook experiments to define the conditions under which hemorrhagic necrosis of the pancreas is produced, and he showed later that the necrosis which develops when bile is introduced into the pancreatic ducts is referable to bile salts. He described hitherto unrecognized thrombi produced by agglutinization of red corpuscles. . . .[24]

Flexner also organized the Ayer Clinical Laboratory at Pennsylvania Hospital and served as its first director. His skills in both administration and research led to an offer to direct the Rockefeller Institute, and he left Penn for that institution in 1903. He went on to contribute significantly to research on poliomyelitis.[25]

HIDEYO NOGUCHI

Hideyo Noguchi was unintentionally recruited for Penn's Department of Pathology.[26] Flexner visited the Kitasato Institute of Infectious Diseases in Tokyo while en route to the Philippines. Noguchi, talking to Flexner, mentioned that he would like to come to the United States. Flexner answered this presumably casual remark by saying, "That would be fine." Noguchi, naive about American idioms, considered this response a formal invitation to work in Flexner's laboratory. After a slight delay due to shortage of funds, Noguchi obtained a steerage passage to San Francisco and arrived in Philadelphia in 1899. Flexner enjoyed recalling that Noguchi arrived "out of the blue, with many Japanese gifts, and wreathed in smiles."

The faculty helped Noguchi find a research project. Weir Mitchell wanted to extend his own work on snake venoms by applying newly developed techniques to the complex proteins that he and Reichert had found in venoms. Mitchell granted Noguchi funds to study them. Noguchi accepted the work but had problems. He knew nothing of the chemistry or immunology of snake venoms. Worse, he had great difficulty communicating with his colleagues and adjusted slowly to American customs and a Western scientific laboratory.[27] Fortunately for him, Flexner's assistants educated him daily. It was evident that their pupil was catching on when the sign "No-touchi, No-guchi" appeared over one of his experiments. He produced significant work. He and Flexner described in detail the hemolysis produced by the venom as well as the specific damage to the endothelium caused by the action of the toxin.

Noguchi followed Flexner to the Rockefeller Institute, where he devised culture techniques to grow the spirochete of syphilis; he demonstrated its presence in brain tissue, thus explaining the well-known neurological symptoms of this disease. He died of yellow fever in 1928 while carrying out research on the disease in Africa.[28]

ALLEN JOHN SMITH

Allen John Smith succeeded Flexner as head of pathology. He was a native Pennsylvanian who had graduated from Penn's medical school and assisted Juan Guiteras.[29] He was also the brother of Edgar Fahs Smith, Penn's distinguished chemistry professor. Allen Smith was ambitious in his own right. He had gone to the University of Texas in Galveston, where he virtually formed the medical school, serving as its dean and primary lecturer in nearly all subjects taught; he also had one of the few microscopes available there.

Smith was a parasitologist. In Texas he found ova of hookworm in an unidentified fecal specimen and then identified the parasite's ova in an Australian sailor. Because he recognized the difference between Old World and New World worms, Smith is credited with establishing the fact that hookworm disease is endemic in the United States. He studied leprosy and was led to evidence that bedbugs conveyed the disease. He made other discoveries as well, publishing his findings in more than 125 papers in journals, some of which he helped found. He translated

Otto von Furth's *Problems of the Physiological Chemistry of Metabolism.* This translation influenced the pioneering work in nutrition of Layafette Mendel and Graham Lusk at Yale University, research later brought to the University of Pennsylvania by Harry M. Vars, who was instrumental in developing intravenous nutrition.

Students gave Smith exceptional respect, and they often stayed past the class hour to hear him elaborate on the relationship between changes in the pathologic anatomy and the function of the organ and the patient's symptoms.

THE FIRST X-RAY PICTURE—ARTHUR W. GOODSPEED, WILLIAM N. JENNINGS, J. WILLIAM WHITE, AND CHARLES LESTER LEONARD

In 1895 Wilhelm Konrad Roentgen, professor of physics at the University of Würzburg, held his hand between a Hittorf tube and a fluorescent screen and became the first person to see the bones of his own hand.[30] But he did not make the first X ray. That had been done five years earlier in a Penn laboratory. Unfortunately the accomplishment was not recognized until Roentgen published his work and a Penn scientist went back to examine what he and a visiting friend had stumbled upon.[31]

It was February 22, 1890, and Arthur W. Goodspeed, a Penn physics professor, was conducting experiments with his guest, William N. Jennings, a British-born photographer. They had been studying the photographic effects of light emitted by the discharge of high-voltage cells. Goodspeed had the equipment ready: the spark gap and the induction coil that amplified voltage for the Crookes tubes used to demonstrate cathode rays to students. Goodspeed connected the coil to the spark gap, and Jennings made a series of photographs of coins, rings, and other small objects with the light from the spark. The evening's planned work completed and the night still young, their conversation turned to other science.[32]

Goodspeed explained to Jennings that the induction coil was usually used to burn Crookes tubes, devices named for Sir William Crookes, who had experimented with them extensively in the 1870s. They consisted of two metal electrodes in a vacuum-sealed glass bulb, which was beautifully pear-shaped. When the negative terminal of a high-voltage supply, as from an induction coil, was attached to one of the electrodes (the cathode) and the positive terminal to another (the anode), the cathode rays (later identified as electrons) were emitted and the glass tube fluoresced.[33]

The physics professor demonstrated the properties of several types of Crookes tubes in Penn's collection and then the properties of the cathode-ray tube. A stack of unexposed photographic plates from the photographic experiments stood nearby; on top of it were two coins Jennings had taken from his pocket for his Woodland Avenue trolley fare. After the demonstrations were finished, Jennings went home, carrying both his exposed and unexposed plates.[34] Several days later, Jennings reported to Goodspeed that some of the unexposed plates were badly fogged, even though they were tightly wrapped in lightproof paper. Furthermore, one of the developed plates was marked with the image of two mysterious discs. Jennings could not offer an explanation. Neither could Goodspeed. They forgot the matter, but Jennings was sufficiently impressed by the disc-shaped shadows that he stored the plate safely away.[35]

In 1895 Goodspeed read Roentgen's report describing X rays, and he immediately tried to obtain deliberate X-ray images of the kind he and Jennings had accidentally secured nearly six years earlier. He was not successful until February 5, 1896. He reported his results in the February 14 issue of *Science*. Goodspeed described how he made his February 5 picture: "A small strip of glass and a piece of sheet lead together with a wedge of wood were held in place upon a sensitive photographic plate by elastic bands. This object was placed horizontally upon a table eight to ten centimeters below the Crookes tube." After he turned on the current, "an exposure of twenty minutes produced upon development a sharp impression of the object. The sight was startling at first, as every experimenter who gets results for the first time can testify." Goodspeed immediately saw the implications for medicine: "Impressions of surgical cases, including deformed fingers, fractures, etc., have been successfully produced."[36]

The same issue of *Science* contains a translation of Roentgen's original report and papers showing X-ray pictures of various objects by Michael Pupin of Columbia University and E. H. Frost of New Hampshire as well as Goodspeed. Goodspeed gave a more detailed report on the X rays to the American Philosophical Society on February 21.

Goodspeed disclosed "Plate 1," as the 1890 X-ray plate by him and Jennings is called. And he was balanced about the circumstances: "The

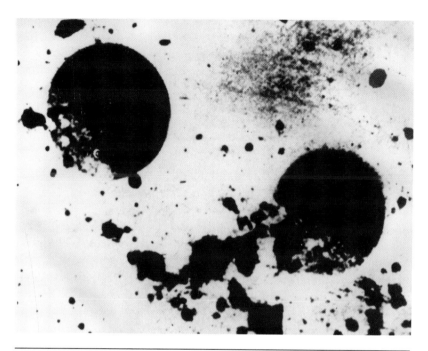

First X-ray picture. The picture of William Jennings's coins for his Woodland Avenue trolley fare, which he laid on the photographic plate exposed to the rays from the Crookes tube Arthur Goodspeed was demonstrating to Jennings in the physics department in 1890. Although Goodspeed failed to realize this picture's importance, it is the first X-ray picture taken. (Brecher and Brecher.)

writer and his associate [Jennings] wish to claim no credit for the interesting accident, but the fact remains, without a doubt, the first Roentgen picture was produced on February 22, 1890, in the physics lecture room at the University of Pennsylvania."[37]

Goodspeed went on to make other contributions. He gave the record produced by the rays the name radiograph because he realized that the image was produced by some type of electromagnetic radiation. Furthermore, he also made extensive studies on the optimal working conditions for the induction coil. He and John Carbutt also produced the first photographic plate designed for X-ray work. The techniques he developed helped him obtain high-quality radiographs of the thorax and abdomen.[38]

By February of 1896, Goodspeed had called J. William White, John Rhea Barton Professor of Surgery, about the possibility of using X rays in surgery. He asked White for patients.[39] White, in turn, enlisted the help of Charles Lester Leonard, a photographer who then was an instructor on the University Hospital's surgical service. Leonard had earlier worked in the Pepper Laboratory on methods of improving photomicrography. He had developed an electrically operated shutter-and-lens system, with which he was able to photograph microorganisms at various stages of their life cycle.[40]

Leonard immediately sensed the possibilities of using Roentgen rays in clinical medicine. He withdrew from his surgical training and began investigating the new science. Shortly he was appointed the hospital's first skiagrapher, or roentgenologist.

It was amazing that he could do anything, considering his facilities. At first, he carried out his X-ray work on an upper floor of the Pepper Laboratory. This site, however, was inaccessible to patients on litters, so he moved his modest equipment to a room partitioned off from the surgical outpatient waiting room on the ground floor of the Agnew Memorial Pavilion. The space was only twenty feet by ten feet, dark, and poorly ventilated, and no bed could be moved through the door. Leonard's darkroom for developing and loading plates was a small closet under the seats of the general surgical amphitheater, two floors above the room containing the X ray. It had a light, a sink with running water, two shelves, and space just sufficient to accommodate Leonard's body.

With these marginal facilities and a 20-volt primary induction coil operated by storage batteries, Leonard was the first person in the United States to demonstrate the presence of stones in the kidney and other parts of the urinary tract. Leonard continued to work under these primitive conditions until he resigned in 1902 to become director of laboratories at other hospitals.

But he had virtually given his life to his work, unaware, like so many early radiographers, of the dangers of X rays and radiation. By the time he left Penn, his hands were so severely burned that his finger had to be amputated, later his hand, and finally his arm. He died in 1923 from a squamous cell cancer produced by X rays in one of his burned fingers.[41]

Like his early colleagues, Leonard believed that tissue damage was caused by the electric magnetic field set up around the electron discharge in the X-ray tube. To reduce exposure to him and to the patient, he shielded his X-ray tubes with aluminum. This offered no protection from the X rays, which Leonard observed as his radiation dermatitis grew progressively worse. Finally he realized that the rays were causing the damage. Prior to his death, he wrote extensively, warning radiologists about the dangers of X rays and urging them to protect themselves with lead shielding.

THE DEPARTMENT OF RADIOLOGY

In his memoir of Henry K. Pancoast, Eugene Pendergrass states that, on the basis of evidence he could find, the Department of Radiology at the Hospital of the University of Pennsylvania began in 1896 and is the first such department established in the United States.[42] When Charles Lester Leonard left the university in 1902, J. William White, chairman of the Department of Surgery, asked Henry K. Pancoast to take the position of skiagrapher. After consulting with Arthur Goodspeed, Pancoast accepted the position.

In 1912 Pancoast became the first professor of roentgenology appointed in the United States. Subsequently this title was changed to professor of radiology to conform with the recommendations of the American Medical Association.

During his thirty-seven-year tenure in this position, Henry Pancoast was a pioneer in developing radiology at Pennsylvania as well as in the United States. He was one of the early radiologists who associated the development of leukemia with exposure to X-ray radiation and a pioneer in using X rays to treat leukemia and Hodgkin's disease. His work for the American Tuberculosis Association established the X-ray picture of the healthy chest.[43] His continued interest in dusty lungs resulted in detailed X-ray studies on pneumoconiosis and silicosis, work that led to the realization that these conditions were industrial hazards.[44] Today he is remembered for pointing out the importance of X rays in the early diagnosis of superior sulcus tumors by the eponym they bear, Pancoast's tumors.[45]

When Pancoast died in 1939, his assistant Eugene Pendergrass succeeded him as professor of radiology. Pendergrass accepted this position only on the condition that radiology be separated from surgery. Thus radiology became an independent department at this time.

JOHN GOODRICH CLARK

When the medical school at Johns Hopkins University was founded, two of its first four faculty members came from Penn: William Osler and Howard A. Kelly.[46] One of the first gifts Penn received in return was John Goodrich Clark. Clark was a Penn graduate who intended to join Osler's service at Hopkins, but when he arrived, he found that his position had been given to someone else. In desperation he went to Kelly, who happened to have an opening. Thus by mere chance Clark became a gynecologist; he turned out to be a creative physician in both the laboratory and the clinics.

As a resident at Hopkins, Clark began an anatomical study of the ovarian cycle as it progressed from follicle to *corpus luteum* to the *corpora albicantia*. He continued his studies in the laboratory of Werner Spalteholz and Wilhelm His at the University of Leipzig. There he demonstrated that the ovary has a single supply of blood, through its pedicle, unlike the male testis, which has a second, peripheral supply. Clark deduced that the sole blood supply, combined with the ovarian scarring from cyclic changes of follicular growth, ovulation, and formation of *corpora albicantia*, provided a self-destructing system; to Clark, this explained why ovarian function ceased earlier in life than testicular function.[47]

Also while he was in Leipzig, Clark studied the blood supply of the uterus. His findings caused Spalteholz to change his anatomical drawings of the uterus. Clark went on to study under Hans Chiari in Prague. His work on the ovary was published in *Archiv für Anatomie* in 1898 and immediately established him as the world authority on that organ.

Clark came to the University of Pennsylvania in 1899. He was a handsome, powerful man with enormous drive. He worked and played with equal intensity. His enthusiasm and pleasant personality stimulated his colleagues to work together and run the excellent gynecological clinic for which he was noted. "Give the credit to my team, not to me," he often said to compliments.[48]

But much was due to him and his acute observations. As early as his days at Hopkins, he noticed that the onset of uterine and cervical malignancies was silent and that many pelvic tumors were well advanced—and therefore inoperable—by the time the gynecologist saw them. Early detection became one of Clark's lifelong projects. To inform the public, he used his subsequent position as chairman of the American

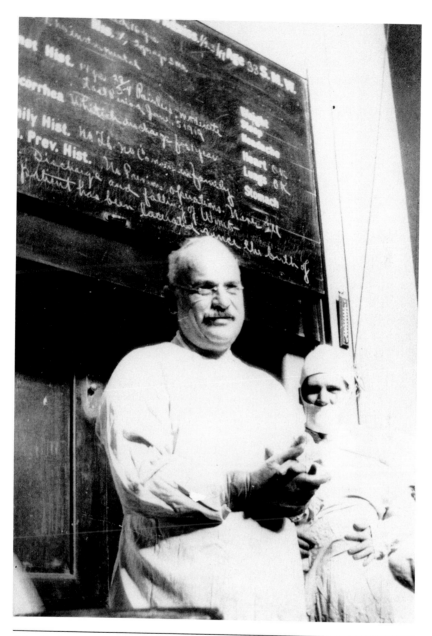

John G. Clark conducting his gynecology clinic. Clark had the history and physical finding written on the blackboard. The patient was prepared and draped behind a screen. When the patient was ready for the operation and the case presentation and discussion had been completed the screen was opened and the operation commenced. (Archives of the University of Pennsylvania.)

Medical Association's committee on cancer of the uterus. He published a pamphlet describing the early signs and symptoms of uterine cancer and mailed it to all physicians in the United States.

It was also during his residency that Clark realized that, contrary to conventional practice, a simple amputation of the cervix or the usual hysterectomy was inadequate in controlling pelvic cancer. He observed that tumor cells remained even when the uterus, cervix, tubes, and ovaries were removed. He felt that a more radical operation would excise the remaining cells.[49]

In 1895 Emil Reis of Chicago developed a radical abdominal operation in which he removed pelvic lymph nodes by dissection, in addition to removing the uterus, cervix, tubes, and ovaries. Reis, however, tried the operation only on animals and cadavers.

Clark introduced a new procedure on women in April 1895. That year he reported on his first two cases, and he pointed out his innovative surgical steps:

first the introduction of the bougies; second the ligation of the upper portion of the broad ligaments, including the round ligament and ovarian arteries, cutting them close to the pelvic walls, opening the two layers before excising any tissue; and excision of a larger portion of the vagina than usual.[50]

Four years later, Ernst Wertheim of Vienna published articles on an extensive series of cases in which he used essentially the same procedure described by Clark. Wertheim popularized the operation in Europe and, to some extent, the United States. For this reason, the radical hysterectomy is usually called Wertheim's operation, although Clark preceded him.[51]

Clark had success with the first fifteen patients he treated with this procedure; but postoperative reports—his own as well as those from Wertheim and others—were not so cheery. Surgical mortality was high, and the cure rate disappointing. To improve the treatment, Clark, along with Charles C. Norris, a junior member of his service, investigated the use of radium to treat the more advanced tumors. After five years, they concluded that radium was better for advanced cases and that surgery should be reserved for early cases.

Clark was also an innovative teacher. To stimulate research by medical students, he organized the Undergraduate Medical Association;

each spring, all regular classes were suspended for a day so that students could read and discuss their basic and clinical research at a symposium sponsored by the organization.

Formal lectures were not Clark's style. He replaced them with conferences and clinical studies, which he enriched by employing lantern slides, anecdotes, reminiscences, blackboard drawings, and anatomical sculptures modeled in plasticine clay. For his surgical clinics, he designed an operating room in which observers were separated from the operating area by a partition that could be raised or lowered. Preparations for the operation were completed behind the closed partition while the audience was given an abstract of the case history, illustrated by slides or a demonstration of the operative steps to follow. The partition was then raised, and the operation began. Such efficiency impressed visiting clinicians from all over the world.[52]

His wife helped him develop Ward K as a model for the postoperative care and convalescence of gynecological patients. He designed cubicles that separated patients according to their stage of recovery. The ward was tastefully decorated, airy, and bright, and always had fresh flowers and recent magazines and books on hand. Ward K is now called the Clark Unit, a tribute from his patients and friends.

SURGERY FOR THE CURE OF PAIN

William G. Spiller, Penn professor of neurology from 1915 to 1932, was the most distinguished American neurologist of his time.[53] Born in Baltimore, he received his medical degree from Penn, then went to Europe for four years, carrying out special studies in medicine and then in pathology. When he returned, he conducted neuropathological research in the William Pepper Laboratory. At the turn of the century, he was appointed to the neurology staff at the Philadelphia Polyclinic Hospital, maintaining a close connection with the Pepper Laboratory.

As time passed he became a fast friend of Charles K. Mills, dean of American neurologists, the two holding frequent sessions to discuss informally new developments in their field. When Mills's vision began to fail, Spiller loyally kept his friend informed by reading important articles to his colleague.

Spiller succeeded Mills and eventually accumulated more than two hundred fifty articles on neurological problems. His source material was

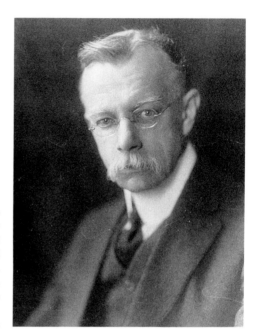

William Spiller, Professor of Neurology and the originator of the operation for tic douloureux and cordotomy for the relief of intractable pain in the lower body. (Historical Collections of the College of Physicians of Philadelphia.)

his large pathological collection and records of cases he had seen at Philadelphia General Hospital.

Spiller was a pioneer in vascular occlusion of the brain stem; he was the first to postulate the medullary syndrome resulting from anterior spinal artery occlusion. He also became an expert on disorders of conjugate extraocular muscle movement.

His patients described him as polite, cool, and abrupt, complaining that he knew them only by their neurological disease. Indeed, Spiller was serious and quiet, without a sense of humor. He was stooped when he walked, and on each side of his large round head the temporal arteries appeared as twin pulsating snakes. He dressed carelessly, and his office was as bare as the cell of an ascetic monk. A frugal man, Spiller never bought a newspaper but searched for one that might be left on the ward or thrown away in the trash. His only interest was neurology, and he knew little of other medical fields. One day he asked a colleague about a new thing called a protein; he mispronounced the word as well.

Spiller did not get along well with Charles Harrison Frazier, the neurosurgeon, even though professionally their paths inevitably crossed.[54] William Erb recalled the stinging inquisition Spiller directed at him when, at the end of his internship, he sought Spiller's advice on specializing in neurosurgery. As Erb had done well on Spiller's service, he felt he could discuss his decision with his teacher and ask for a recommendation. Erb broached the subject. Spiller was silent for a moment, then inquired, "Erb, are you sure you want to be a neurosurgeon?" Erb said yes. Spiller asked, "You know Frazier?" Erb said yes. "You know [Francis] Grant [a distinguished Frazier protégé]?" Again yes. Then Spiller said, "You want to be like them?" Erb became a prominent general surgeon.

Yet Spiller's and Frazier's names have been linked in treatments based on the former's research and the latter's surgical skill. The facial pain known as "tic douloureux," or trigeminal neuralgia, probably was described, albeit vaguely, by early Greek and Roman physicians. But it was not until the nineteenth century that the fifth nerve was implicated as the source of the pain, and then surgeons resected the entire gasserian ganglion of the fifth nerve. The operation was difficult, and postoperative complications, keratitis, and motor defects were common.[55]

In 1901 Spiller showed that the sensory root of the gasserian ganglion did not reunite after its fibers were divided. Frazier advanced that idea by showing that retroresection of the ganglion was not only technically possible but easier to perform than ganglionectomy. The Spiller-Frazier solution was used throughout the world for twenty years to treat the problem; it has since been modified, but the principle is the same.[56]

Spiller and Frazier are also linked in the relief of intractable pain by cordotomy. From the 1880s, posterior rhizotomies were usually done, but, according to a critical review by Frazier in 1918, they gave relief to only 19 percent of the patients. The problem basically was that surgeons could not pinpoint the pain tracts because the functional anatomy of the spinal cord was not known.

Spiller provided the earliest clear understanding of the location of the pain tracts. He reported a case in which a patient lost pain and temperature sensation in the lower part of the body without losing motor or bowel function. Spiller determined that the patient had bilateral tubercular abscesses of the lower spinal cord at the area of the anterolateral spinothalamic tracts. This brilliant diagnosis was confirmed by autopsy. Other neurologists later observed that those tracts carried pain impulses to the brain. Spiller suggested to Frazier that the neurosurgeon could relieve lower-body pain by cutting the anterolateral tracts. Frazier did not believe it and refused to attempt such an experimental operation.

Undeterred, Spiller went over Frazier's head and persuaded Edward Martin, John Rhea Barton Professor of Surgery and chairman of the department, to do the procedure. Martin performed the first cordotomy in January 1911. Frazier subsequently took it up and developed it. In 1920 he reported that he had found the optimal site for section of the spinothalamic tract in the upper thoracic region.[57]

At the start of his career, Charles Harrison Frazier studied pathology and neurology in Europe. He was especially influenced by Rudolf Virchow and Ernst G. von Bergmann, from whom he learned the new aseptic and surgical techniques then being developed.

He started at Penn as an instructor in surgical pathology in 1896, was elevated to clinical professor of surgery in 1901, then succeeded John B. Deaver as the John Rhea Barton Professor of Surgery in 1922. He was always interested in surgery of the central nervous system. He not only trained himself in the field but is also one of a small group of pioneers who created neurosurgery as a branch of surgery. During World War I, he gained experience treating soldiers who had suffered wounds to their nervous systems.[58]

Frazier was also one of the first thyroid surgeons in the United States. He conceived of the idea of a thyroid clinic at the University hospital, staffed by surgery, radiology (then a division of surgery), and medicine. By 1936, knowledge of the management of endocrine diseases had so advanced that the clinic was expanded to cover general endocrine disorders.

The tension of neurosurgery impelled physicians who conducted it to take on less stressful surgery as well. Frazier's interest in the thyroid apparently originated in some departmental vindictiveness. As I. S. Ravdin told the story, Deaver did not like Frazier because the younger colleague had once tried to improve the medical school by reforming the clinical faculty. When Deaver became the Barton Professor in 1915, he held a meeting at which he assigned the parts of the body upon which each member of the department was permitted to operate. Deaver assigned the peripheral parts and fractures to younger members of the staff and kept the more desirable general surgery for himself. He might have preferred to close Frazier out altogether, but could not because of Frazier's clinical appointment as well as his strong political and family ties to Penn. (Frazier's uncle Charles C. Harrison was the University provost from 1894 to 1912.) But Deaver made it clear to Frazier that he could not operate on anything below the clavicle. Frazier obeyed the order until operating only on the brain and spinal cord began to get on his nerves. He went to Deaver and requested that he be allowed to operate on other parts of the body. Deaver relented and allowed Frazier to operate on the thyroid—within the boundary originally assigned.[59]

Frazier was sturdily built and had a ruddy complexion. His piercing blue-gray eyes stared from under a full head of hair arranged as orderly as he was precise. He had a fiery temper; his resounding voice and commanding disposition struck fear in many colleagues as well as interns and residents, who considered him autocratic and tyrannical. Some who knew him more intimately feel that he was only superficially harsh; they describe him as a gentleman who was gracious, charitable, and helpful. Before his death Julian Johnson wrote in a letter that Frazier could be an S.O.B. in the operating room but otherwise he was very nice and concluded that was where he learned some of his habits.[60]

Throughout his career he had deep concern for the academic reputation of Penn's medical school. He established and edited the *University of Pennsylvania Medical Magazine* and established one of the first laboratories of surgical pathology in the country. He reorganized the

J. William White giving an anatomy lecture in Medical Hall. (Nadine Landis.)

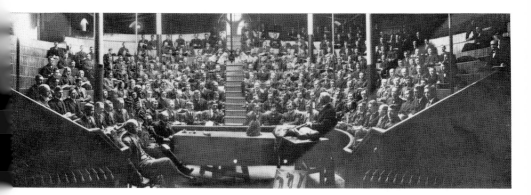

surgery department, bringing clinical and research activities closer together, and stressed the importance of applying the principles of physiology, physiological chemistry, and pathological physiology to the management of surgical patients. He trained a number of neurosurgeons who went on to occupy important chairs at Penn and elsewhere.[61]

Determined throughout his life, Frazier operated to the end, even though, when he developed his final illness, he had to be strapped to the operating table to keep from falling.[62]

NOTES

1. H. Cushing, *The Life of Sir William Osler* (Oxford: Oxford University Press, 1940), pp. 220–22; C. G. Roland, "William Osler, 1849–1919," Commemorative Issue, *Journal of the American Medical Association*, 210(1969):2213–71; W. Osler, *Aequanimitas, with Other Addresses to Medical Students, Nurses and Practitioners of Medicine* (Philadelphia: P. Blakiston's Son & Co., 1932); H. E. Sigerist, *The Great Doctors* (1933, reprint ed., New York: Dover, 1971); A. M. Chesney, *The Johns Hopkins Hospital and The Johns Hopkins School of Medicine—A Chronicle*, vols. 1 and 2 (Baltimore; Johns Hopkins University Press, 1943).

2. H. Cushing, *Life of Osler*, pp. 220–21.

3. *Ibid.*, p. 221.

4. *Ibid.*, p. 222.

5. *Ibid.*, p. 233.

6. *Ibid.*, p. 235.

7. *Ibid.*, pp. 235–36.

8. *Ibid.*, pp. 237; 296–97; 683–85.

9. R. Friedman, *A History of Dermatology in Philadelphia* (Fort Pierce Beach, Fla: Froben Press, 1955) This collection contains the following articles: H. W. Stelwagon, "Memoir of Louis A. Duhring, M.D.," pp. 81–127; "Bibliography of Dr. Duhring's Most Important Papers," pp. 127–34; "A Character Study of Louis A. Duhring," pp. 233–69 "The Will of Louis A. Duhring, M.D.," pp. 245–56; A. Van Harlingen, "Sketch of Louis A. Duhring," p. 266; L. C. Parrish, *Louis Duhring* (Springfield, Ill.: Charles C. Thomas, 1967); *Leaders in Dermatology, Louis Duhring* (Palo Alto, Calif.: Syntex, 1966).

10. H. Beerman and E. S. Beerman, "A Meeting of Two Famous Benefactors of the Library of the University of Pennsylvania—Louis Adolphus Duhring and Theodore Dreiser," *Transactions and Studies of the College of Physicians of Philadelphia* 4th. ser., 42(1974):43–48.

11. G. B. Roth, "An Early American Pharmacologist, Horatio C. Wood (1841–1920)," *Isis* 30(1939):38–45; G. E. De Schweinitz, "Horatio C. Wood as a Medical Teacher," *Transactions and Studies of the College of Physicians of Philadelphia* 3d ser., 42(1920):235–57.

12. H. C. Wood, "Harrison Allen (1841–1897)," *Transactions and Studies of the College of Physicians of Philadelphia* 3d ser., 20(1898):xxxix–lii.

13. *History of the American Physiological Society, 1887–1937* (Baltimore, 1938); newspaper obituary, University of Pennsylvania Archives.

14. "Tracing Heredity by Means of Blood Crystals," *New York Sun*, June 8, 1913; H. F. Judson, *The Eighth Day of Creation: The Makers of the Revolution in Biology* (New York: Simon and Schuster, 1979), pp. 511–12, 610.

15. E. T. Reichert, *Differentiation and Specificity of Corresponding Proteins and Other Vital Substances in Relation to Biological Classification and Organic Evolution: The Crystallography of Hemoglobins* (Washington, D.C.: Carnegie Institute, 1909 Report No. 116); E. T. Reichert, *The Differentiation and Specificity of Starches in Relation to Genes of Starches, etc.: Stereochemistry Applied to a Protoplasmic Process and Product; and as a Strictly Scientific Basis for Classification of Plants and Animals* (Washington, D.C.: Carnegie Institute, 1913 Report No. 173, vols. 1 and 2).

16. A. C. Abbott, "Lunching with Reichert," *Scope* (1924):63–70; G. W. Corner, *Two Centuries of Medicine* (Philadelphia: Lippincott, 1965), pp. 179–80, 186, 215.

17. E. F. Smith, "Prof. Theodore G. Wormley," *Journal of the American Chemical Society* 29 (1897):275–79; John Ashurst, Jr., "The Late Professor Theodore G. Wormley," *Transactions and Studies of the College of Physicians of Philadelphia* 3d ser., 19(1897):lxxix–lxxxviii; W. M. MacNevin, "Theodore G. Wormley—First American Microchemist, 1826–1897," *Journal of Chemical Education* (April 1948):182–86; *Philadelphia Inquirer*, January 3, 1897.

18. T. G. Wormley, *The Microchemistry of Poisons* (New York: Bailliere Bros., 1867).

19. MacNevin, "Theodore Wormley."

20. E. R. Long and D. T. Rowlands, *The Development of the Department of Pathology in the School of Medicine at the University of Pennsylvania* (Philadelphia: privately printed 1977), pp. 1–6.

21. *Ibid.*,pp. 6–13.

22. *Ibid.*,pp. 14–19.

23. E. L. Opie, "Simon Flexner—1863–1946," *Archives of Pathology* 42(1946):234–42; A. E. Cohn, "On Simon Flexner, 1863–1946," in *Retreat from Reason and Other Essays* (New York: Harcourt Brace and Co., 1948), p. 243; Long and Rowlands, *Development of the Department of Pathology*, pp. 20–28; S. Flexner and J. T. Flexner, *William Henry Welsh and the Heroic Age of American Medicine* (New York: The Viking Press, 1941), pp. 280–82; J. T. Flexner, *An American Saga* (Boston: Little Brown, 1984), pp. 317–33, 330–33.

24. Opie, "Simon Flexner," pp. 243–42.

25. S. Flexner,"Poliomyelitis, Mode of Infection and Means of Prevention," *Transactions and Studies of the College of Physicians of Philadelphia* 3d ser., 54 (1932):11–32.

26. G. Eckstein, *Noguchi* (New York: Harper and Bros., 1931); P. F. Clark, "Hideyo Noguchi," *Bulletin of the History of Medicine* 33(1959):1–19; G. Williams, *The Plague Fighters* (New York: Charles Scribner and Co., 1969) pp. 185–326; T. Smith, "Hideyo Noguchi," *Bulletin of the New York Academy of Medicine* 5(1929):877–84.

27. S. W. Mitchell, *Researches Upon the Venom of the Rattle Snake* (Washington: Smithsonian Institution, 1861); S. W. Mitchell and E. T. Reichert, *Researches Upon the Venoms of Poisonous Serpents* (Washington: Smithsonian Institution, 1886); H. Noguchi, *Snake Venoms* (Washington, D.C.: Carnegie Institute, 1909).

28. Williams, *Plague Fighters*, p. 248.

29. Members of the Medical Department of the University of Pennsylvania, "Allen John Smith—A Tribute," *Journal of Parasitology* 13(1927):157–61; "Allen J. Smith," *American Journal of Medical Sciences* 173 (1927), unpaged section of four pages with portrait following p. 752; newspaper clippings, Archives of the University of Pennsylvania.

30. R. Brecher and E. Brecher, *History of Radiology* (Baltimore: Williams and Wilkins, 1969); H. A. Kelley and W. L. Burrage, *A Dictionary of American Medical Biography* (Boston: Milford Press, 1928); E. R. W. Gregg, *The Trail of Invisible Light from X-Strahlen to Radio(bio)logy* (Springfield, Ill.: Charles C. Thomas, 1965); O. Glasser, *William Conrad Roentgen and the Early History of Roentgen Rays* (Springfield, Ill.: Charles C. Thomas, 1895).

31. Brecher and Brecher, *History of Radiology.*

32. *Ibid.*, p. 3.

33. *Ibid.*, pp. 4–5.

34. *Ibid.*, p. 3.

35. *Ibid.*, pp. 4–5.

36. M. Pupin, "Röntgen Rays," *Science* 3 (1896):231–35; E. H. Frost, "Experiments on the X–Rays," *Science*, 3(1896): 235–36; A. Goodspeed "Experiments on the Röntgen Rays," *Science* 3 (1896):236-37; W. K. Röntgen, "On a New Kind of Rays, *Science* 3(1896):227–31. From a translation in *Nature* by Arthur Stanton from the *Sitzungberichte der Wurtzberger Physik-medic. Gesellschaft* (1895).

37. Goodspeed, "Experiments," pp. 236–37.

38. Brecher and Brecher, *History of Radiology*; L. Leopold, *Radiology at the University of Pennsylvania.* (Philadelphia: University of Pennsylvania Press, 1981), pp. 3–18; A. W. Goodspeed, "Remarks Made at the Demonstration of the Röntgen Ray, at Stated Meeting, February 21, 1896," *Proceedings of the American Philosophical Society* 35, 150(1896):17–24; A. W. Goodspeed, *Medical News* 68(1896):169; A. W. Goodspeed, *International Medical Magazine* 5(1896): 319.

39. A. W. Goodspeed, C. L. Leonard, and J. W. White, "Case Illustrations of the Practical Application of the Roentgen Rays to Surgery," *American Journal of Medical Sciences* 112 (1896):125–47.

40. Leopold, *Radiology at the University of Pennsylvania*, pp. 8–9.

41. *Ibid.*, pp. 9–16.

42. E. P. Pendergrass, "Memoir of Henry Kunrath Pancoast," *Transactions and Studies of the College of Physicians of Philadelphia*, 4th ser., 8(1940–1941):47–52.

43. "The Normal Chest and Tuberculosis," *American Journal of Roentgenology and Radium Therapy* 17 (1927): 557–65. Authors: H. K. Pancoast, H. R. M. Landis, University of Pennsylvania; F. H. Baetjer, C. R. Austrian, Johns Hopkins University; H. K. Dunham, K. D. Blackfan, University of Cincinnati.

44. H. K. Pancoast, T. G. Miller, H. R. M. Landis, "A Roentgen Study of the Effects of Dust Inhalation upon the Lungs," *American Journal of Roentgenology* 5 (1918):129–39; H. K. Pancoast, "Roentgenologic Study of Pneumoconiosis and other Fibrosing Conditions of the Lung," *Annals of Clinical Medicine* 2(1923):8–21; H. K. Pancoast, E. P. Pendergrass, A. R. Riddell, A. J. Lanza, W. J. McConnell, R. R. Sayers, H. L. Sampson, and C. U. Gardner, "Roentgenological Appearances in Silicosis and Underlying Pathological Lesions," *Public Health Reports*, Reprint no. 1696 (Washington, D.C.: U. S. Government Printing Office, 1935), pp. 2–8.

45. H. K. Pancoast, "Importance of Careful Roentgen Investigation of Apical Chest Tumors," *Journal of the American Medical Association* 83 (1924):1407–11.

46. A. McG. Harvey, "Early Contributions to the Surgery of Cancer: William S. Halstead, Hugh H. Young and John G. Clark," *Johns Hopkins Medical Journal* 135(1974):399–417; J. G. Clark, "Ursprung, Wachstum und Ende des Corpus Luteum" *Archiv für Anatomie und Physiologie (Leipzig)*, (1898):95–134; J. G. Clark, "The Origin, Development, and Degeneration of the Blood Vessels of the Human Ovary," *Johns Hopkins Hospital Reports*. Dedicated by His Pupils, W. H. Welch, vol. 7 (Baltimore:

Johns Hopkins University Press, 1899), pp. 181–221; J. J. Mikuta, "John Goodrich Clark, M. D., Tribute," presented at the President's Address before the Obstetrical Society of Philadelphia, May 6, 1976.

47. Mikuta, "Clark, Tribute".

48. "Dr. John G. Clark," 1891. *Alumni Register* 19(1916): 150–57.

49. *Ibid.*, p. 154.

50. J. G. Clark, "A More Radical Method of Performing Hysterectomy for Cancer of the Uterus," *Johns Hopkins* Hospital Bulletin, 6(1895):4.

51. *Ibid.*,

52. Mikuta, "Clark, Tribute."

53. A. M. Ornsteen, "William Gibson Spiller (1863–1940)," in *The Founders of Neurology*, ed. Webb Haymaker (Springfield, Ill.: Charles C. Thomas, 1953), pp. 388–92.

54. Personal conversations with Edward Rose, William Erb, and Julian Johnson.

55. F. H. Lewey, "Charles Harrison Frazier (1870–1936)," in *The Founders of Neurology*, ed. Webb Haymaker (Springfield, Ill.: Charles C. Thomas, 1953), pp. 426–28; G. Horrax, *Neurosurgery: An Historical Sketch* (Springfield, Ill.: Charles C. Thomas, 1952), pp. 77–80; A. E. Walker, *A History of Neurological Surgery* (Baltimore: Williams and Wilkins, 1951), pp. 309–20.

56. W. G. Spiller and C. H. Frazier, "The Divison of the Sensory Root of the Trigeminal Nerve for Relief of Tic Douloureux," *University of Pennsylvania Medical Bulletin* 14 (1901):341–52; C. H. Frazier, "A Refinement in the Radical Operation for Trigeminal Neuralgia," *Journal of the American Medical Association* 76(1921):107.

57. W. G. Spiller, and E. Martin, "The Treatment of Persistent Pain of Organic Origin in the Lower Part of the Body by Division of the Anteriolateral Column of the Spinal Cord," *Journal of the American Medical Association* 58 (1912): 1489–90: C. H. Frazier, "Rhizotomy for the Relief of Pain," *Journal of Nervous and Mental Diseases* 47 (1918):343–62; C. H. Frazier, "Section of the Anterolateral Columns of the Spinal Cord for Relief of Pain," *Archives of Neurology and Psychiatry* 4 (1920):137–47.

58. Lewey, "Charles Harrison Frazier."

59. Statements of I. S. Ravdin and personal conversations with William Erb and I. S. Ravdin.

60. Lewey, "Charles Harrison Frazier."

61. Letter to David Y. Cooper from Julian Johnson, March 30, 1984.

62. Personal conversations with Julian Johnson and Edward Rose.

7
A CHAIR FOR SURGERY

The good surgeon is a physician and something else.

I. S. Ravdin

The John Rhea Barton Professorship of Surgery, established in 1877, was the first fully endowed surgical chair in America. Permanent endowments answered an increasingly important question as the nineteenth century progressed: how to support an improved faculty. During this period, the status of surgeons advanced. Scientific discoveries led to new surgical techniques that decreased both the suffering of patients and the rate of death due to either surgery or disease.

At the same time, the medical school budget was strained. There was an increasing demand for research facilities, equipment, and personnel. The medical school admitted greater numbers of students, but course fees, traditionally paid directly to the teacher, did not suffice. And surgeons engaged in research could not readily supplement their incomes by private practice, as they once had.[1]

Thus $50,000 given by Sarah Rittenhouse Barton, widow of John Rhea Barton, was a timely blessing.[2] Barton himself never held a position on the Penn faculty, although both his uncle Benjamin Smith Barton and his brother William P. C. Barton were Penn professors. John Rhea graduated from the medical school in 1818. He served first as surgeon at the Philadelphia Almshouse and in 1823 joined the surgical staff at Pennsylvania Hospital, where he worked for the remainder of his long career.[3]

He developed what is still known as the Barton head bandage, a strip of muslin two inches wide and five yards long, tied in a figure-eight design around the head and under the jaw to support an injured mandible and to cover other head injuries.[4] He also described and developed the treatment of the fracture of the distal end of the radius, called the Barton fracture.[5]

In addition, he devised an ingenious operation for treatment of ankylosis by intentionally forming artificial joints. He divided the femur near its upper part with a saw. After placing it in a straightened position, he moved the lower portion to prevent union of the bone and to establish a false joint. The operation enabled a previously bedridden patient to stand and walk. He went on to treat ankylosis of other joints successfully. The surgery was an amazing accomplishment because it was done without anesthesia or antibiotics. It was also a brilliant example of surgical reasoning. In devising the operation, Barton anticipated every problem that such a procedure would present. No structures later required to support the pseudoarthrosis were damaged by the incisions.[6]

D. HAYES AGNEW

The first incumbent of the Barton chair was D. Hayes Agnew, a master surgeon who entered the specialty after mastering anatomy.[7] The son of a Lancaster, Pennsylvania, physician, Agnew received an M.D. degree from Penn in 1838. He spent much of his student time carrying out anatomical investigations in a rented, private dissecting room. After practicing medicine briefly near Noblesville, Pennsylvania, then unsuccessfully entering the iron foundry business of his late father-in-law, Agnew set up a medical practice in Cochransville, in Chester County. His zeal to learn anatomy and surgery led him to a rather desperate scheme. He purchased bodies in Philadelphia, had them delivered to a dissecting room at his home, then engaged a farmer to sink the remains in a local pond, where the eels finished the dissection and prepared perfect bone specimens. The eels were said to be noted locally for their flavor, size, and snappiness—until the secret got out.[8]

Agnew finally found his calling in 1853. He purchased the Philadelphia Anatomical School from Jonathan M. Allen for $600. He toiled diligently to teach the medical students anatomy, keeping his rooms open twelve to eighteen hours a day. In 1854 he opened the Philadelphia School of Operative Surgery on the third floor of his building so that he could demonstrate new procedures on cadavers. Agnew sold the school in 1862.[9]

Reputed as an anatomist and teacher, Agnew joined the staff of Philadelphia Hospital and shortly afterwards was appointed a surgeon there. In 1863 he was appointed as a demonstrator in anatomy, subordinate to Joseph Leidy, at Penn. He brought with him many of his paying anatomical students. After six years without a promotion, he threatened to quit unless he was given faculty status. University officials feared that Agnew and his pedagogical flair, along with his students, would decamp to Jefferson. They appointed him professor of clinical surgery with the additional title of demonstrative surgeon, so that he could continue to teach his course in cadaver surgery. In 1871 he succeeded to the senior chair and stepped into the Barton professorship in 1877.[10]

Among his surgical innovations, Agnew devised operations for dividing webbed fingers and for repairing vesicovaginal fistulae; he also improved several amputation techniques. Among surgical instruments, he invented clamps that made surgical procedures easier or possible for the first time; his most important device was the artery forceps.[11] He also carried out experiments on animals, especially to observe the behavior of clots and the healing of bone, which he noted were similar in humans.

Bone fractures, he reported, formed callus in a sequence of stages. At first, the body "brooded quietly" over the disorder for up to thirty-six hours. Then a reactionary period of inflammation set in, "an increase of determination of blood to the part. . . ." After a period of "vascularity, . . . the real work of repair begins, that in which the true fibrogenous matter, swarming with cellular elements, assumes the appearance of order." Finally, "the differentiation of this constructive material into cartilage or fibro-cartilage and intracellular substance and the subsequent deposition of the bone salts, ultimately permeating the mass and imparting solidity to the bone, are the work of four to five weeks."[12] The cellular processes involved in bone healing have been explained more accurately since then, but many of Agnew's ideas remain valid.

Agnew's most famous patient was President James A. Garfield, shot by a madman on July 2, 1881. Garfield rallied despite his own physicians' failure to remove the bullet with their fingers and long forceps. By the time Agnew was summoned, the damage had been done, so he recommended conservative management. Garfield died of infection on September 19.[13]

The medical class of 1889 commissioned Thomas Eakins to paint Agnew to honor him at Commencement in 1889, on his seventieth birthday. Eakins had painted Samuel Gross of Jefferson fourteen years earlier. In the intervening time, advances in surgical asepsis made the latter work seem several generations ahead of its predecessor. Blood was still part of the scene, however, and Eakins painted Agnew accordingly. When Agnew complained about the bloody hands and gowns, protesting that he did not want his operations so depicted, Eakins reluctantly complied with his subject's revisions.[14]

J. WILLIAM WHITE

J. William White, the third incumbent of the Barton chair, was independently wealthy and brought to his field the fiery, aggressive spirit of the growing industrial nation.[15] Although primarily a clinical surgeon, he understood the importance of research in surgery. In 1906 he appointed J. Edwin Sweet as an associate in experimental surgery, the first such position in the world. And in his will he provided funds to endow a professorship in research surgery.[16]

White received both a Ph.D. and an M.D. from Penn in 1871. He explored the waters of the South Atlantic with a Harvard naturalist before accepting posts, successively, at Philadelphia Hospital, then Eastern State Penitentiary, and then with the First City Troop.[17] His temper gained him national notoriety as a participant in the last pistol duel in America. Fortunately it was bloodless. White insisted that he should be permitted to wear the uniform of the First City Troop, but he was challenged by a Trooper Adams. At fifteen paces on the Delaware-Maryland border, White shot in the air, Adams's gun missed White, and the principals shook hands.[18] White liked fairness. He helped relocate the riot-prone Army-Navy football game to the neutral ground of Franklin Field in 1899.[19]

His career on the Penn faculty began in genitourinary surgery, where he made two advances. One was his use of X-rays to detect fractures and bone deformities.[20] The other was his treatment of prostatic enlargement by orchectomy. He had observed that uterine fibroids as well as the uterus became atrophied after an ovariectomy. Reasoning that the prostate and testicular function were similarly related, he proposed removing the testes to reduce prostatic enlargements and relieve urinary obstructions. It worked in dogs. In humans, White reported dramatic relief of the obstruction in some cases, but felt that surgical mortality was higher than it should be. Unfortunately, as he did not examine the prostatic tissues of these cases at autopsy to determine whether cancer had caused the hypertrophy, it was impossible to evaluate his therapy. Not for forty years would orchidectomy be shown to be effective in treating carcinoma of the prostate.[21]

EDWARD B. MARTIN

Edward Martin succeeded White in the Barton chair.[22] He was a handsome Hicksite Quaker who graduated from Swarthmore College and then from Penn's medical school. He had an early interest in aviation and before the Wright brothers' accomplishments conducted experiments that proved heavier-than-air flight was possible.

As a surgeon Martin was the first to use morphine to relieve postoperative pain at the University hospital. He also introduced breathing exercises and carbon dioxide inhalation to combat the respiratory depression associated with the use of narcotics. He published original papers on such topics as ambulatory treatment of fractures of the lower extremity, occlusive dressings for war wounds, the use of adrenaline to treat shock, and acacia as a blood substitute. In the classroom, Martin introduced motion pictures to add to lantern slides as pedagogical devices. Martin's legacy is not exclusively medical.[23] Debonair and married, he fancied himself a ladies' man and admitted female admirers to the hospital for long stays.[24] The director of the hospital entered Martin's office one day and shot him in the back for philandering with his wife. The episode is recorded in Martin's inkstand, which was perforated by a stray bullet; the inkstand is part of the permanent historical exhibition in the John Morgan Building.[25] Later in life, when his vanity was scarred by carcinoma of the left lower part of his nose, Martin ordered a gelatin prosthesis that was renewed from time to time and tinted to match his skin to disguise the deformity.[26]

JOHN BLAIR DEAVER

Martin unexpectedly resigned the Barton chair in 1918, and John B. Deaver succeeded him.[27] Deaver probably operated more than any surgeon in Philadelphia. Scheduling eighteen to twenty-four cases in a single day was not unusual for him. His clinic was well organized, and there were few delays, even though he did not use his assistants to their full capabilities. He felt that his obligation to the patient and the referring physician required his performing the operation himself. Late in life he allowed his residents to do more, but he still held a tight rein. In hysterectomies the resident was not permitted to begin the operation until Deaver had safely placed the clamps alongside the uterus so that the ureters would not be cut. He called a Caesarean section "his" operation. [28]

John B. Deaver's Clinic at Lankenau Hospital. (Historical Collections of the College of Physicians of Philadelphia.)

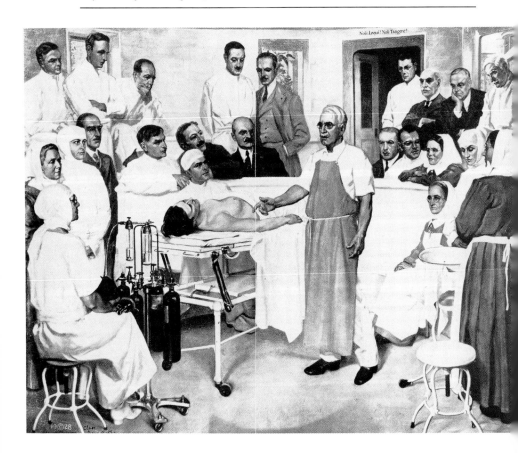

With the scalpel Deaver was rapid and impatient, a "great slasher." He may have lacked the patience for fine dissections; but in the abdomen, where meticulousness is less critical, he was confident and met accidents with perfect poise. He also expressed contempt for pathology, seeming to doubt a science of disease. At the operating table he challenged others by demanding, "What is the pathology?" or "Demonstrate the pathology!" as if it either could be shown at once on a tray or else did not exist.[29]

His name is associated with a retractor whose use can make anyone seem clumsy. Every intern, resident, or surgical assistant has been rebuked by an operating surgeon for not holding the Deaver properly. Something about this instrument contains the spirit of its inventor.[30]

As a teacher, Deaver established operative clinics on Saturday afternoons, drawing medical students and students of surgery from all over the world. He played to his large audiences. He would exclaim, "What this case needs is the aseptic scalpel at the earliest possible moment!" and then lay open an abdomen with a single stroke.[31] He had a formula for the length of incision, the duration of an operation, and the period of a hospital stay for an appendectomy: "an inch and a half, a minute and a half, and a week and a half." To remind students that surgical treatment, unlike medical management, was definitive, he insisted, "Sew well, get well, stay well." If residents were too vigorous with patients, he advised, "Let the patient get well."[32]

NOTES

1. Minutes of the Faculty Meeting (the guarantee).

2. W. A. Damon, "A Brief History of the John Rhea Barton Chair of Surgery," *Transactions and Studies of the College of Physicians of Philadelphia*, 4th ser., 23 (1955):94–104; R. H. Ivy, "Personal Recollections of Holders of the John Rhea Barton Professorship of Surgery at the University of Pennsylvania School of Medicine," *Transactions and Studies of the College of Physicians of Philadelphia*, 4th ser., 42 (1975): 239–62.

3. Damon, pp. 94–95; Ivy, pp. 240–41.

4. J. R. Barton, "A Systematic Bandage for Fracture of the Lower Jaw," *American Medical Recorder* 2 (1819):153.

5. J. R. Barton, "Views and Treatment of an Important Injury to the Wrist," *Medical Examiner* 1(1838):365–69.

6. J. R. Barton, "On the Treatment of Ankylosis by Formation of an Artificial Joint," *North American Medical Journal* 3 (1827): 279–92.

7. J. H. Adams, *History of the Life of D. Hayes Agnew, M.D., L.L.D.* (Philadelphia:

F. A. Davis, 1892); DeF. Willard, "D. Hayes Agnew, M.D., L.L.D.," read by invitation to the County Medical Society, April 13 1892; DeF. Willard, "D. Hayes Agnew, M.D., L.L.D.," *University of Pennsylvania Medical Bulletin* (April 13, 1892); S. X. Radbill, "David Hayes Agnew (1818–1892)," *Transactions and Studies of the College of Physicians of Philadelphia* 4th ser., 33 (1965–66):252–60.

8. Adams, *Life of D. Hayes Agnew*, pp. 71–72.

9. *Ibid.*, pp. 84–92.

10. *Ibid.*, pp. 136–40.

11. *Ibid.*, pp. 174–77.

12. *Ibid.*, pp. 182–92.

13. *Ibid.*, pp. 220–49.

14. *Ibid.*, pp. 332–35.

15. A. Repplier, *J. William White, M.D.* (New York: Houghton Mifflin, 1919); H. A. Kelley and W. L. Burrage, *A Dictionary of American Medical Biography* (Boston: Milford Press, 1928).

16. G. W. Corner, *Two Centuries of Medicine* (Philadelphia: Lippincott, 1965), pp. 242, 273.

17. Ivy, *Personal Recollections of Holders of John Rhea Barton Chair*, p. 245; Repplier, *J. William White*, pp. 8–28.

18. Repplier, pp. 45–46.

19. G. Schoor, *The Army and Navy Game—A Treatise of the Football Classic* (New York: Dodd and Mead, 1967), pp. 401–403, [game statistics, 415; riot described, 421; last game played at Annapolis; *Philadelphia Inquirer*, Dec. 3, 1982 statement that this would probably be the last game between the academies because of injuries to players and time diverted from studies; Repplier, *J. William White*, pp. 87–89.

20. A. W. Goodspeed, C. L. Leonard, and J. W. White, "Case Illustrations of the Practical Application of Roentgen Rays to Surgery," *American Journal of Medical Sciences* 112(1896):125–47; R. Brecher and E. Brecher, *History of Radiology* (Baltimore: Williams and Wilkins, 1969); L. Leopold, *Radiology at the University of Pennsylvania* (Philadelphia: University of Pennsylvania Press, 1981).

21. Damon, pp. 98–99.

22. *Ibid.*, pp. 99–101.

23. *Ibid.*, p. 99.

24. Conversation with T. Grier Miller.

25. Conversation with T. Grier Miller. Inkstand with bullet hole in museum located in the front hall of the John Morgan Building.

26. Conversation with Julian Johnson and T. Grier Miller; Ivy, *Personal Recollections of Holders of the John Rhea Barton Chair*, p. 249.

27. I. S. Ravdin, "John Blair Deaver, Master Surgeon." *Philadelphia Medicine* 56 (1960):741–85; A. P. C. Ashurst, "Memoir of John Blair Deaver, M.D.," *Annals of Surgery* 95 (1932):637–40; D. B. Pfeiffer, "Memoir of John Blair Deaver, M.D.," *Transactions and Studies of the College of Physicans of Philadelphia* 3rd ser., 54(1932):lxxvii–lxxix; Damon, pp. 99–100; Ivy, pp. 249–51.

28. Ashurst, "Memoir," 637–40.

29. *Ibid.*

30. *Ibid.*

31. *Ibid.*

32. *Ibid.*

8

SPECIALIZED INSTITUTES

If "Ye shall know the truth, the truth shall set you free," not from change or from grief, or from final passage beyond the vail but free from careless fears, from useless labor; and this is a part of wisdom "which passeth and goeth through all things."

John Shaw Billings
Address at the Opening of the School of Hygiene, 1892

The development of cities in an industrialized America brought new problems to the attention of this country's physicians. Infectious diseases required not only cures but also greater understanding of how diseases spread and how to prevent them through clean water supplies, adequate waste and sewage disposal, and good housing and food. European clinics had begun systematic scientific studies of diseases, which produced important advances in understanding and treatment. Penn was the site of some of the first American institutes to mass a large frontal attack on particular health problems.[1]

THE SCHOOL OF HYGIENE

An early example was the School of Hygiene. The single course that had begun in 1865 in the Auxiliary School of Medicine was hardly sufficient for the material two decades later, when the University hospital's facilities were steadily increasing. Plans for a school were discussed in the spring of 1888, shortly after a fire destroyed most of the fourth floor of Medical Hall. Provost Pepper was surveying the damage with Henry C. Lea, the wealthy publisher and philanthropist, and learned of Lea's interest in public health. Lea offered $10,000 to promote the study of hygiene.[2]

Pepper's flair for fund-raising was aroused. He began negotiating with John Shaw Billings from Johns Hopkins Hospital to direct the new department. Then he approached Lea, who increased his proposal to $50,000 for a laboratory if Billings would come and if an additional $250,000 was secured for equipment and an endowment; Lea also insisted that hygiene be made a required course.

Pepper started by subscribing $10,000 and made his estate "personally responsible for the entire amount." Within four hours he had five other donors, but then his march to success slowed. Pepper was $60,000 short as Lea's deadline approached. Pepper wrote: "I felt a sense of anxiety that I cannot overstate. It seemed to me that my health must break down under the strain. At this time a near relative . . . at my earnest solicitation inserted in his will a clause leaving $60,000 to the University for the establishment of a professorship. . . ."[3]

Billings and Lea jointly oversaw the design and construction of the building; and the school, on 34th Street north of Spruce Street, was formally opened on February 22, 1892. It did not escape Billings that externally the building was plain compared to the unusual library building, designed by Frank Furness, which Lea had given to Penn three years earlier. At the dedication, Billings noted that the hygiene building had been "planned from within outward, which is the reason why it looks like a laboratory and not like a castle or cathedral. . . . It is fit and proper that it should be so. The library represents the garnered experience and wisdom of the past: the laboratory is the workshop of the future. One is fruit, the other is seed."[4]

Bad seed, however, had already been sown. In bringing Billings to Philadelphia, Pepper hurt the ambitions and the feelings of Samuel G. Dixon, who was already teaching hygiene. Dixon was a practicing attorney when, because of his health, he turned to medicine. He earned a degree from Penn in 1886 and then traveled to Europe to study bacteriology. When he received his professorial appointment, he opened a small laboratory in Medical Hall, the first in the United States devoted to hygiene.

In 1889 Dixon wrote to Pepper that Billings's appointment in effect abolished his own professorship, and Dixon left Penn. He transferred his research to the city's Academy of Natural Sciences and eventually became its president. In addition, he had a distinguished career in city and state public health.[5]

When Billings came, he brought Alexander C. Abbott, M.D., a bacteriologist who had helped William H. Welch at Hopkins both teach

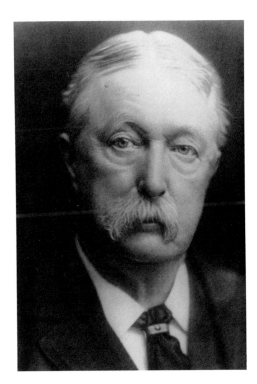

*John Shaw Billings, first Director
of the School of Hygiene. (Historical Collections of the College of
Physicians of Philadelphia.)*

in the school and organize and run it.[6] Billings taught "practical hygiene," covering such subjects as water supplies, garbage disposal,
house drainage, methods of ventilating and heating homes, food inspection and adulteration, "offensive and dangerous trades," and "san-
itary jurisprudence."

In bacteriology, Abbott covered methods of isolating pure colonies
of bacteria, techniques of the microscope, immunity, disinfection, antisepsis and asepsis, and bacteriological investigations of air, sewer,
and water.[7] Within four years, Billings's enrollment dwindled to almost
zero, while the size of Abbott's classes steadily rose. Abbott was so
successful that by 1896 bacteriology was required for all Penn medical
students.[8] Bacteriology in the School of Hygiene was considered practical or applied rather than the pure science it was in the medical
school; there, it was included in Tyson's Department of Pathology and
taught by Juan Guiteras, who held one class a week in the subject.

When Simon Flexner became head of pathology in 1899, he wanted bacteriology to be taught by a pure scientist. He brought Abbott into the medical school. A new wing, containing an improved student laboratory and a lecture hall, was added to the school.[9]

Even by the mid-1890s, Billings felt frustrated. He resigned and went to New York, where he created the New York Public Library.[10] His departure discouraged Lea, who abandoned his plans to support an enlargement of the school. Abbott was named head of the school, but because he knew little about public health and preventive medicine, the institution languished.[11] In 1898 a vain effort was made to offer the services of the school to communities in the Commonwealth of Pennsylvania. The provost wrote to mayors of 160 municipalities describing the laboratory's services. Only eight replied, of whom two accepted the offer.[12]

In 1903 the school received another blow when Abbott became head of the city's Bureau of Health. He stayed on as director of the school and taught hygiene for the few who enrolled.[13] Subsequently the course was taught by faculty members from various University departments. In 1914, on Abbott's recommendation, the director's title was discontinued and the school was officially incorporated as a division of the medical school.

A few years later, the Rockefeller Foundation decided to establish a fully equipped school of public health at a leading medical school. Harvard, Hopkins, and Penn were the front-runners, but Penn's case was substantially weakened because of the wavering support it seemed to give the subject. Hopkins was chosen—Welch's revenge, perhaps, for having his earlier plans interrupted when Pepper recruited Billings and Abbott.[14]

Penn's trustees responded to the Rockefeller rebuff by designating Abbott's course in hygiene the School of Hygiene and Public Health. All but three of the faculty of the so-called school were members of Abbott's department. This effort at organizing a separate entity ended with Abbott's resignation in 1928.[15]

There was little stability. In 1931, the medical-school administration formally separated bacteriology and hygiene. Stuart Mudd was appointed as chief and professor of bacteriology. In retrospect, the most important contribution of the Pepper-Lea endeavor was introducing this subject to Penn.[16]

But the professorship of hygiene was left vacant through the 1930 s until 1939, when it was renamed the George S. Pepper Professorship of Public Health and Preventive Medicine. The department's name was changed accordingly, and the University conferred its first degree in public health.[17] In 1967 the name was changed once more, to the Department of Community Medicine, but soon afterward the department was phased out completely. Its chaired professor remains, and its endowment has been incorporated into the Department of Human Genetics.

THE WISTAR INSTITUTE

The same year that the School of Hygiene opened its doors, the Wistar Institute for Anatomy and Biology was opened at 36th and Spruce Streets, bounded on the north by the diagonal slant of Woodland Avenue as it traveled west. The institute began as a museum for Caspar Wistar's anatomical collection; the museum had been expanded by Horner and Leidy as a teaching and research resource. It was given new life by General Isaac J. Wistar.[18]

Wistar was prodded by James Tyson, dean of the medical school, to found the institute, chiefly to display the Caspar Wistar collection. Wistar responded by establishing a trust fund of $20,000, to which he added $125,000 at Pepper's behest. The resulting structure was the first fire-proof building in the United States. The institute is independent from Penn but the University trustees elect its board of managers; one of the nine managers must be the oldest and nearest male heir of Caspar Wistar, and two must be members of the city's Academy of Natural Sciences.

In its first decade, the institute improved the museum and organized a machine shop.[19] In 1905, Milton Jay Greenman became its third director. He wanted it to became a research institute, and the board agreed. Its initial work focused on embryology, neurology, and comparative anatomy. Between 1906 and 1914, the brains of some 250 people, Presidents and Supreme Court justices among them, were collected and studied at Wistar.[20] In 1908 the institute acquired a printing press and shortly became a publisher of learned biological and anatomical journals.[21]

The institute became the medium for the dissemination of the albino rat as the main laboratory animal throughout the world.[22] The rat came

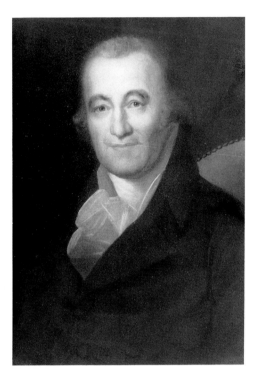

Caspar Wistar, Professor of Anatomy, Surgery and Midwifery. The Wistar Institute was founded by his nephew Isaac Wistar to house the Wistar-Horner anatomical collection. (Historical Collections of the College of Physicians of Philadelphia).

to the institute in 1906 with Henry Donaldson, the institute's first scientific director. Donaldson was a professor of neurology and dean of the Ogden School of Science at the University of Chicago, when Greenman called him to Philadelphia.[23] Donaldson brought with him Shinkishi Hatai, a research associate with whom he had studied the rat. Four albino rats came to the institute as well.

They were descended from an albino mutant of *Epimys norvegicus*, a brown or gray rat originating in Asia. The brown or gray ones were used for baiting with trained terriers, a popular sport in France and England that spread to America before being stopped in 1870 or so. The sport required the capture of hundreds of rats, which were held in pounds until their contest. Albino rats appeared from time to time; they were removed from the colony and kept for show or breeding and tamed by frequent handling. Specimens had likely been transported by the

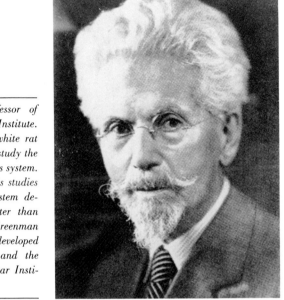

Henry Donaldson, Professor of Neurology of the Wistar Institute. Donaldson brought the white rat to the Wistar Institute to study the development of the nervous system. He used white rats for his studies because their nervous system developed thirty times faster than that of humans. Milton Greenman and Helen Dean King developed the Wistar rat colony and the inbred rat strains. (Wistar Institute.)

Swiss zoologist Adolf Meyer when he joined Donaldson's department at Chicago in 1890.[24]

When Donaldson arrived at the Wistar Institute, he carried out what was for that time a huge research program on the development of the albino rat. Donaldson noted that "the nervous system of the rat grows in the same manner as that of man, only 30 times as fast." In addition, from birth to death, the rat's development is equivalent to that of a human of the same age, so that "observations on the nervous system of the rat can be transferred to man and tested."[25]

From the first, the institute maintained a randomly bred colony in addition to one maintained by strict brother-sister matings. The latter was carried through the 135th generation and became known as the King albino. The former served as the commercial stock sold to other research institutions. Serious losses of the animals to toxicity, respiratory infections, and infectious diseases spurred development of breeding facilities made of brick, concrete, steel, and glass, materials that did not harbor dirt and could be easily cleaned. Diets advanced from local restaurant scraps to recipes for "wheat and peas with milk" and "hominy grits, vegetables, and eggs" until dry dog and fox diets became available in 1950. Many books on the rats grew from the institute's research program. The seminal one was Eunice Chase Green's *Anatomy of the Rat.*[26]

Edmund J. Farris succeeded Greenman as acting director in 1937. He served for 20 years in that capacity and distinguished himself through fertility studies. Hilary Koprowsky, a virologist at Lederle Laboratories, was appointed director in 1957.[27]

Koprowsky initiated the institute's current interest in cell biology, cancer research, and immunology. A pioneer in the development of polio vaccines, Koprowsky developed an improved vaccine against rabies. In other research, a vaccine that protects a pregnant mother from rubella has been developed and successfully tested by Stanley A. Plotkin, who is currently developing a vaccine against cytomegalovirus, another producer of birth defects.[28]

THE HENRY PHIPPS INSTITUTE

The Henry Phipps Institute, like the School of Hygiene and the Wistar Institute, was founded by a wealthy benefactor who gave building and research monies. The Phipps Institute, which opened in 1903, targeted its effort at the contemporary health crisis of tuberculosis; it was the first institution organized solely for treating and studying a single disease. Ironically its scientific success led it to close its doors 76 years later.[29]

In 1901 Andrew Carnegie sold his steel firm and overnight created several multimillionaires, including Henry Phipps Jr. of Pittsburgh. Influenced by Carnegie's philanthropy, Phipps turned to supporting charitable causes.[30] He heard of the work of Lawrence Flick at the White Haven Sanatorium in Pennsylvania. After meeting with Flick, he decided to found a dispensary. The two traveled abroad in 1902 to see how tuberculosis was managed in Europe. The next year, the Henry Phipps Institute for the Study, Treatment, and Prevention of Tuberculosis formally opened under Flick's directorship. Phipps gave $50,000 a year for seven years to support the institute. In 1910 he secured its future by having it affiliate with Penn. He gave $54,000 a year until

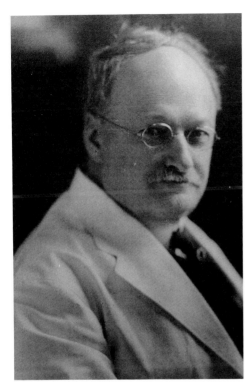

Lawrence Flick, founder of the Henry Phipps Institute, crusader against tuberculosis. (Historical Collections of the College of Physicians of Philadelphia.)

1916, then, in a final gesture, gave $500,000 in 1926 to establish an endowment fund for the institute.[31]

The institute was first located in the 200 block of Pine Street, in ordinary townhouses converted into a hospital complete with an autopsy room, laboratory, and nurses' training school. Eventually it moved to one of the most degraded spots in Philadelphia, at Seventh and Lombard Streets. Flick chose the location because he wanted to place there an institution consecrated to uplifting human beings.[32] Flick was evangelistic in his fight against tuberculosis.[33] He assembled a competent staff of clinicians, pathologists, and bacteriologists, most of them working part-time. The staff devised and practiced rigid rules for the care of the patients.[34] To find competent nurses, Flick hired women who had been patients at the White Haven Sanatorium and showed signs of improvement; then he trained them in his own school. This method of recruiting became common practice. The recruits were eager for the activity and the opportunity to defray some of their expenses, even though the salary was low. Flick was a better director of clinical work than of research. Impetuous and lacking a research background, he had difficulty finding and maintaining competent scientific investigators, because he did not realize that research cannot be hurried.

MAZYCK PORCHER RAVENEL

The major scientist of the institute's early period was Mazyck Porcher Ravenel, a bacteriologist at Penn's School of Veterinary Medicine.[35] He and his Phipps Institute colleagues demonstrated the ineffectiveness of an anti-TB serum prepared by Edoardo Maragliano.[36]

But Ravenel's main interest was in tracing the route of the bovine strain of the bacillus into humans. In the 1800 s, Robert Koch discovered the tubercle bacillus. Koch thought that infection of humans from cattle was so insignificant that cattle inspection was not necessary (the most common route of infection was the respiratory tract). At an international TB congress in 1908, Ravenel challenged Koch's opinion about the cattle but without proof. He created a stir; eight years later, he was able to publish evidence that children frequently acquired the bacillus through the alimentary tract.[37]

PAUL A. LEWIS

Paul A. Lewis, a graduate of the medical school and professor of experimental pathology, was the first director of the institute's laboratories after it came under University control in 1910.[38] Lewis's studies focused on hereditary factors in guinea pigs that are associated with the resistance of animals to TB. He also made other experimental contributions. With John Auer he demonstrated that acute anaphylactic death in guinea pigs is caused by severe broncho-constriction, which reduces air exchange in the lungs and produces asphyxia. Lewis and Simon Flexner found that experimental poliomyelitis could be transferred from monkey to monkey for generations by a filterable virus—thus further establishing polio's viral origin.

EUGENE L. OPIE

Eugene L. Opie succeeded Lewis as director of the Phipps Institute laboratories in 1923.[39] Over the next nine years, he and his associates proved that the "spread of tuberculosis occurs in large part by long, drawn-out family or household epidemics in which the disease is slowly transmitted from one generation to the next." He also found that the bodies of persons who had died following "galloping consumption" did not show evidence of having tuberculous infections in childhood. With this knowledge of how the disease spread, Opie began studying the prevalent strain of TB in rural black Jamaicans who had not been exposed to tuberculosis until they flocked to crowded towns for work. Having no immunity, they contracted virulent tuberculosis and died about three times as rapidly as the white population. Opie also carried out extensive studies on the nature of the tuberculosis antigen and other sensitivity reactions.[40]

ESMOND R. LONG

Esmond R. Long succeeded Opie in 1932. He had contracted the disease in 1913 while a medical student at the University of Chicago.[41] When his active tuberculosis was arrested, he traveled to Prague where, under Anton Gohn, he studied the primary lesions of tuberculosis, called Gohn's complex.

At Chicago, he had begun collaborative research with biochemist Florence Seibert, and they were reunited at the Phipps Institute, where they continued their work on the chemical nature of TB. Correctly reasoning that Koch's earlier infection tests of tuberculin extracted from tubercle bacilli were unreliable because the active principle of the extracts was not known, they set out to isolate the active principle. By 1926 Long and Seibert had determined that tuberculin was a protein.

Seibert eventually purified and crystallized tuberculin to such a degree that it could be standardized and used clinically. This protein, prepared from Koch's "old tuberculin," was called the purified protein derivative of tuberculin (PPD). In 1952, after further purification, PPD became the official standard of the United States Public Health Service. The availability of PPD gave means to standardize a TB test for the first time.

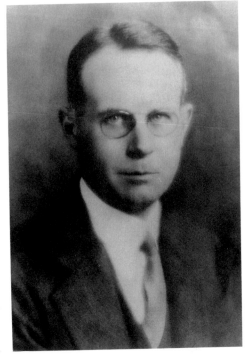

Esmond R. Long, Director of the Phipps Institute. He and Florence Seibert purified the antigen of the tubercle bacillus (purified protein derivative, PPD) thereby making the PPD test more specific as a screening procedure for tuberculosis. (Historical Collections of the College of Physicians of Philadelphia.)

Long's retirement in 1955 signaled the end of tuberculosis research in Philadelphia. Streptomycin, the first specific therapeutic agent for the disease, had been introduced in the late 1940s. Such chemotherapeutic agents as isoniazid, rifampin, and ethambutol followed quickly. There was no further need for prolonged rest and major surgical procedures—or for research in this field.

In the late 1960s the Phipps Institute was directed toward supporting community medicine. The old buildings were sold and a smaller institute built at 42nd Street and Chester Avenue. This attempt met with limited success, and in 1979 the trustees applied the assets of the Henry Phipps Trust Fund—amounting to more than $1.5 million—to research in human genetics. The facility was sold to the City of Philadelphia for use as a health-care and counseling center.

NOTES

1. G. W. Corner, *Two Centuries of Medicine* (Philadelphia: Lippincott, 1965), pp. 181–82.

2. F. N. Thorpe, *William Pepper, M.D., LL.D.* (Philadelphia: Lippincott, 1904), p. 278.

3. *Ibid.*, pp. 278–79.

4. Opening Exercises of the Institute of Hygiene of the University of Pennsylvania. Philadelphia, 1892. Address of John Shaw Billings, p. 15. Published as a pamphlet.

5. Corner, *Two Centuries of Medicine*, pp. 181–82.

6. S. Flexner and J. T. Flexner, *William Henry Welsh and the Heroic Age of American Medicine* (New York: Viking Press, 1941), p. 341.

7. *Ibid.*, p. 342.

8. Corner, p. 182.

9. Announcement of the Course of Instruction in the Laboratory (of Hygiene), February 1, 1892. In folder containing the program of the opening exercises of the School of Hygiene, College of Physicians of Philadelphia.

10. F. B. Rogers, *Selected Papers of John Shaw Billings* (Baltimore: Waverly Press, 1965), pp. 1–15.

11. Corner, p. 183.

12. *Ibid.*

13. *Ibid.*

14. *Ibid.*

15. *Ibid.*, p. 184.

16. *Ibid.*, p. 183.

17. *Ibid.*, p. 184.

18. *Ibid.*, p. 183.

19. *Twentieth Anniversary of the Organization of the Advisory Board of the Wistar Institute of Anatomy and Biology* (Philadelphia: Wistar Institute, April 13, 1825); M. J. Greenman, "The Wistar Institute of Anatomy and Biology," in I. J. Wistar, *Autobiography of Isaac J. Wistar* (Philadelphia: Wistar Institute of Anatomy, 1937, pp. 164–65.

20. *Twentieth Anniversary*, p. 31.

21. *Ibid.*, p. 32.

22. *Ibid.*, pp. 37–39.

23. J. R. Lindsay, "Historical Foundation," in *The Laboratory Rat*, vol. I, ed. H. J. Baker, J. R. Lindsay, and S. H. Weisbroth (New York: Academic Press, 1979), pp. 2–36.

24. Baker et al., *Laboratory Rat*, pp. 2, 5; H. H. Donaldson, "The Rat. Reference Tables and Data from the Albino Rat (*Mus norvegicus albimus*) and the Norway Rat (*Mus norvegicus*)," 1st ed., *Memoirs No. 6*, Wistar Institute of Anatomy and Biology (Philadelphia: Wistar Institute, 1915). pp. 7–9, 10–15.

25. *Ibid.*, p. 6; p. 10; pp. 10–11; E. C. Green, *The Anatomy of the Rat*, *Transactions of the American Philosophical Society* (Philadelphia: American Philosophical Society, 1835); M. J. Greenman and F. L. Duhring, *Breeding and Care of Albino Rats for Research Purposes* (Philadelphia: Wistar Institute, 1923); 2d ed., 1931.

26. Baker et al., *Laboratory Rat*, p. 11; E. J. Farris and J. Q. Griffiths, Jr., *The Rat in Laboratory Investigations* (Philadelphia: Lippincott, 1949); E. J. Farris, ed., *The Care and Breeding of Animals* (New York: Wiley, 1950), p. 11.

27. W. L. Purcell, "An Outline of the History of the Wistar Institute," *Wistar Institute Biannual Report* (1971).

28. "At the Forefront of Medical Research," *The 1984 Annual Report of the Wistar Institute,* p. 2; *American Men and Women of Science,* 16th ed. (New York: R. R. Bowker, 1986), p. 440.

29. *Ibid.,* p. 18.

30. C. Hatfield, Jr., "The Henry Phipps Institute for the Study and Treatment of Tuberculosis," in F. P. Henry, A.M., M.D., *Founders Week Memorial Volume* (Philadelphia, 1909), pp. 840–44; F. A. Craig, *Early Days at Phipps* (Philadelphia: Henry Phipps Institute, 1952); *University of Pennsylvania Twenty Second Annual Report of the Henry Phipps Institute for the Study, Treatment, and Prevention of Tuberculosis* (Philadelphia: Henry Phipps Institute, 1930), pp. 1–12.

31. E. G. Price, *Pennsylvania Pioneers Against Tuberculosis* (New York: National Tuberculosis Association, 1952), p. 152.

32. F. L. Flick, "The Crusade Against Tuberculosis in Pennsylvania." Annual Address of the President of the Free Hospital for Poor Consumptives and Whitehaven Sanitorium Association. Fourth Annual Report, 1907–1908, pp. 22–23.

33. Flick, *Crusade Against Tuberculosis,* p. 25; Henry, et al., *Founders Week Memorial Volume,* 840.

34. E. M. F. Flick, *Beloved Crusader: Lawrence Flick, Physician* (Philadelphia: Dorrence, 1944), pp. 9–15, 20–22.

35. Craig, *Early Days at Phipps,* p. 38.

36. *Ibid.*

37. *Ibid.,* pp. 29–30; M. P. Ravenel, "Present Views in Respect to Modes of Infection in Tuberculosis," *Journal of the American Medical Association* 66(1916):613–18.

38. H. R. M. Landis, "Paul A. Lewis, 1879–1929," *American Review of Tuberculosis* 21(1930):587–92.

39. P. Rous, M.D., "An Inquiry into Certain Aspects of Eugene L. Opie," *Archives of Pathology* 34(1942):1–12; J. G. Kidd, "Citation and Presentation of the Academy Medal to Eugene L. Opie," *Bulletin of the New York Academy of Medicine* 36(1960);228–34; D. M. Angevine, M.D.,"Eugene Lindsay Opie, M.D.," *Archives of Pathology* 92(1971):145–46; D. M. Angevine, M.D., "Comments on the Life of Eugene Lindsay Opie," *Laboratory Medicine* 12(1963):3–7.

40. Kidd, Celebration and Presentation of Academy Medal to Opie, p. 233.

41. P. C. Nowell, M. D. and L. B. Delpino, "Esmond R. Long, June 16, 1890–November 11, 1979," *Biographical Memoirs of the National Academy of Sciences, U.S.A.* 56(1987):285–310; George W. Corner, "Esmond Ray Long (1890–1979)," *Year Book of the American Philosophical Society* (Philadelphia: American Philosophical Society, 1980), pp. 613–17.

9
REFORM, GENTLEMANLY AND OTHERWISE

American universities are not properly constructed. They should be built like Hagenbeck's Tiergarten in Hamburg: with large enclosures in which the professors are placed so they can roar to their hearts' content and not bite each other.

Otto Rosenthal

In 1906, national concern over the quality of education stimulated the formation of the Carnegie Foundation for the Advancement of Teaching. The foundation began by investigating medicine with a survey headed by Abraham Flexner, the brother of Penn's former pathology chairman. Flexner's committee visited every medical school in the United States and Canada and issued its report in 1910.[1]

A sense of urgency was real. Medical education nationwide varied widely. Admission requirements were low; many students entered medical school immediately after graduating from high school. Curricula had little uniformity and fewer standards.

The report's assessment of Penn was not negative. But, it pointed out, other schools had more stringent admissions requirements, better facilities, a greater percentage of full-time, preclinical laboratory instructors, and more established research scientists. What especially galled the Penn faculty was that the Johns Hopkins School of Medicine received higher ratings in all of the categories evaluated in the report.[2]

Penn was certainly alert to a potential problem even before the Flexner group began its survey. In 1907, Daniel J. McCarthy, a neurologist, and C. Y. White, a pathologist to Children's and Episcopal Hospitals, gathered nine other physicians and formed the John Morgan Society to stimulate faculty research. The members also discussed research in formal meetings twice a year in order to promote interaction between younger and older members of the faculty. In addition they held an annual dinner to promote conviviality. Some compulsion to meet the goals of the group was imposed by fines: for instance, members were fined $30 if they failed to publish two papers a year or $5 for missing a business meeting and $25 for missing the annual meeting. Membership was so exclusive at first that the society grew slowly. Eventually entry was liberalized, and more recently even interested clinicians on the hospital staff have joined.[3]

Such an organization, needless to say, was not a deep solution to such a pervasive problem. Penn, of course, did have some stellar research initiatives. Moreover some of the foundation's complaint applied to medical academe generally, not to Penn alone. Yet the perception in some quarters was that the University had indeed fallen behind, that its malaise was self-inflicted. In 1919 William Ashton wrote in the *Alumni Register:*

> Forty years ago Philadelphia was the center of medicine and surgery in America. . . . But forty years ago Philadelphia fell asleep; and while she slept, peacefully dreaming of her past achievements, the great modern impulse of scientific thought and practice was gradually making itself felt throughout the world.[4]

The problems of medicine at Penn can be encapsulated in two events, unique in its history, which validated the sense that even the august University could stand for reform.

One event was a cheating scandal. It suggested that the goal of at least some medical students was the degree to practice rather than a knowledge of medicine.[5] Fifteen members of the class of 1899 paid an employee of the medical department $175 to let them submit fraudulent answer books. The usual arrangement was that students took their exams in Medical Hall, after which the employee carried the papers to the professors' residences for grading. The guilty fifteen persuaded the courier to substitute papers written outside the examination room for those they had written inside. The answers substituted were on operative and clinical surgery by E. R. Kirby (formerly J. William White's assistant and the individual giving the anesthetic in Thomas Eakins's painting *The Agnew Clinic*) and on medicine and clinical medicine by John D. Target and George Robinson, 1898 Penn graduates.[6]

The ruse succeeded, and graduation took place in June. Some time later in the month, a member of the graduating class informed J. William

White of the conspiracy. White reported it to Dean John Marshall. Marshall confronted the accused students, but they denied they had cheated. In the fall, however, one of them apparently had a fit of conscience and confessed. The others then broke as well, and the faculty revoked their degrees.[7]

The faculty had its own expression of turmoil, instigated by a reform drive that preceded the issuance of the Flexner report. The University administration had already been shaken up when Charles C. Harrison succeeded William Pepper as University provost. As an M.D., Pepper enjoyed a congenial working relationship with Dean Marshall. Harrison was a businessman, so successful in his sugar refinery that he was able to retire at the age of 42 and devote himself to philanthropy. He was appointed acting provost when Pepper stepped down in 1894, and some early accomplishments led the trustees to make the appointment permanent.[8] But Marshall had difficulty working with him.

Nor did Marshall like the growing influence of Harrison's aggressive nephew, the surgeon Charles Harrison Frazier. Frazier encouraged his uncle to foster original experimental work at Penn and, along the way, to reorganize the medical faculty. Marshall resigned in 1902, and Frazier succeeded him.[9]

Frazier proceeded to preempt any concerns the Carnegie Foundation, still years away from birth, might have had about standards at Penn. He upgraded entrance examinations, stimulated scientific research, sought out new practitioners for positions on the clinical faculty, and kept his uncle aware of developments in the profession generally. As it was provocatively put, Frazier was intent on "dragging the medical school out of the atmosphere of self-satisfied complacency and scientific stagnation."[10]

Some members of the faculty opposed Frazier, fearing that professors more oriented toward science would displace what they considered an excellent tradition in clinical practice and teaching. Thus the faculty were already disposed to fall into opposing factions when the so-called Edsall affair occurred.[11]

This episode began when David L. Edsall, the professor of pharmacology, was offered the chair of medicine at Washington University in St. Louis in 1910. A petition signed by five hundred Penn alumni urged the administration to keep him at Penn. Meanwhile, Frazier drew up a reorganization plan of the faculty, and Harrison concurred with it. Edsall, who benefited from the plan, was so pleased with it and with the likelihood of its being implemented that he declined the call to St. Louis.[12]

Harrison took action by getting the trustees to approve the changes, skirting steps in the consultative process that even the self-interested Frazier and Edsall would have taken. On March 25, Harrison convened the medical faculty and announced the reorganization as a fait accompli. James Tyson would retire from the chair of medicine and Edsall would succeed him—a must if Penn were to keep Edsall. Further, it was expected that the professor of medicine would devote half of his time solely to the work of the school; other clinical faculty members were expected to do the same.[13] A. N. Richards was brought from Northwestern University to fill the pharmacology chair vacated by Edsall; of all the new faces, Richards's turned out to be the most significant.[14]

In addition, Marshall, under threat of demotion and a 25 percent salary cut, would retire from the chemistry chair. Alonzo E. Taylor, recruited from the University of California, would head a new Department of Physiological Chemistry (Harrison announced that he had received $100,000 from an anonymous donor to establish a chair in this field).

Allen John Smith would move from patholology to comparative pathology; he was being groomed as the dean to succeed Frazier. Howard Taylor Ricketts, a biologist from Chicago, was appointed to succeed Smith, but Ricketts died of typhus in Mexico City just weeks after accepting the Penn offer. Harrison offered the chair to George H. Whipple, but was so overly cautious (he made the appointment only probationary) that Whipple declined; he later won the Nobel Prize. Richard Pearce, who had been at Penn but left for the Rockefeller Institute, returned to take the position temporarily. It might be supposed that Louis Duhring was untouchable; indeed, White, in his usual flamboyant way, announced that if the distinguished dermatologist were removed, there would be dire consequences. Duhring was not removed, but his health was failing, and he was persuaded to retire within a year, to be replaced by Milton Bixby Hartzell.[15]

In some circles Edsall was *persona non grata*. When he tried to take over the hospital service under his new post, he was told with "considerable violence" that he had been assigned no hospital beds at all and that he was requested to keep out of the wards until the hospital's board of managers acted upon the matter. This issue was settled in time, but a more painful one emerged. He asked Alfred Stengel, the director of the Pepper Laboratory, to supply him with space and equipment for his research projects. This request should have caused no problem, because the laboratory director serves under the professor of medicine. But Stengel had old-guard ties. He was the cousin of William Pepper Jr., and he did not see fit to fulfill Edsall's request.[16]

Edsall was so discouraged by this treatment that he did not teach in the fall of 1910. Moreover, he lost his chief support. Harrison bore heavily the mounting criticism by the faculty and resigned suddenly. Weir Mitchell, who was eighty-two years old, resigned four months later; he wrote to Osler that he was tired "of constant hot water in the faculty." Edsall had had enough. He accepted the offer from Washington University. Curiously, he stepped into another seething cauldron there and then, in 1912, went to Harvard, where he had a distinguished career.[17]

To succeed Harrison, the trustees appointed Edgar Fahs Smith, who

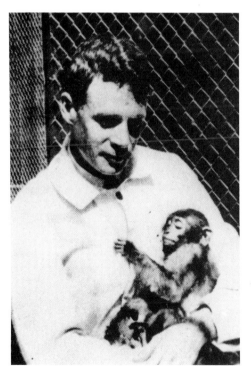

Howard Taylor Ricketts, the pathologist for whom Rickettsia *are named. In 1906, he settled the problem of the transmission of Rocky Mountain spotted fever by demonstrating it could be transferred from one guinea pig to another by a tick. A few weeks after accepting his call to Philadelphia, he died from typhus in Mexico City. (Archives of the University of Pennsylvania.)*

was the vice provost. "The things which had been done in the medical school were undone," he was able to state shortly; for one, he reappointed his brother Allen John Smith to the pathology chair.[18]

In a letter to Simon Flexner in 1912, Edsall wrote:

> Pennsylvania is doing badly enough. They have legislated Pearce and Taylor out of the Medical Council by making a new executive faculty, thus eliminating all of the "Young Turk" element except Richards, who is not aggressive; and they split Dr. Musser's chair between Riesman and Sailer, after vainly trying to get Thayer. The latter act they have kept quiet. . . . That act of Edgar Smith's was, however, the only suggestion of the recognition of the need of regeneration I have heard of. They all seem outwardly deeply satisfied with themselves.[19]

No doubt Penn's medical faculty lost a valuable academician in Edsall, but their erstwhile colleague may have been too eager to write their epitaph. Academic medicine was changing; Penn was able to change with it, often leading the way.

NOTES

1. G. W. Corner, *Two Centuries of Medicine* (Philadelphia; Lippincott, 1965), p. 221; J. C. Aub and R. K. Hapgood, *Pioneer in Modern Medicine: David Lynn Edsall of Harvard* (Boston: Harvard Alumni Association, 1970), pp. 67–68.
2. Corner, *Two Centuries of Medicine*, pp. 229–32.
3. A. N. Richards, An address given November 8, 1957 at the fiftieth meeting of the John Morgan Society held in the Lenape Club, University of Pennsylvania.
4. W. E. Ashton, "The Merger of the Medico-Chirurgical College with the University of Pennsylvania," *Pennsylvania Alumni Register* 19(1916–1917):387–400.
5. Minutes of the Medical Faculty, book 10, 1898, pp. 158, 176 (hereafter MFM)
6. MFM, January 8, 1900, book 11, pp. 22–42, describes events associated with the cheating scandal.
7. MFM, pp. 40–42.
8. E. P. Cheyney, *History of the University of Pennsylvania, 1740–1940* (Philadelphia: University of Pennsylvania Press, 1940), pp. 334–37.
9. Corner, *Two Centuries of Medicine*, pp. 196, 210–11.
10. *Ibid.*, pp. 211–12.
11. *Ibid.*, p. 219.
12. *Ibid.*, p. 223; Aub, *Pioneer in Modern Medicine*, pp. 80–83.
13. Aub, pp. 84–85.
14. *Ibid.*, p. 89.

15. *Ibid.*, pp. 87–88; Corner, *Two Centuries of Medicine*, 225,
16. Aub, pp. 92–93.
17. Corner, pp. 234–35; Aub, pp. 103–20.
18. Corner, pp. 234–35.
19. Aub, p. 102.

10

A NEW BUILDING AND NEW RESEARCH GROUPS IN SURGERY AND DERMATOLOGY

Good judgement is usually the result of experience, and experience is frequently the result of bad judgment.

Lovett

Every age has its myths and calls them higher truths.

Anonymous

Within a short time after the medical faculty moved to its new facilities west of the Schuylkill River in the 1870s, they realized that both the Hospital of the University of Pennsylvania and Medical Hall were inadequate for teaching the recent medical advances. Just as the University was moving westward, experimental medicine—bacteriology and gross and microscopic pathology—was developing in Europe. Other changes were in the wings. For one thing, lengthening the medical curriculum strained space. For another, asepsis was being increasingly accepted and the surgical amphitheaters of the University Hospital, constructed of wood, were therefore not easily adaptable to use of the new aseptic surgical techniques. And even though, when Medical Hall was opened in 1877, it contained more laboratory space than Penn physicians had ever enjoyed and was the most advanced facility for medical teaching in the United States, its usefulness was clearly already limited.[1]

Pushed, in part, by competition at Johns Hopkins and elsewhere, the medical faculty persuaded the trustees to construct new research and teaching space, which opened in 1904 as the Medical Laboratories Building (renamed the John Morgan Building in 1987). It had four large lecture halls; physiology and pharmacology settled in on the first floor, and pathology and bacteriology on the second.[2] It proved adequate until 1929, when a wing for anatomy and chemistry was added.[3] From the move west until then, those subjects were housed in the Laboratory (Hare) Building, built in 1879.[4] Separating anatomy and chemistry from the other sciences maintained a Penn medical tradition that had existed since Shippen taught anatomy in the shed on his father's property and Woodhouse taught and experimented in chemistry in a laboratory in Surgeon's Hall.

The requirements for aseptic surgery and orthopedic surgery were met by the construction of the Agnew Pavilion, opened in 1897, which contained tile operating rooms with steel amphitheaters and modern orthopedic facilities.

SURGICAL RESEARCH

Over the years, J. William White, who had fought for reform with Agnew and Pepper, had become more conservative. He feared that the University's demand for full-time salaries would prevent it from recruiting the ablest physicians. Ironically he could have easily served under the provost's plan because he was independently wealthy. But he was perceived as one of those who defeated Harrison, and he was elected to the board of trustees.[5]

Yet White was far from being an enemy of the direction Dean Frazier wanted for the school. He fully realized the importance of research, and when the Medical Laboratories were constructed in 1904, White funded a laboratory for surgical research which was located in four rooms on the second floor at the southern end of the pathology laboratory. He also outfitted a suite in the tower over the main entrance of the new building for his administrative offices.[6]

In 1906, White invited J. Edwin Sweet of the Rockefeller Institute to join the Department of Surgery with the title of associate in experimental surgery; thus was begun America's first surgical-research department.[7] Sweet had earlier served in Penn's Laboratory of Hygiene. After his return to Philadelphia, his research was productive in such areas as the use of Eck's fistula, gastric pouches, experimental colitis, the influence of extracts of ductless glands (including the adrenal gland)

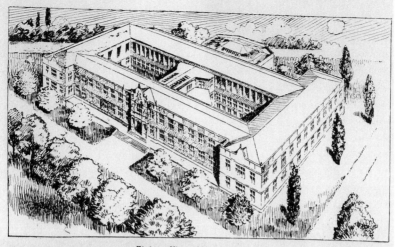

Birdseye View of New Laboratories

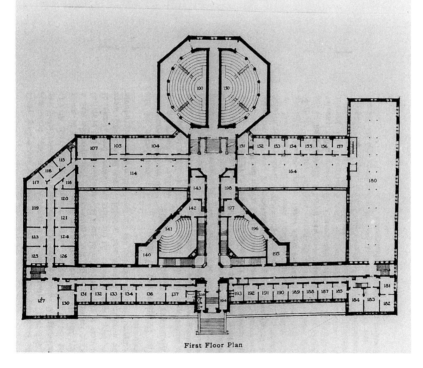

First Floor Plan

The New Medical Laboratories Building (John Morgan Building). TOP: sketch of the new laboratories from the program of the opening exercises; BOTTOM: plan of the interior of the Medical Laboratories. (Archives of the University of Pennsylvania.)

on pancreatic function, the effects of tension on steel plates to fix fractures, surgery on blood vessels, and the influence of diet on the growth of experimental tumors. In 1917 he entered the Army and studied the effectiveness of dichloramine-T on wound healing and the pathogenesis and treatment of trench foot. After the war he resumed his work on the pancreas and initiated studies on the pathogenesis of renal infection and the physiology of the gall bladder.[8]

Much of his experimentation was conducted on dogs. In fact, an increasing amount of research across the nation made use of animals, a legacy of the renewed recognition and reorganization of basic sciences at the beginning of the century. That trend was fought by antivivisectionists, who lobbied state legislatures to outlaw research on animals. In the Commonwealth of Pennsylvania, the medical schools of Philadelphia sent a delegation, which included Reisman, Stengel, and Taylor, to argue against the bill. The bill was defeated, as was a similar one in New York.[9]

The antivivisectionists then tried direct legal action against scientists. Sweet was vulnerable. He was in charge of the animal house as well as the Laboratory of Experimental Surgery.[10] To care for the animals and maintain the animals' quarters, Sweet brought Samuel Geyer, an experienced animal caretaker, from the Rockefeller Institute. For some time Geyer had complained to Sweet that the table scraps from the hospital kitchen, which he was feeding to the dogs, were little more than garbage and an unfit diet for any animal, much less dogs convalescing from surgical procedures. Geyer also told Sweet that researchers in other departments did not care for their animals properly. Although Sweet promised to speak to the dean about the deplorable conditions, he always reminded Geyer that there was no money for improvements.[11]

Geyer also procured the dogs. Since he knew these animals were for the most part obtained by doubtful means, Geyer usually held the dogs for two weeks or so to allow time for the owners of stolen pets to retrieve them. He ended up with a large number of dogs, some of which he sold to supplement his salary.[12] In 1911, Henrietta and Bertha Ogden, who were sisters, began buying dogs from Geyer for $.50 to $1 each to save them from experimentation. After about two years, they gained Geyer's confidence, and he took them through the animal house, showing them dogs recovering from surgery.[13] The Ogdens also entered on their own during the night through loose boards in the fence of the medical department; they made their own unguided inspections with a "pocket electric light."[14]

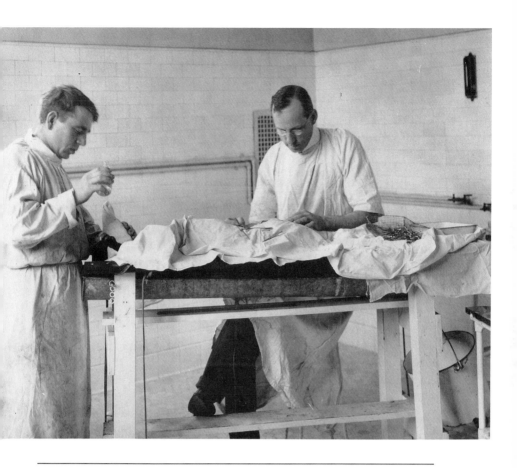

J. Edwin Sweet operating on a dog in the laboratory of surgical research. (Archives of the University of Pennsylvania.)

As a result of the Ogdens' investigations, the Women's Society for Prevention of Cruelty to Animals secured magistrate's warrants against Sweet and five other professors, whom a grand jury charged with "wanton cruelty" to animals.[15]

Sweet was brought to trial on April 15, 1914. Evidence was generally polarized.[16] The prosecutor brought up an experiment in which, as he described it, a weight was dropped with a gibbet on the back of unanesthetized dogs to break their spines. In defense of the work, Frazier testified that the dogs were anesthetized and their spines were not fractured. The spinal cord was exposed by a laminectomy and injured by the dropped weight, he said; the purpose was to see whether permanent spinal injury could be prevented by decompressing the swelling of the injured region with an appropriate incision.[17]

The three-day trial was intense. Henrietta Ogden collapsed and Bertha Ogden broke down under the defense attorney's interrogation.[18] Three women were ejected for disorder in the court room, and one man was hailed to the bar for hissing at a lawyer. The newspapers felt that the judge had predisposed the jury by stating that "any physician whose experiment caused pain or discomfort was guilty of a crime." Not all of the jurors were convinced by him. The jury could not reach a verdict, remaining hung after being sent back three times.[19] The case was dismissed. Sweet was not retried, nor were the other professors brought to trial.[20]

After his stint in the Army, Sweet returned to his Penn work. In 1926 he was about to step into the White chair when he accepted a comparable post at the Cornell University Medical School.[21] He had soured on Frazier's attitude toward research; as Sweet reportedly put it, "Frazier thinks you can grab a research problem by the seat of the pants and shove it into print."[22]

THE HARRISON DEPARTMENT OF SURGICAL RESEARCH

I. S. Ravdin, who had started as a junior fellow in the department, rose to the White chair and head of surgical research.[23] But the department lacked an endowment until 1935, when George Leib Harrison, a chemical manufacturer, left a $2.24 million bequest to Penn. Harrison had already been a generous friend to Penn medicine.[24] He was one of three donors who helped raise money for the Red Cross Base Hospital No. 20, which was staffed by volunteers from the University Hospital and Graduate Hospital during World War I. Private subscription was necessary because the government provided no funds for such units. The head of one of the two surgical divisions of the unit was John Berton Carnett, who became a close friend of Harrison as well as his personal physician. As a token of his appreciation of Carnett's services, Harrison

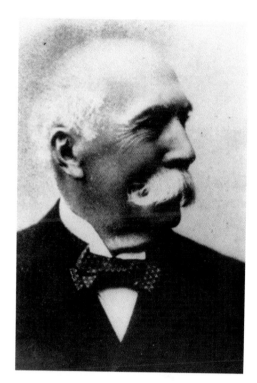

George Leib Harrison, benefactor of the Hospital of the University of Pennsylvania, Red Cross Base Hospital No. 20 in France in World War I, and the Harrison Department of Surgical Research. (Archives of the University of Pennsylvania.)

left his fortune (if no other heirs were surviving) to the University of Pennsylvania to support Carnett's research.

However, Carnett died before Mr. Harrison. When the terms of Harrison's will were announced in the papers the University suddenly found it had received a huge bequest of which it had been unaware, to be managed by the professors of surgery of the University of Pennsylvania.[25]

I. S. Ravdin reacted promptly to the news, met with the trustee in charge of medical affairs, and informed his chief Frazier of the windfall. Frazier advised Ravdin to "keep in touch with the probation of the Harrison bequest and see that we are not euchred out of our just share."[26] Ravdin did his work so well that top University officials agreed to put control of the funds "in the hands of those individuals interested in the truly academic phase of surgery." The upshot was that the endowment was earmarked for the Department of Research Surgery,

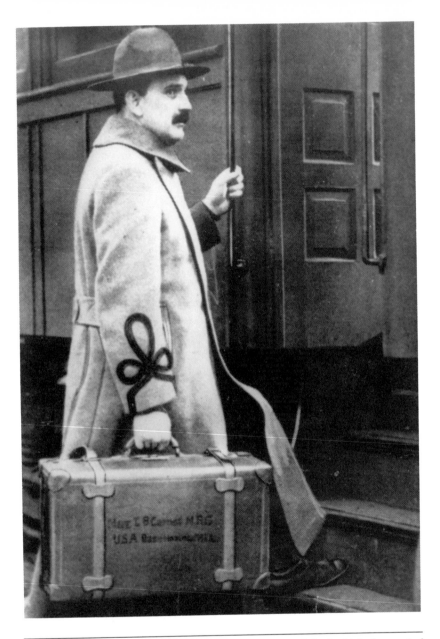

John Berton Carnett, Professor of Surgery in the Graduate School, chief of a surgical division of the Red Cross Base Hospital No. 20 in France in World War I, and physician of George Leib Harrison. The money for a research department was bequeathed to John Berton Carnett, but when he predeceased Mr. Harrison the bequest became the responsibility of the Professor of Surgery of the University of Pennsylvania. (Archives of the University of Pennsylvania.)

which received income to pay not only for scientific investigations but also for fellows, an artist, a statistician, and support staff. The department was renamed for Harrison and his wife, Emily McMichael Harrison. A surgical professorship bearing their names was also established, but the word research in the chair was deliberately avoided "to establish the conviction . . . that surgical research does not necessarily imply dog surgery."[27]

Ravdin was named to the chair. His original group of fellows turned out to be choice. Among them Jonathan E. Rhoads was instrumental in introducing total intravenous feeding. He eventually became (as, in fact, did Ravdin as well) the John Rhea Barton Professor of Surgery and president of the American College of Surgeons. Julian Johnson became chief of thoracic surgery at Penn's hospital. John Gibbon developed the heart-lung machine at Jefferson Medical College. Norman Freeman later headed neurosurgery at the University of California. And Robert B. Brown became Surgeon General of the Navy.[28]

RESEARCH MEDICINE

A few years after surgical research started, Penn established the first Department of Research Medicine. The school wanted to extend the function of the Pepper Laboratory. The medical faculty realized the need to apply scientific methods to the study of the alterations that disease produces in the body's physiology and chemistry. It was also felt that a trained researcher on the hospital wards and clinics, with sufficient assistants, would not only make important discoveries but also stimulate the spirit of investigation throughout the faculty.

John Herr Musser, a clinical professor of medicine, was in a position to help implement the idea. An 1877 Penn medical graduate, he contributed regularly to medical journals, and various memoirs call him one of the most beloved and distinguished physicians of his day. He had a patient and friend, Harriet C. Prevost, the wife of a railroad executive, who wanted to pay tribute to him. He persuaded her to give money to the new project. She gave $100,000 at the time and promised to give an equal amount later for a professorship.[29]

She imposed so many stipulations on her gift that the University worried that, in the future, they would be "conditions difficult of fulfillment."[30] For one thing, she specified both the diseases which the department should concentrate on and the means it should use:

> the application of the methods of bacteriology, pathology, physiology, chemistry, and pharmacology in the investigation of diseases of the kidneys, gout, rheumatism, and of conditions of the environment and of disorders of the organism which have any bearing on the case, the nature, mode or recognition, and the treatment of these diseases.[31]

She also directed that lectures and publications disseminate the discoveries and ordered that Musser direct the department until he stepped aside or died. When Musser died in 1912, the trustees renegotiated the conditions of her gift to better fit the policies of the University. At first, the site of the department was in the Medical Laboratories Building. It was moved to the Maloney Clinic when that facility opened in 1929, thus physically moving closer to yet one more aim of the benefactor, who expressly wanted the research to benefit patients.

Richard M. Pearce, Musser's son-in-law, was the first John Herr Musser Professor of Research Medicine. A Harvard University medical graduate, he had served under Simon Flexner's direction at Penn from 1900 to 1903 until leaving for various appointments in New York State.[32]

Pearce was one of America's early experimental pathologists, and not long after he returned to Penn, he was indicted in the animal-research trial.[33] The experience disturbed him because of the problems he felt it would cause for medical science. He developed a lecture, later published as "The Arguments For and Against Experimentation on Animals." In it, he stated:

> Scientific men are under definite obligation to experiment upon animals so far as that is the alternative to random and possibly harmful experimentation upon human beings, and so far as such experimentation is a means of saving human life and of increasing human vigor and efficiency. Opponents reply [that] . . . animal experimentation is useless and . . . has not added to our knowledge [and is] . . . therefore indefensible. If, therefore, it can be shown even in a single instance that life has been saved or human happiness . . . increased as the result of such experimentation, the basic moral issue is settled in the affirmative.[34]

Pearce then recited a brief history of medicine which, in case after case, emphasized the benefits of animal research to humans. Pearce's own research interests were varied. He wrote papers on diseases of the spleen, hemolytic jaundice, anemia, the nature of anaphylactic reaction, pancreatitis, nephritis, and the value of renal-function tests. But his studies did not lead directly to new discoveries. His contributions lay in establishing the investigation of clinical disease as a scientific discipline and in improvements to medical education.

He left Penn to direct medical education at the Rockefeller Institute in 1922 and was succeeded by J. Harold Austin, who had come from that institute. An expert statistician and clinical chemist, Austin improved techniques for studying blood and urine in disease.[35] In 1941 he moved on to head the Pepper Laboratory.

WILLIAM C. STADIE

William C. Stadie also came from the Rockefeller Institute, in 1924, and worked with Austin until he succeeded him as the Musser Professor.[36] Trained in chemistry, engineering, and mathematics as well as medicine, Stadie specialized in the transportation of blood gases. He was not reluctant to use himself as a test object, after a procedure had been tested on dogs but before human volunteers were enlisted. His quantitative studies were the first to relate anoxemia to decreased arterial oxygen and to demonstrate that cyanosis was caused by the dark red color of unsaturated blood.

To study the effects of oxygen on the anoxemia of patients with pneumonia, Stadie designed and built a chamber in which he could manage patients in an atmosphere that controlled oxygen and carbon dioxide. His was one of the first uses of an oxygen chamber for the treatment of respiratory diseases.[37]

At Penn, Stadie did important work on the buffering capacity of hemoglobin. He collaborated with Helen O'Brien in 1932 to purify an enzyme from red blood cells that speeded up the carbon dioxide hydration reaction. They reported its properties, and shortly thereafter, Andrew N. Meldrum and F. J. W. Roughton reported that they isolated the same enzyme and named it carbonic anhydrase. This discovery explained how bicarbonate was formed at rates that agreed with in vivo observations. Stadie also helped explain the role of carbamino compounds in the transportation of carbon dioxide from the tissues to the lung.[38]

He continued to invent or enhance instruments. He designed and built a controllable, sensitive, and stable electron-tube potentiometer, which improved on the colorimetric methods of measuring pH then in

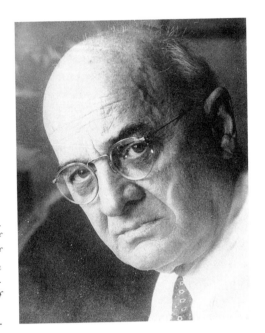

William C. Stadie, Professor of Research Medicine, discoverer of carbonic anhydrase and pioneer in studying oxygenation of hemoglobin and the buffering capacity of blood. (Joseph C. Touchstone.)

use. Elements of his original principles were modified and used in instruments developed by others and can be found, modified even further, in pH meters today.[39]

As World War II approached, Stadie turned his attention to the new field of cell physiology, especially in examining the biochemical mechanism of oxygen toxicity. Stadie and his colleagues looked at slices of brain tissue and found that high oxygen pressure inactivated enzymes that contained sulfhydryl groups. They also demonstrated that high pressure did not interfere with the function of cytochrome oxidase; thus it did not destroy itself as well as other enzymes by generating active oxygen radicals, as had been once supposed. Stadie's main goal in this work eluded him—the mechanism of oxygen toxicity remains unexplained to this day—but he and a colleague are memorialized in the Stadie-Riggs tissue slicer, which not only facilitates the cutting of tissue but standardizes the slices.[40]

Stadie's final major project involved the mechanism of insulin action. He and Ella and Niels Haugaard used radioisotope labeling to learn that insulin bound to cells in close association with tissue enzymes that metabolize carbohydrate or fat. They speculated that, when insulin binding took place, a new system was formed, qualitatively and quantitatively altering the metabolic activity.[41]

Stadie was succeeded by Colin M. MacLeod, a Canadian. He worked with Oswald T. Avery, whose laboratory at the Rockefeller Institute was studying pneumococci and trying to develop vaccines to treat pneumonia. MacLeod was one of the first to test the effectiveness of sulfa-pyridine as a chemotherapeutic agent. But all of this work was done prior to his coming to Penn in 1956 from New York University.[42]

When he returned there in 1960, Robert Austrian succeeded him as the Musser Professor. Austrian was trained at Johns Hopkins and became involved in the work on pneumococci when he served on MacLeod's service at New York University. At Penn, Austrian made the first general vaccine for pneumonia, utilizing the body's immune system to prevent bacterial infection rather than relying on chemotherapy for treatment.[43]

DERMATOLOGICAL RESEARCH

Penn's Laboratory of Dermatological Research was the first in the country to devote its entire effort to skin diseases. Duhring provided for it in his will (and for much more: his bequest of $910,000 was the largest single gift the University had received up to 1913, when he died), but not specifically. He had left money for free beds in the University hospital to treat "cutaneous, cancerous, and allied diseases and for a system of baths and general hydropathic treatment." His other gift to his professional field was an equal amount to the "Department of Cutaneous Medicine" (as it was then called) for the study and treatment of skin diseases.[44]

Milton Bixby Hartzell, who had succeeded Duhring as department chairman in 1910, decided as early as 1916 that the money should be applied to a research laboratory.[45] The laboratory received $260,000 from Duhring's bequest and space, four flights up, in the tower of the Medical Laboratories Building; it officially opened on July 1, 1917. Hartzell was the director.[46] Frederick D. Weidman, an expert on animal parasitology, was hired as assistant director. He had served as an instructor in Penn's pathology department and as pathologist at the

Philadelphia Zoological Society. World War I interrupted his new duties. He took over as acting chairman of pathology when the chairman, Allen J. Smith, was called into the service.[47]

The dermatological laboratory was restarted in 1919. As his first project Weidman collected, classified, and filed the dermatologic material at Penn: Duhring's papers, photographic negatives of skin diseases, and pathological slides and specimens, as well as pertinent material in the histological section of the Department of Surgical Pathology.[48] Henry Stelwagon had a significant collection, too, and it was added to the laboratory when he died. Weidman never stopped cataloging fungi that caused dermatoses. His work was aided when Raymond Sabourad gave the laboratory his type-culture collection of cutaneous fungi. By the time Weidman retired in 1946, the laboratory had a descriptive file of more than 5,000 histological studies and mycological preparations. It maintained the loan collection of slides used by candidates preparing for certification by the American Board of Dermatology until the Armed Forces Medical Museum took over this duty.

Hartzell, an excellent pathologist, made photomicrographs of pathological-histological sections. He took all of the classic photomicrographs that illustrate his dermatology textbook. One of his secrets was to use a Welsbach gas lamp to illuminate the slides. Since the lamp had low intensity, long exposures were needed. To overcome boredom and prevent shortening the exposure time through impatience, Hartzell took walks timed to the length of the exposures.[49]

He and Weidman worked well together, but Hartzell was a clinician rather than a scientist. At one point he complained to his assistant director, "Isn't it time that you were having publications from this department?" Weidman, astounded by the remark, replied, "There's been no time." Allen Smith witnessed this exchange and replied characteristically, "I think, Milton, the proper order of things is that the work must precede the publication. Give your man time, and you will get the output you're asking for."[50]

Nevertheless, Weidman understood his superior's point. The first publication from the laboratory followed shortly thereafter; it was a paper on pemphigus in an orangutan—based on work Weidman had done at the zoo, before he came to Penn.

Weidman did provide the output Hartzell expected, but Hartzell was not present to appreciate it. He suffered a stroke in 1921 and resigned in June of that year. Weidman was appointed professor of research dermatology and director of the laboratory, becoming the first American dermatologist to devote his full time to research.[51]

From the outset Weidman was interested in classifying and studying fungi that produced skin lesions, and he extended the work to cover various yellow dermatoses or xanthomas, published in 1941 as the pioneering monograph *Xanthoma and Other Dyslipoidoses*.[52]

In other work, Weidman, with Stanley Chambers, noted that many saprophytic fungi over-grow ringworm growing in culture tubes. It happened so often that they wondered whether organisms living on normal skin might act as biological protectors against ringworm infection. In an extensive study Weidman and Chambers concluded that *Bacillus subtilis* was frequently found on normal skin; growth of 11 species of fungi, including *Trichophyte interdigitale*, were completely inhibited by the bacillus in culture; and clinical trials in which the bacillus was applied to toes infected with ringworm showed sufficient promise to warrant further trials. Subsequently, however, they could never obtain preparations that were therapeutically reliable.[53]

Weidman and White studied epidermal hyperplasia that occurred in chronic skin ulcers, the first systematic work on this problem. They found that every gradation of hyperplasia, as well as early epithelioma or cancerous degeneration, was present in the regenerating skin of these ulcers. They distinguished some of these changes from those of a developing epithelioma and felt that proliferative changes should not be assumed to be malignant unless they had infiltrated the dermis to the level of the sweat glands. In their papers they pointed out that careful evaluation of the changes prior to radical surgery for leg ulcers would avoid many destructive surgical procedures.[54]

When Hartzell resigned early in Weidman's career in the laboratory, Dean Pepper knew that Weidman was not interested in heading a clinical department. He broke with tradition by appointing John Hinchman Stokes from the Mayo Clinic and the University of Minnesota. Furthermore, the dean took the unusual step of offering him a larger full-time salary than most chairmen had in order to protect his income when he moved his practice to Philadelphia.[55]

Stokes assumed the chairmanship in 1924 and began to reorganize the department. At first he tried to coordinate clinical activities with those of Weidman's laboratory; he placed a small research laboratory in his hospital clinic and assigned departmental assistants to the laboratory. The start was friendly, but the two groups gradually drifted apart.

Weidman began looking to Philadelphia General Hospital and Graduate Hospital for his clinical material.

For his part, Stokes could not afford the research because the expenses of his clinic absorbed the hospital's share of the Duhring bequest. To seek other avenues of support, he organized the Institute for the Study of Venereal Disease, which drew grants from government and other agencies. The new institute integrated the work of other departments—for instance, bacteriology and neurology—related to dermatology and syphilology. But by the 1930s, the medical school was somewhat embarrassed by having two divisions in one department, led by two men with contrasting personalities and different aims.[56]

Syphilis was Stokes's major focus.[57] When he entered the field, most practitioners felt that the major advances in understanding and treating the disease had already been made. But Stokes defied this conventional thinking from the start. His first book was called *Modern Clinical Syphilology*; in 1,200 pages, he emphasized the fact that physicians could neither diagnose nor treat syphilis intelligently by relying on laboratory studies alone. They had to study the patient carefully as an individual and know the biology of the infection in humans. This book established Penn as the primary clinic for syphilis therapy.[58]

When penicillin first became available, Stokes helped evaluate it. When it became the treatment of choice for syphilis, he converted a small red-brick building, located behind the hospital and known affectionately as the "pest house," into a treatment center. During World War II Stokes kept the activities of this clinic secret because he did not want the public to know that penicillin was being used to treat syphilis rather than the wounds of soldiers overseas.[59]

Stokes also studied the relationship of psychogenic factors to skin diseases. Patients with asthma, eczema, and hay fever had a personality he called the "tension frame of mind," and he went on to describe their tremendous drive, restlessness, and overambition. Dermal and eczematoid eruptions on the hand, he and some associates felt, clearly illustrated the importance of psychogenic factors in a complex that included dermatitis, allergy, and infection.

Stokes was a superb dermatologist in general. He felt that a skin disease could be managed only by considering the medical condition of the patient as a whole. His first step with patients was to stop all previous medications and use the simplest soaks until he could appraise their problems. Because he was persuaded that many skin diseases had psychological origins, he tried to evaluate the emotional status of his patients. He insisted on a good history, and generations of his students praised his skill in taking one.

Radiation therapy was so dangerous, Stokes felt, that he used it only to treat some inoperable skin cancers. He was sensitive toward possible litigation and took cautious therapeutic approaches and avoided experiments on patients, even any treatment that could be construed as an experiment.[60]

His classes reportedly drew students "in complete force, in sickness, in health, in fair weather and foul. The reading assignments were prodigious, and the class requirements rigid," according to Clarence Livingood, one of his students.[61] Stokes was also a creative instructor. He knew that serious and lasting complications could result from intra-

John H. Stokes conducting his Thursday dermatology class, known as Stokes's Circus. (Photograph album of Norris Smith, Archives of the University of Pennsylvania.)

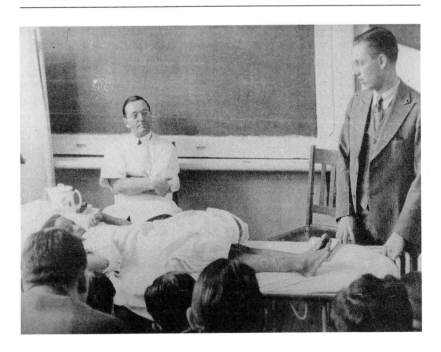

venous arsphenamine if the drug escaped into tissue or was injected outside the vein; yet novices could not learn the procedure without practice. So he and Herman Beerman, his assistant, developed manikins for students to practice intramuscular as well as intravenous injections. Three dollars' worth of plaster of paris, rubber tubes, gauze, cotton, water colored amaranth red, and some clever tucks were fashioned into "a more or less attractive arm," Livingood reported. He added, "No student in Stokes's class failed to learn a great deal, and none of them has forgotten the experience, because he had served under an incomparable but unrelenting taskmaster."[62]

The rivals Stokes and Weidman retired within a year of each other. Donald M. Pillsbury succeeded Stokes as chairman in 1945. By this time, federal funds had enabled the department to establish laboratories devoted to bacteriology, histochemistry, histology, mycology, pathology, and virology. Weidman retired in 1946, and Pillsbury discontinued the Laboratory of Dermatological Research the next year. He consolidated the various research areas under the name of the Duhring Laboratory. It was located at first in the penicillin treatment center, then was moved to elegant quarters on the second floor of the new Clinical Research Building.

NOTES

1. G. W. Corner, *Two Centuries of Medicine* (Philadelphia Lippincott, 1965), pp. 130–31.

2. Minutes of the Medical Faculty, b. 12, pp. 533, 535, 536, 537, 538, 539, 541; Program of the Opening of the Medical Laboratories in 1904.

3. E. R. Clark, "Department of Anatomy University of Pennsylvania School of Medicine," in *Methods and Problems of Medical Education*, 17th ser. (New York: Rockefeller, 1930).

4. Corner, *Two Centuries of Medicine*, pp. 157–58.

5. Corner, p. 234; J. C. Aub and R. K. Hapgood, *Pioneer in Modern Medicine* (Boston: Harvard Medical Alumni Association, 1970), p. 93.

6. According to R. L. Gilman, "The History of the Laboratory of Dermatological Research, University of Pennsylvania," in R. Friedman's *A History of Dermatology in Philadelphia* (Fort Pierce, Fla.: Froben Press, 1955). The administrative offices of Prof. J. William White were located in the Tower of the Medical Laboratories over the main entrance. This space was subsequently the apartment of Alonzo Taylor, Benjamin Rush Professor of Physiological Chemistry. In 1917, the Laboratory of Dermatological Research moved into this small suite of rooms. Julian Johnson stated to the author that J. Edwin Sweet was brought from the Rockefeller Institute in 1906 as an associate in experimental surgery by J. William White. Space for his work was provided in a group

of four rooms located at the southern end of the hall that passes through the pathology museum at the end of the western wing of the new Medical Laboratories.

7. Corner, p. 219; *Commonwealth v. Joshua Sweet, Court of Q.S. No. 2, September Session, 1913, No. 950, Charge Cruelty to Animals*, Philadelphia, Pennsylvania, April 14, 1914, p. 118.

8. Corner, p. 219.

9. *Ibid.*, p. 242.

10. *Ibid.*, p. 242.

11. Transcript of Antivivisectionist trial, pp. 118–19.

12. *Ibid.*, pp. 7–9.

13. *Ibid.*, pp. 37–38.

14. *Ibid.*, p. 11.

15. Transcript, p. 73.

16. Corner, p. 242.

17. Transcript, p. 115.

18. *Ibid.*, pp. 184–86.

19. Transcript, p. 214.

20. Corner, p. 242.

21. *Ibid.*, p. 273.

22. *Ibid.*, p. 273; concerning Frazier's understanding of science, personal conversation of David Y. Cooper with Jonathan E. Rhoads.

23. Corner, pp. 275–76.

24. *Philadelphia Inquirer*, March 13, 1935.

25. Ravdin Papers, found in a file in the Harrison Department, which include the correspondence between Dr. I. S. Ravdin and the medical trustees concerning the probation of the George L. Harrison will and the setting up of the George and Emily McMichael Harrison Department of Surgical Research. From Ravdin's justification for using the bequest to support the research already in progress, it is evident that it had been difficult for him to obtain funds. The picture of George Leib Harrison on the Annual Report of the Harrison Department of Surgical Research, July 1, 1964–June 30, 1965 is not the picture of the department's benefactor. George Leib Harrison (1836–1935) was one of two George Leib Harrisons, both of whom lived on Locust Street. The other George L. Harrison (1811–1885) is the one whose picture is on the cover of the annual report of the Harrison Department. A picture of the donor of the money that formed the Harrison Department of Surgical Research is found in a *History of the 20th Base Hospital*. When George L. Harrison died on March 6, 1935 he was ninety-nine years old, and for several years prior to his death he was blind. In order to get around his home without being constantly aided by his servants, he had wires suspended from the ceilings which led from his chair in the living room to important chambers in his house—the bedroom, the toilet, the dining room, and the hall. When he wanted to go to these areas, he hooked the handle of his cane over the appropriate wire and thus was guided to where he wished to go (personal conversation with J. E. Rhoads).

26. Ravdin Papers, letter from Dr. Charles Harrison Frazier to I. S. Ravdin, dated Friday.

27. Ravdin Papers, Dr. Ravdin's notes on a conversation with Mr. John Zimmerman; Minutes of the Executive Board of the Trustees for Medical Affairs of the University of Pennsylvania, November 8, 1935; Minutes of the Executive Board, December 9, 1935; Board of Medical Affairs, Trustees of the University of Pennsylvania, March 23, 1936; Board of Medical Affairs, March 23, 1936; Board of Medical Affairs Minutes, April 13, 1936. Appendix regarding The George and Emily McMichael Harrison

Foundation; Ravdin Papers, Minutes April 7, 1938, Two typewritten pages dictated by "AS" (Alfred Stengel) and typed by ECS (Stengel's secretary); Board of Medical Affairs, April 13, 1936; Minutes Board of Medical Affairs, April 13, 1936; Minutes Board of Medical Affairs, April 13, 1936; Ravdin papers, letter from Mr. John Zimmerman to I. S. Ravdin.

28. Ravdin papers, Budget of Harrison Department of Surgical Research.

29. G. A. Piersol, "Memoir of John Herr Musser, M.D.," *Transactions and Studies of the College of Physicians of Philadelphia* 3d ser., 34 (1912):lxxii–lxxx; R. M. Pearce, "The Teaching of Experimental Pathology and Pathological Physiology to Large Classes," *Johns Hopkins Bulletin* 22(1911):1–10.

30. Minutes of the Trustees of the University of Pennsylvania, vol. 14 (March 12, 1909), p. 605.

31. Trustees Minutes, p. 605.

32. Obituary Richard M. Pearce, folder Archives of the University of Pennsylvania.

33. R. M. Pearce, "Research in Medicine," Reprinted from *Popular Science Monthly*, (May 1912):503–15; (June 1912):548–62; (July 1912):1–18; (August 1912):115–32; (September 1912):209–26. The annual Charles C. Hitchcock Lecture, delivered at the University of California, January 23–26, 1912.

34. R. M. Pearce, "The Argument For and Against Experiments on Animals," *Old Penn* (1913–1914):421–30.

35. O. H. P. Pepper, "Memoir of James Harold Austin (1883–1952)," *Transactions and Studies of the College of Physicians of Philadelphia* 4th ser., 21(1953–1954):25–26.

36. I. Starr, "Memoir of William C. Stadie (1886–1959)," *Transactions and Studies of the College of Physicians of Philadelphia* 4th ser., 28 (1960–61):50–51.; J. Stokes, "William Christopher Stadie (1886–1959)," *Year Book of the American Philosophical Society* (Philadelphia: American Philosophical Society, 1962), 176–78.

37. W. C. Stadie, "The Oxygen of the Arterial and Venous Blood in Pneumonia and its Relation to Cyanosis," *Journal of Experimental Medicine* 30(1919):215–40, three color plates; W. C. Stadie, "The Treatment of Anoxemia in Pneumonia in an Oxygen Chamber," *Journal of Experimental Medicine* 35(1922):337–60; W. C. Stadie, "Construction of an Oxygen Chamber for the Treatment of Pneumonia," *Journal of Experimental Medicine* 35(1922):323–35.

38. W. C. Stadie and H. O'Brien, "The Catalyst of the Hydration of Carbon Dioxide and the Dehydration of Carbonic Acid by Enzymes Isolated from Red Blood Cells," *Journal of Biological Chemistry* 103(1933):521–29; W. C. Stadie and H. O'Brien, "Uber die Zustandsformen des Kohlendioxide im Blut," *Biochemische Zeitschrift* 237(1931):290–302.

39. W. C. Stadie, "An Electron Tube Potentiometer for the Determination of pH with the Glass Electrode," *Journal of Biological Chemistry* 83(1929):477–92; W. C. Stadie, "Determination of the pH of Serum at 38° C with the Glass Electrode and an Improved Electron Tube Potentiometer," *Journal of Biological Chemistry* 91(1931):243–69.

40. W. C. Stadie and B. C. Riggs, "An Apparatus for Determination of the Gaseous Metabolism of Surviving Tissue in vitro at High Oxygen," *Journal of Biological Chemistry* 154(1944):666–69; William C. Stadie, B. C. Riggs, and N. Haugaard, "Oxygen Poisoning VI. Effects of High Oxygen Pressure Upon Enzymes: Pepsin, Catalase, Cholinesterase, and Carbonic Anhydrase," *Journal of Biological Chemistry* 161 (1945):175–80; W. C. Stadie and N. Haugaard, "Oxygen Poisoning X. The Effect of Oxygen at Eight Atmospheres upon the Oxygen Consumption of the Intact Mouse," *Journal of Biological Chemistry* 164(1946):257–63; N. Haugaard, "Oxygen Poisoning XI. The Relationship Between Inactivation of Enzymes by Oxygen and Essential Sulfhydryl

Groups," *Journal of Biological Chemistry* 164(1946):265–70; W. C. Stadie and B. C. Riggs, "Microtome for Preparation of Tissue Slices for Metabolic Studies *in vitro*," *Journal of Biological Chemistry* 154(1944):687–90.

41. W. C. Stadie, N. Haugaard, J. B. Marsh, and A. G. Hills, "The Chemical Combination of Insulin with Muscle (Diaphragm) of Normal Rat," *American Journal of Medical Sciences* 218(1949):265–74; W. C. Stadie, N. Haugaard, A. G. Hills, and J. B. Marsh, "Hormonal Influence on the Chemical Combination of Insulin with Rat Muscle (Diaphragm)," *American Journal of Medical Sciences* 218 (1949):275–80; W. C. Stadie, N. Haugaard, and M. Vaughn, "The Quantitative Relation Between Insulin and its Biological Activity," *Journal of Biological Chemistry* 200(1953):745–63.

42. M. McCarthy, "Colin Munroe MacLeod (1909–1972)," *Year Book of the American Philosophical Society* (1972):222–30.

43. R. H. Austrian, *Life with the Pneumococcus: Notes from the Bedside, Laboratory, and Laboratory* (Philadelphia: University of Pennsylvania Press, 1985).

44. Friedman, *History of Dermatology*, pp. 245–56; *Leaders in Dermatology: Louis Duhring, The Man and His Work* (Palo Alto, Calif.: Syntex Laboratories, 1966), p. 20.

45. *Ibid.*, p. 281.

46. R. L. Gilman, "The History of the Laboratory of Dermatological Research, University of Pennsylvania," in Friedman, pp. 443–57; Herman Beerman and Gerald Lazarus, *Tradition of Excellence* (Philadelphia: privately printed, 1986), p. 32.

47. Herman Beerman, "Frederick DeForrest Weidman, M.D., An Evaluation of his Influence on Dermatology and Dermatologic Research," *Journal of the American Academy of Dermatology* 9 (1983):479–86.

48. *Ibid.*

49. Friedman, pp. 449–50.

50. *Ibid.*, p. 451.

51. *Ibid.*, p. 452.

52. *Ibid.*, p. 456.

53. Beerman, "Frederick DeForrest Weidman"; S. O. Chambers and F. DeF. Weidman, "A Fungistatic Strain of Bacillus Subtilis Isolated from Normal Toes," *Archives of Dermatology and Syphilology* 18(1928):568–72.

54. C. White and F. D. Weidman, "Pseudoepitheliomatous Hyperplasia at the Margin of Cutaneous Ulcers," *Journal of the American Medical Association* 88(1927):1959–63.

55. Beerman, *Tradition of Excellence*, pp. 44–45.

56. *Ibid.*, pp. 45–46.

57. Friedman, pp. 473–78; Herman Beerman, "John Hinchman Stokes, M.D., An Appreciation," *Journal of the American Academy of Dermatology* 9(1983):321–34.

58. Beerman, "John Hinchman Stokes," 1983.

59. *Ibid.*

60. *Ibid.*

61. *Ibid*; J. H. Stokes, *Archives of Dermatology and Syphilology* 17(1928):466–488.

62. John H. Stokes and Herman Beerman, "Manikins for Teaching Intravenous and Intramuscular Injection Technique," *Journal of the American Medical Association* 94 (1930):1658–60.

11
MERGERS AND GRADUATE EDUCATION

Don't descend into the well with a rotten rope.

Turkish proverb

When Edgar Fahs Smith succeeded Charles Custis Harrison as provost in 1910, he sought a way for Penn to regain its lost medical leadership, at least as the Flexner report and some observers had intimated it had. He took a hint from the Flexner report, that medical education in the United States could be improved by bringing many of the private medical schools under the control of schools with academic connections.[1]

MERGER DISCUSSIONS WITH WOMEN'S MEDICAL COLLEGE AND JEFFERSON MEDICAL COLLEGE

Smith cast his eye upon three local possibilities—the Women's College of Medicine of Pennsylvania, Jefferson Medical College, and the Medico-Chirurgical College.[2] Women's seemed interested, for the Flexner report had given it a bad rating. In 1915 Smith began discussions, but it was soon evident that Women's did not want to join the University.[3]

Discussions with the other institutions were more promising. Smith was encouraged to pursue them by Henry Pritchett, president of the Carnegie Foundation, who was eager to implement the merger recommendation of the Flexner report. Pritchett wrote, none too subtly, that he had recently visited Chicago, where mergers were being explored: "and it occurred to me to wonder whether the time has not come when the University of Pennsylvania could bring into its jurisdiction the other [independent] medical schools of Philadelphia."[4]

Smith agreed that medical education in Philadelphia amounted to a "confused pattern." He informed Pritchett that he was "awake to the subject" and continued to report his progress and setbacks to Pritchett, hoping, in his subtext, that the Carnegie Corporation or another benefactor would help finance any definite plans.[5]

Pritchett liked the looks of Jefferson and told Smith that he, as the Penn provost, should go "frankly after the Jefferson people" to sound out their interest. But he was elusive about suggesting that the Carnegie Corporation would help fund the merger.[6]

In the negotiations between Penn and Jefferson, Penn was the more enthusiastic partner, but an agreement did inch closer. Still, the document setting forth the union that the respective representatives drew up in 1916 was well short of a merger:

> The identity of two institutions, with maintenance of the inherited values of the respective names, and without change in the rights, powers, and authorities vested in them by their respective charters and organic laws, is hereby recognized and preserved inviolate.[7]

The proposed name was the Medical School of the University of Pennsylvania and Jefferson Medical College. Jefferson's board would continue to control the college's internal affairs. A layer of administration would be added, one dean with two assistant deans, presumably one from each school. Finances would be jointly administered, but the endowments would remain separate.[8]

Pritchett deplored these arrangements. In a letter to William Potter, Jefferson's chief representative, he said that he could envision physicians proposing a double- or triple-headed organization, but not a businessman. He also predicted that Jefferson would die as an independent school. What died was further attempts at a merger.[9]

MERGER WITH MEDICO-CHIRURGICAL COLLEGE AND HOSPITAL AND THE POLYCLINIC COLLEGE AND HOSPITAL

Just as the union with Jefferson was disintegrating, Provost Smith turned his attention to the third merger possibility, the Medico-Chirurgical

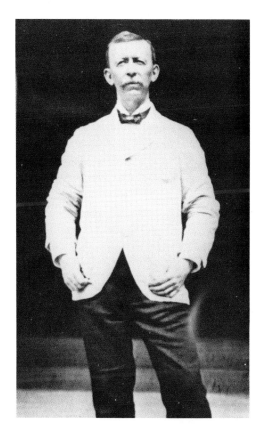

*Edgar Fahs Smith, Professor of
Chemistry and Provost of the University of Pennsylvania. (Archives
of the University of Pennsylvania.)*

College and Hospital. This institution, located on the southwest corner
of Broad and Market Streets, was anxious to join the University because
it had received a bad rating in the Flexner report and also because it
was losing its property at 18th and Cherry Streets, which had been
condemned to make way for the Benjamin Franklin Parkway. This
medical college originated as a society founded by James Bryan in 1849
for "the dissemination of medical knowledge [and] the defense of the
rights and the preservation of the repute and dignity of the medical
profession." It began accepting students in 1881; it was the first medical
school in the United States to have a three-year curriculum, which was
later extended to five years.[10]

Smith's idea in the merger was to relocate the college to the University campus and turn it into a graduate school, where experts would investigate health problems full-time. On campus, he felt, they would be in the company of other scientists and working in dedicated scientific facilities, so that the enterprise would be academic rather than vocational.[11] The official agreement outlining the details of this merger was signed July 31, 1916.

In 1917 the Polyclinic Graduate College and Hospital indicated it also wanted to join this merger with the University. An agreement was signed in 1918 merging the University with the Polyclinic College and Hospital, the only postgraduate medical school in the state. It had been founded by John B. Roberts, a surgeon who had reopened the Philadelphia School of Anatomy and realized that medical graduates needed practical experience. He opened the graduate college at 13th and Locust Streets in 1883; by 1890, pressured for space, he had a new building constructed on Lombard Street between 18th and 19th Streets. At first the name Polyclinic confused some people, who thought it was a public hospital because the old German name for a city hospital is *Poliklinic*. In a presage of computer-generated blunders, one creditor billed the hospital as "Polly McClintoc."[12]

Under its initial agreement with Medico-Chirurgical, Penn agreed to build a hospital of two hundred ward beds and fifty private beds. After the Polyclinic joined the merger, it increased the total capacity to 497 beds and located the hospital next to the existing Polyclinic Hospital. The building was completed in 1927. Three more institutions were folded into it: Diagnostic Hospital (formerly known as Charity) in 1926, Howard Hospital in 1929, and the assets of the North American Sanitorium in Ventnor, New Jersey, in 1930. The new Graduate Medical School and Hospital did not wait for the completion of the new beds to start operation, although its opening was delayed by America's entry into World War I in 1917 and the enlistment of many of the faculty. By the fall of 1919, enough had returned for them to offer a short preliminary course to physicians returning from Europe. This historic course was the most comprehensive one in graduate medical education ever offered in the United States.[13]

THE RICHARDS-MILLER REPORT

Trends in medical education had already begun to make the graduate school obsolescent, however. Rapid medical advances and the rise of specialties and subspecialties affected the medical undergraduate. This development was recognized by A. N. Richards and T. Grier Miller, a gastroenterologist, who were appointed by Penn President Thomas S. Gates to survey medical affairs at the University and recommend directions for the future. They submitted their confidential report in March 1931. In it, they stated that most medical observers feel "that the chief medical research activities of universities should be centered in the schools and hospitals for undergraduate teaching"—just the opposite of Smith's and Pepper's intentions.

FATE OF THE GRADUATE SCHOOL OF MEDICINE OF THE UNIVERSITY OF PENNSYLVANIA

Financially Richards and Miller saw little hope of foundation or other outside grants for Graduate Hospital; in fact, they added, the sorry state of its finances seemed like "evidence of bad educational and administrative judgment" on Penn's part. Furthermore, undergraduate medical education, they pointed out, was so demanding clinically that students "do not feel they are part of an organization which accepts as a major responsibility the enlargement of medical knowledge by modern experimental methods. . . . At present we have not the means to give to the young physician who has the intellect to become a leader the years of unhampered study and inspired guidance needed in preparation for his career." They recommended, among other things, that the University concentrate its assets in the undergraduate medical school.[14]

The Graduate School of Medicine received a fresh breath of life after World War II, when hundreds of medical officers were discharged from the Armed Services. Older ones wanted refresher courses before they returned to practice. Younger ones, who often had entered the service after their internship, wanted to obtain board certification in a specialty. There were too few residency positions in hospitals around the country to accommodate them. The two-year course offered by the Graduate School of Medicine, combined with the G.I. Bill of Rights, offered a solution; specialty boards cooperated by allowing the graduate courses to count toward fulfilling board requirements. Further easing the customary financial plight was the emergence of the National Institutes of Health as a large resource for grants for both clinical research and basic science.

The years between 1946 and 1953 constituted the school's most glorious era.[15] Prosperity even eased, temporarily, the tensions between the graduate and undergraduate faculties. Julius Comroe and Seymour Kety were two among many superb clinical and basic-science teachers who transferred their academic positions from the undergraduate school to the Graduate School of Medicine. Comroe also organized the first correlated course in basic science in the United States, one of the best courses ever offered anywhere. Comroe organized a clinical pharmacology correlation course, which combined ophthalmology, neurology, basic science, and advanced clinical instruction.

But in the early 1950s, the backlog of war veterans requiring residency positions dropped, and specialty boards withdrew approval of the Graduate School's courses.[16] National Institutes of Health grants began to be given for basic science in the undergraduate medical schools, where research facilities boomed. And advanced clinical training was done in residency programs in hospitals connected to undergraduate medical schools. Time seemed to have passed the Graduate School of Medicine by. It won a reprieve when foreign students, especially from Central and South America, took its seats. They would help spread modern medical techniques abroad. The program was only partly successful, however, because of language difficulties between teachers and students and, it was short-lived.

In 1955 Comroe and Henry Bockus suggested changes to meet the crisis of falling enrollment. They recommended constructing facilities for clinical offices and teaching on the grounds of Philadelphia General Hospital. If clinicians conducted their practice close to where they taught, they reasoned, an effective teaching program could be established. It would be a refresher course of five months of basic sciences and five months of advanced clinical work; it would fill the needs of residency training programs in community and municipal hospitals distanced from large medical centers.

To John McKay Mitchell, dean of the medical school, the proposal sounded like the start of a second medical school at Penn. It had other important opponents as well, including Norman Topping, vice president for medical affairs. The discussions became quite heated. One morning Comroe gave his secretary a check for $2,000 and told her to obtain two $1,000 bills at the bank. At a meeting that afternoon, Topping made a statement against the plan. Comroe stood up, exclaiming, "What you have just said is a damn lie!" He then pulled out the two bills and threw them on the table, saying, "Topping, if you can prove what you said isn't a lie, the two thousand is yours!" Topping quietly and sheepishly sat down and said no more. The plan, nevertheless, was not approved; the medical administrators preferred not to strain the school's limited resources by founding a new teaching institution.[17]

Comroe was disheartened and felt that Penn held no future for him. In 1957 he attended a professional meeting in San Francisco, which he found so beautiful that he decided to accept an offer if one came. Shortly thereafter, he was named head of a new Institute for Cardiovascular Diseases at the University of California Medical School. He remained there until he died in 1984.[18]

In 1964 the faculty of the Graduate School was officially merged with that of the undergraduate medical school. That relationship remains; in 1979, the hospital was sold off, and currently has no formal ties to Penn.

NOTES

1. A. Flexner, *The Carnegie Foundation for the Advancement of Teaching Medical Education in the United States and Canada* (New York: Carnegie Foundation, 1910).

2. Papers of Edgar Fahs Smith (hereafter EFSP) in the Archives of the University of Pennsylvania, which include correspondence with Abraham Flexner and Henry Pritchett; letter of Henry Pritchett to Edgar Fahs Smith, April 2, 1915; letter of Edgar Fahs Smith to Henry Pritchett, April 6, 1915; July 25, 1915 mentioning possibilities for mergers.

3. EFSP, correspondence with Women's Medical College; letter from E. F. Smith to Henry Pritchett April 6, 1915; letter from E. F. Smith to Henry Pritchett July 23, 1915; These papers are also collected and bound in a volume, "An Account of the Union of Medical Schools in Philadelphia," September 15, 1916, Edgar Fahs Smith.

4. EFSP, correspondence regarding merger with Jefferson Medical College: letters from Henry Pritchett to E. F. Smith, August 13, 1915; December 30, 1915.

5. EFSP, letter to Henry Pritchett, April 6, 1915.

6. EFSP, letter of Henry Pritchett to E. F. Smith, August 13, 1915.

7. EFSP, Report to the Trustees of the University of Pennsylvania and the Jefferson Medical College of Philadelphia [on the merger of the two institutions]; Document of Merger, there is no date on the printed report. E. F. Smith, "An Account of the Union of Medical Schools in Philadelphia," indicates this document was circulated to those concerned in late May or early June 1916.

8. *Ibid.*, p. 2.

9. EFSP, letter from Henry Pritchett to William Potter, esq., July 11, 1916; Henry Pritchett to Edgar Fahs Smith, July 11, 1916.

10. F. P. Henry, *Founders Week Memorial Volume* (Philadelphia: City of Philadel-

phia, 1909), pp. 366–76; J. T. Scharf and T. Wescott, *History of Philadelphia 1609–1884* (Philadelphia: L. H. Evert, 1884), pp. 1651–52.

11. "The Medical Merger," *Old Penn* 14(1916):1204–1205.

12. "Petition of the Medico-Chirurigical College of Philadelphia, The Medico-Chirurgical Hospital of the City of Philadelphia and the Trustees of the University of Pennsylvania for leave to merge and the court decree effecting the merger, Common Pleas No. 5 for the County of Philadelphia, No. 2147, June 16, 1916; Petition of the Philadelphia Polyclinic Hospital and College for Graduates in Medicine and the Trustees of the University of Pennsylvania for leave to merge and the court decree effecting the merger, 2075, December Term, 1917.

13. A Synoptic report upon the History, Aims, Plans, and Organization of the Graduate School of Medicine. Archives of the University of Pennsylvania, May 19, 1921.

14. A. N. Richards and T. G. Miller, *Survey of Medical Affairs of the University of Pennsylvania Prepared for President T. S. Gates and Submitted to him on March 5, 1931.* Annotated on the title page "This is one of three copies, T.G.M."

15. Memo for the Record to Mr. Blanshard, October 8, 1957, from D.T.S. Background on the Graduate School of Medicine–School of Medicine Unification Program, p. 2.

16. *Ibid.*, p. 3.

17. Conversation with George Koelle, March 1986.

18. *Ibid.*

12
ESTABLISHING TWENTIETH-CENTURY PRACTICE OF SCIENCE

The beginning of wisdom is to call things by their right name.

Chinese proverb

David Riesman was the William Osler that the University of Pennsylvania trained. Osler's motto was "litterae, scientia, praxis," and surely Riesman was his spiritual descendant.

Riesman, born in Germany, was raised in Ohio. As a young adult, he considered a business career but decided that he did not have the personality for the marketplace. He turned to medicine, enrolling at the University of Michigan medical school, then transferring to Penn.[1]

After graduating, he served as an intern at Philadelphia General Hospital, then became an assistant instructor in pathology. He started at once publishing numerous clinical and pathological descriptions of the interesting diseases he encountered, a practice he continued throughout his career. When Alfred Stengel was made professor of medicine after the departure of David Edsall, he appointed Riesman clinical professor in charge of Philadelphia General's medical service. Riesman, like his predecessor Osler, made no discoveries in medical science but gained renown as a superb clinician and teacher thoroughly identified with Philadelphia General. Medical students stated repeatedly that Riesman had no peer as a teacher, and he is credited with developing the next generation of brilliant clinicians, including John Barnwell, David A. Cooper, and Thomas Fitzhugh.

Among Riesman's other official titles was professor of the history of medicine. He wrote *Medicine in the Renaissance* and numerous articles

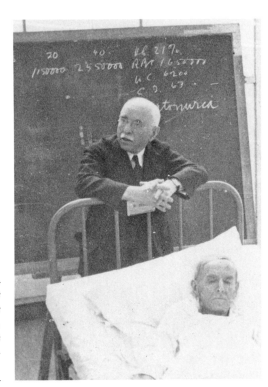

David Riesman lecturing in the Medical Lecture Room in the Medical Clinic Building. (Photograph Album of Norris Smith, Archives of the University of Pennsylvania.)

on topics that interested him, including extinct diseases, a physician in the Vatican, and doctors in Dublin.[2] He was an encourager of science generally, ranging as far as astronomy and physics; he convinced soap manufacturer Samuel Fels to build a planetarium in Philadelphia.

EDWARD B. KRUMBHAAR

Edward B. Krumbhaar served as chairman of pathology from 1934 to 1948, during which time the department distinguished itself with its analyses of diseases, especially cancer.[3] His own most important contribution to medical science was a chance discovery about cancer, although he and others did not realize it at the time. Krumbhaar started in research medicine at Penn under Richard Pearce. His early papers, published between 1912 and 1917, describe the pathology of white blood cells. In the Army during World War I, he was sent to France and assigned the task of conducting autopsies on victims of mustard gas. Their deaths followed a stormy clinical course, characterized by a low white blood cell count, gastrointestinal hemorrhage, and broncho-pneumonia. On further investigation of these symptoms, Krumbhaar found that, in addition to causing eye, skin, and pulmonary lesions, the gas produces a profound systemic intoxication that manifests itself some hours after the initial exposure. In 1919, Krumbhaar and his wife reported that death due to sulfur mustard

> is characterized by leucopenia, and in cases that come to autopsy, by aplasia of bone marrow, dissolution of lymphoid tissue and ulceration of the gastrointestinal tract.[4]

The dissolution of the lymphoid tissue that he had attributed to sulfur mustard gas turned out to be a clue to the development of a chemotherapeutic agent for treating leukemias and lymphomas. But this step had to await World War II, when the United States Army renewed its interest in chemical warfare, this time in nitrogen mustards. Army scientists observed that these mustards created toxic effects on tissues other than the lymphatic system; in addition, proliferating cells were selectively vulnerable to their toxic action.

Alfred Gilman, Louis Goodman, and T. F. Dougherty figured that the mustards could be used to treat neoplasms of lymphoid tissue. When the nitrogen mustard was administered, it rapidly dissolved the trans-planted lymphomas, although the dose required was close to toxic and the tumor invariably recurred. But encouraged, the three made a clinical trial of nitrogen mustard on patients in the terminal stages of various cancers. The most favorable results occurred in Hodgkin's disease, in which there were remissions similar to those following X-ray therapy.[5]

Krumbhaar pursued the pathology of blood cells and the reticulo-endothelial system throughout his active scientific life. He introduced the term "reticulocyte," the concept of "leukemoid blood pictures," and the "hemolytopoietic system." He also made contributions in other fields. He edited the *American Journal of Medical Sciences* for years. In medical history, he edited *Clio's Short History of Medicine* and translated Castiglioni's *History of Medicine* into English. He helped reorganize and catalogue the historical collections of the College of

Physicians of Philadelphia and helped found the Association of the History of Medicine and the International Association of Medical Museums.

JAY FRANK SCHAMBERG

Jay Frank Schamberg, who received his medical degree from Penn in 1892, was an ardent student of dermatology.[6] While he waited for his practice to grow, he wrote a compendium of skin diseases. To learn more about the cutaneous lesions associated with infectious diseases, he gained an appointment to the Philadelphia Hospital for Infectious Diseases. His work there led to his color-illustrated text *Acute Contagious Diseases* in 1905. At that hospital, he also studied five thousand cases of smallpox. Appalled by the ravages of a preventable disease a century after Edward Jenner discovered vaccination, he became a proponent of mandatory vaccination.

Schamberg was tall and dignified and known for his dress; he wore pince-nez glasses attached to a black ribbon around his neck, a white-laced vest, a dark suit, and spats. He was courteous, kind, unemotional, and coldly logical. At international professional meetings he impressed his colleagues because he delivered and discussed papers in French or German as well as English. He chaired dermatology at Temple University and the Jefferson Medical College prior to Graduate Hospital. He railed against socialized medicine, which he felt could be prevented if medical care were improved.

Schamberg has the distinction of having his name attached to two diseases. In 1899, early in his practice, he became intrigued by a spotty series of lesions in the pretibial skin of a fifteen-year-old boy.[7] The dermatitis started as red dots that slowly enlarged; similar eruptions appeared subsequently on the wrists. In time these flat, asymptomatic spots became brownish-red or brownish-yellow and finally disappeared. Schamberg, who had done postgraduate studies in Europe at Duhring's urging, knew that he had not seen lesions of this nature in clinics there. Nor had Duhring or his colleagues seen them. To be certain that he was describing a condition not previously observed, Schamberg followed the patient for two years before he published his initial case report in the *British Journal of Dermatology*. The lesion was progressive pigmented purpuric dermatitis, still known as Schamberg's disease.

There was to be yet another Schamberg's disease, one that died out as the home environment became cleaner. Schamberg first noticed it in 1901, when he reported on an epidemic of a disease resembling chickenpox and accompanied by intense itching. But he could not determine its etiology until 1909.

In that year the disease broke out again, frightening Philadelphia citizens much as Legionnaires' disease alarmed them in the 1970s. The epidemic started on the steam yacht of P.A.B. Widener, when many of the crew developed severe and generalized urticarial and vesicular eruptions. It spread to other ships anchored in the harbor and to homes near the wharfs, then to homes throughout the city. Most of the cases occurred among the poor, and groups of patients contracted the disease at the same time, ruling out person-to-person contagion. It also disappeared immediately after the patients were hospitalized.

Schamberg recognized the condition as the one he had seen in 1901. When the epidemic spread to fashionable Center City hotels, city health officials called upon the United States Public Health Service to investigate. Joseph Goldberger, who later would discover the cause of pellagra, was sent. He joined his background in parasitology to Schamberg's knowledge of skin lesions, and together they discovered that the cause of the rash was an ascarine mite that infested straw mattresses.[8]

In 1912 or so, P.A.B. Widener developed psoriasis and became a patient of Schamberg. This association led to Widener's giving financial support to Schamberg to organize a research group. In 1914 Schamberg opened the Dermatological Research Laboratories with John Kolmer, a bacteriologist and serologist, and George Raiziss, a chemist. They occupied meager space in two basement rooms of Philadelphia Polyclinic College for Graduates in Medicine (eventually Graduate Hospital).[9]

At first they focused on psoriasis. Figuring that they could broaden their investigations without unduly increasing their expenses, they entered the newly established field of chemotherapy. They synthesized compounds designed to destroy the germs of various diseases and tested their effectiveness on animals. Making no progress with mercury compounds, they tried arsenic compounds. World War I forced another project upon them. When the British blockaded German ships from American harbors, the researchers realized that the supply of Salvarsan, a valuable remedy for syphilis made by a German pharmaceutical firm, might be cut off. After some months of experimenting in the spring of

1915, Raiziss succeeded in synthesizing Salvarsan. He and his colleagues revealed the details of the synthesis at the May meeting of the American Dermatological Association; the association and the American pharmaceutical industry expressed their awe at the small, independent laboratory.[10]

Throughout the fall of 1915, Schamberg received an increasing number of requests from physicians and hospitals for Salvarsan, which they could not otherwise obtain. But Schamberg feared that selling it in the United States would infringe on the German patents. He met with the American distributor of the German drug, who tried to persuade him that ample supplies could skirt the blockade. Schamberg doubted that, and he also felt morally obliged to see that America had adequate quantities of the arsenical. To clear the situation, he suggested that the German licensee obtain a court order restraining distribution of the drug. The licensee refused, knowing that no court would enjoin Dermatological Research Laboratories from furnishing a lifesaving drug when the original supplier could not or would not furnish it. He finally agreed not to interfere if the laboratory went ahead and distributed its product, as long as it stopped when the German supplies arrived.

Schamberg's laboratory marketed its drug as Arsenobenzol and sold it at $2.50 a tube, two dollars less than Salvarsan cost. In June 1916 the German submarine Deutschland broke the blockade and brought Salvarsan to the United States, and Schamberg ceased production. But the shipment was soon exhausted, and Schamberg resumed making his product. In November 1917, when the United States entered the war, Congress passed the Trading with the Enemy Act, authorizing the Federal Trade Commission to license American citizens to operate foreign patents. The Dermatological Research Laboratories was granted license number one to produce and market Arsenobenzol. The demand was so great that the laboratory subcontracted two other laboratories to make it.

The sale of Arsenobenzol, even at its cut-rate price, brought profits sufficient to make the laboratory self-sustaining, even to allow a move to a larger facility, despite the death of Widener and the loss of his support. Schamberg was careful about how the profits were handled; he established a special fund for salaries and laboratory expenses. But when the war ended, Schamberg faced a difficult problem. His laboratory had been created for research rather than for financial gain, and critics harped that he had commercialized his work. To escape what he called "innuendoes of this character," he established another institute for dermatological research from the more than $500,000 of profits from Arsenobenzol. He told a newspaper reporter:

> Republics are notoriously ungrateful, and the fact that we sold the government Salvarsan at one-half the price we could have legitimately charged them and, moreover, at a time when they could have got it nowhere else, is either soon forgot or else never known by the general public. In our own hearts we are satisfied that we have carried out in the best interests of our country and of the people's health. We have gained nothing personally from the rewards of our work. The war has ended between nations, but the war against disease must go on; and it is for this purpose that we have dedicated our financial rewards.[11]

Newspaper advertisement announcing that the Submarine Deutschland *had broken the British blockade and brought a new supply of Salvarsan and other drugs to America from Germany. (Schamberg Papers, College of Physicians of Philadelphia.)*

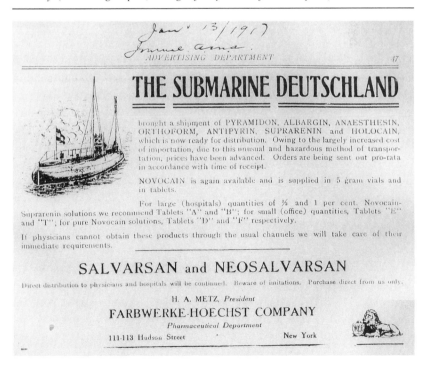

Jan' 13/1917

Journal Comm.

ADVERTISING DEPARTMENT 47

THE SUBMARINE DEUTSCHLAND

brought a shipment of PYRAMIDON, ALBARGIN, ANAESTHESIN, ORTHOFORM, ANTIPYRIN, SUPRARENIN and HOLOCAIN, which is now ready for distribution. Owing to the largely increased cost of importation, due to this unusual and hazardous method of transportation, prices have been advanced. Orders are being sent out pro-rata in accordance with time of receipt.

NOVOCAIN is again available and is supplied in 5 gram vials and in tablets.

For large (hospitals) quantities of ½ and 1 per cent. Novocain-Suprarenin solutions we recommend Tablets "A" and "B"; for small (office) quantities, Tablets "E" and "T"; for pure Novocain solutions, Tablets "D" and "F" respectively.

If physicians cannot obtain these products through the usual channels we will take care of their immediate requirements.

SALVARSAN and NEOSALVARSAN

Direct distribution to physicians and hospitals will be continued. Beware of imitations. Purchase direct from us only.

H. A. METZ, *President*

FARBWERKE-HOECHST COMPANY
Pharmaceutical Department

111-113 Hudson Street   New York

He added:

> We are living up to the immemorial traditions of medicine that make it
> incumbent upon medical men to give their inventions and discoveries freely
> to the world.[12]

But the criticisms did not stop until Schamberg, on the advice of
his counsel, sold Dermatological Research Laboratories. The German
licensee offered $50,000 more than any other bidder, but Schamberg
turned him down because of his previous behavior and his affiliation
with Germany. Schamberg accepted a bid from Abbott Laboratories,
which paid $150,000 plus $31,000 for the stock of Arsenobenzol.
Schamberg used the money to organize the Institute for Cutaneous
Medicine for the exclusive purpose of research.

GEORGE RAIZISS

George Raiziss was born in Odessa, Russia, earned his doctorate from
Albert Ludwig University in Germany, and came to the United States
in 1910.[13] He served as a fellow at the Rockefeller Institute and worked
for private firms before coming to Philadelphia in 1913. He was in
physiological chemistry at Polyclinic Hospital when he started collab-
orating with Schamberg. In 1918 he was appointed professor of chemotherapy at Graduate Hospital, the first to hold this title in the world.

When Dermatological Research Laboratories was sold to Abbott
Laboratories, Raiziss stayed on as its director. He also maintained his
academic appointment. In 1923, he prepared Metaphen, a potent mer-
curial antiseptic for nose and throat infections and abrasions, used too
to sterilize surgical fields and instruments. Shortly thereafter, he synthesized Bismarsen and Aldarsone, low-toxic agents against neurosy-
philis and trichomonas vaginitis.

When sulfa drugs were shown to be effective against streptococci
and staphylococci, Raiziss tried to synthesize and improve them. He
synthesized Sulfapyrazine and Sulfathiazoline. Later he synthesized
Diasone; Diasone and Dapsone are the only sulfones licensed in the
United States for treating leprosy. Raiziss also experimented with oil
suspensions of various drugs and developed the penicillin-in-oil preparation used in experimental syphilis.[14]

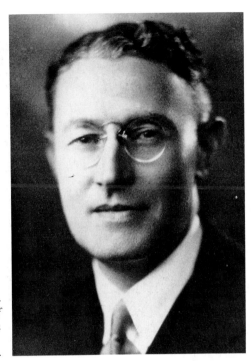

George Raiziss, first Professor of Chemotherapy in America. (Sonia Raiziss.)

ALFRED NEWTON RICHARDS

Alfred Newton Richards directed the medical school's policies for almost half a century and helped mobilize American science during World War II.[15] But his most significant contribution was discovering how the kidney makes urine. His work settled an old controversy: Was urine formed by filtration and resorption of the glomerular filtrate, or through secretion by the tubules?

Richards was headed toward this question before he quite knew it. In 1903–1904 he was teaching experimental pharmacology at the College of Physicians and Surgeons in New York. In conducting work on the hepatic detoxification of drugs, he decided that an improved and more reliable perfusion system could provide answers to many circulatory and hepatic problems.

Called to Penn as head of pharmacology during the Edsall episode, he constructed, as his first project, a perfusion system. With Cecil K. Drinker, who had just graduated from Penn's medical school, Richards perfused the brain of a cat for nearly two hours with no detectable damage.

When Drinker left to study physiology at Johns Hopkins, Oscar Plant joined the laboratory and suggested to Richards that the system be used to maintain a constant flow of blood through the kidney and thereby gain evidence on the mechanism of the diuretic action of xanthenes.[16]

---

*A. N. Richards with his students at a meeting of the International Physiological Society in Boston in 1929. Seated: A. N. Richards (then 53 years old). Standing, left to right: Arthur Walker, Leonard Bayliss, Isaac Starr, Joseph Wearn, Carl F. Schmidt, Cecil Drinker, Oscar Plant, John Barnwell, A. E. Livingston, Joseph Heyman, and Howard Florey. (*Annals of Internal Medicine, *Supplement 8, 71[1969].)*

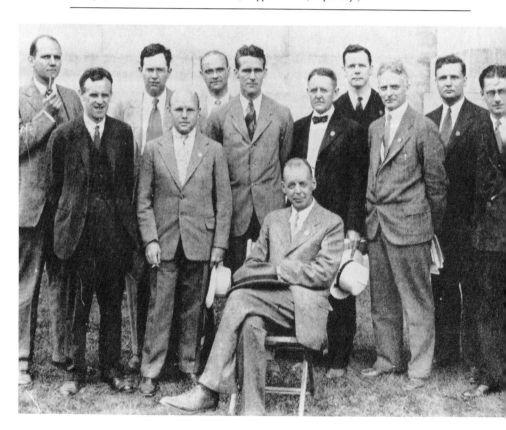

Accomplishing the goal was more difficult than expected. Richards worked long before the discovery of heparin, and the only anticoagulant approximating a physiologically inert one was hirudin—leech-head extract—which was expensive, not entirely nontoxic, and practically impossible to obtain during World War I. Richards, however, received some from an anonymous friend and carried out a small series of experiments using his new perfusion system. He showed that the formation of urine increased after caffeine was injected into a rabbit's kidney that had been perfused with a constant volume of blood, despite a marked fall in blood pressure. This result supported the secretory theory.

Richards's work was interrupted by World War I, during which he joined Henry H. Dale in England to study the mechanism of wound shock.[17] He and Dale published an article on the action of histamine, a classic in medical literature. After the war, Richards, drawing on his histamine study, felt that a rise in glomerular filtration would occur with a rise in renal arterial pressure. He raised perfusion pressure by partially obstructing the renal vein, stimulating the splanchnic nerves, and adding minimally effective doses of adrenaline in the perfusing blood. Diuresis resulted in every case, which Richards regarded as strong support for the filtration-resorption theory.[18]

A visitor to Richards's laboratory suggested that he gather data with an oncometer, which Richards used after injecting a kidney with adrenaline. The blood pressure rose, diuresis occurred, and blood volume in the kidney increased.

A major step was taken after the arrival of Joseph Wearn, who came to Penn after an internship at Peter Bent Brigham Hospital and army service.[19] Wearn helped prepare the animal experiments in pharmacology for the medical students. Richards taught him how to prepare a living frog so that its glomerular circulation could be observed. Richards had also visited Robert Chambers at Cornell and had seen Chambers inject red blood cells with a minute glass pipette. Wearn suggested that they puncture Bowman's capsule with a Chambers pipette and obtain some glomerular fluid. The fluid could be analyzed for protein, sugar, chloride, urea, dyes, and other substances; and the results could be compared with those of similar analyses of the blood and urine.[20]

Richards enthusiastically approved the idea. He assigned Wearn to a quiet laboratory in the basement of the Medical Laboratories Building, and they proceeded to gather equipment, much of which they had to build themselves. The test showed that a protein-free filtrate is separated from the blood stream as it passes through the glomerular capillaries. Sodium and glucose, both normal constituents of blood plasma, were found in the glomerular fluid but not in urine in the bladder, proving beyond doubt that the renal tubule reabsorbed these substances. Richards reported this work at the 1921 annual meeting of the American Physiological Society and shared the limelight with Frederick J. Banting and Charles H. Best's report of the first isolation of insulin (insulin was actually first successfully isolated the following January by James B. Collip in the Department of Biochemistry at the University of Toronto).[21] Critics, noting that the work was done on amphibia, questioned whether the mechanism was similar in higher mammals. Richards felt that it was, but his intuition was confirmed only some twenty years later when scientists demonstrated essentially the same mechanism in rats, guinea pigs, and opossums.

Richards's discovery not only laid the groundwork for understanding renal function in general but also was fundamental to the development of new diuretics and systems of dialysis for patients who have no renal function. Scientific method was an ancillary beneficiary. Richards noticed that the human eye can distinguish small color differences in fluids contained in thin glass tubes. These color differences could be expressed quantitatively by comparing them with a series of standards contained in similar tubes. Painstakingly modifying the analytical procedures of the time, Richards and his colleagues made quantitative measurements of eleven separate urinary components in fluid, then made similar measurements of foreign substances. The microtechniques they developed introduced a quantitative dimension to their studies and pioneered the development of microbiochemistry.[22]

SIMON S. LEOPOLD AND CHARLES S. LEOPOLD

In 1925 the Pepper ward was opened in the Gibson Wing of the hospital. The ward was especially designed for metabolic studies and the care of patients with renal disease. It contained an advanced diet kitchen and a unusual room in which the the temperature, humidity, and particulate matter in the air could be controlled. It was probably the first climate-controlled room in a hospital.

The "air-conditioned" room was made by Simon Leopold and his brother Charles, who was a graduate of Penn's Towne School of Engineering. Simon Leopold wanted to evaluate the effect of inhaled substances and atmospheric conditions on bronchial asthma and other respiratory diseases. In his studies Leopold found changes in barometric pressure, temperature, and humidity had no effect on the clinical symptoms of his patients. He discovered, however, that house dust contains one or more groups of specific, antigenic substances capable of producing immediate onset of asthma.[23]

EDMUND B. PIPER

Edmund B. Piper succeeded Hirst as professor of obstetrics. He graduated from Princeton University and entered business before going to medical school, graduating from Penn in 1911.[24] During World War I he treated severe machine-gun and shrapnel wounds in France, gaining vast experience in managing septicemia (and, incidentally, diligently fighting the army on how military surgery should be practiced).

On returning to Philadelphia, Piper studied the use of Mercurochrome in treating urological infections, especially blood poisoning after childbirth. His experiments showed him that Mercurochrome injected intravenously sterilized the bloodstream of rabbits with experimental septicemia, and he became the chief local consultant on severe bloodstream infections. When he treated patients with puerperal sepsis by injecting Mercurochrome intravenously, he had some apparent successes but also many failures. Small doses of the compound caused marked renal damage, so that effective levels of it could not be maintained for periods long enough to sterilize the bloodstream.[25]

Piper had better luck with instruments. He developed the aftercoming head forceps used in delivering babies with breech presentations and modified these for use as axis-traction forceps. He also invented the adjustable leg holders for obstetrical tables, modifications of which are still used today.[26]

It was his extracurricular hobby of sports cars, however, that brought him to public attention. He increased the driving range of his Packard convertible by fitting it with an oversize gas tank; he also cut a hole in the floor and carried a funnel and tube so that he could relieve himself. He liked to race trains from city to city. In 1928, to regain the center of attention of his family which had been seized by his daughter, who was getting married, he raced from Philadelphia to Los Angeles and

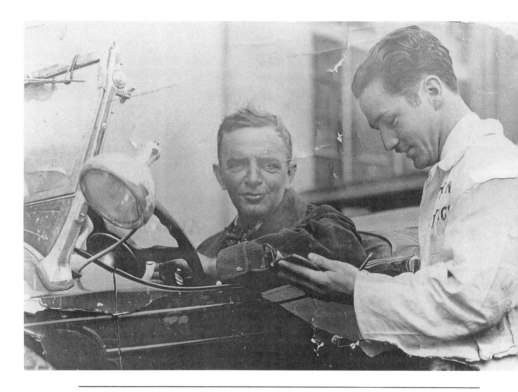

Edmund Piper, Professor of Obstetrics, and his automobile in which he raced a train across the United States and arrived ahead of it in Los Angeles. (Mrs. Donaldson Cresswell, Edmund Piper's daughter.)

beat the train, and his story and picture ran in newspapers all over the United States.[27]

NOTES

1. D. A. Cooper, "David Riesman," *Weekly Roster and Medical Digest* 36(1940–41):494–95; S. R. Kagan, "David Reisman," in *The Modern Medical World. Portraits and Biographical Sketches of Distinguished Men in Medicine* (Boston: Medical-Historical Press, 1945), p. 23; H. A. Christian, Remarks Made by Dr. Henry Christian at the Dinner to Honor Dr. Riesman's 70th Birthday, March 25, 1937.

2. D. A. Cooper, *David Riesman, High Blood Pressure and Longevity and Other Essays* (Philadelphia: John C. Winston, 1937).

3. E. R. Long and D. T. Rowlands, *The Development of the Department of Pathology in the School of Medicine of the University of Pennsylvania* (Philadelphia: privately printed, 1977), pp. 41–46.

4. E. B. Krumbhaar and G. D. Krumbhaar, "The Blood and Bone Marrow in Yellow Cross Gas (Mustard) Poisoning." *Journal of Research Medicine* 40(1919):497–506; E. B. Krumbhaar, "Role of the Blood and the Bone Marrow in Certain Forms of Gas Poisoning, I. Peripheral Blood Changes and their Significance," *Journal of the American Medical Association* 72(1919):39–41.

5. A. Gilman and F. S. Philips,"The Biological Actions and Therapeutic Applications of b-Chloroethyl Amines and Sulfides," *Science* 103(1946):409–15.

6. R. Friedman, *A History of Dermatology in Philadelphia* (Fort Pierce Beach, Fla.: Froben Press,1955); H. Beerman, "The Rise of Dermatology in Philadelphia," *Transactions and Studies of College of Physicians of Philadelphia* 4th ser., 40(1972):39–54; obituary of Jay Frank Schamberg, *New York Times*, March 30, 1934.

7. J. F. Schamberg, "A Peculiar Progressive Disease of the Skin," *British Journal of Dermatology* 13(1901):1–13.

8. J. F. Schamberg, "An Epidemic of a Peculiar and Unfamiliar Disease of the Skin," *Philadelphia Medicine* (1901):5–6; J. Goldberger and J. F. Schamberg, "Epidemic of an Urticaroid Dermatitis Due to a Small Mite (*Pediculosis Ventriculosis*) in the Straw of Mattresses," *Public Health Report* 24(1909):973–75; J. F. Schamberg, "Grain Itch: Acro-Dermatitis Urticaroides: A New Disease in this Country," *Journal of Cutaneous Disorders* 28(1910):67–89.

9. W. B. Shelley and H. Beerman, "Jay Frank Schamberg: 1870–1934," *American Journal of Dermatopathology* 6 (1984):441–44.

10. Report of the Dermatological Research Laboratories to the Board of Trustees of the Philadelphia Polyclinic and College for Graduates in Medicine, Status of Production and Distribution of Arsenobenzol; Dermatological Research Laboratories, Inc. Abstract of Meeting of Organization, 1921; H. Kogen, *The Long White Line* (New York: Random House, 1963), pp. 108–13; Papers of the Dermatological Research Laboratories. Historical Collections of the College of Physicians of Philadelphia.

11. Papers of Jay Frank Schamberg, College of Physicians of Philadelphia.

12. *Ibid.*

13. "George W. Raiziss, Chemotherapist," *Encyclopedia of Biography*, vol. 26, p. 607; Obituary of George Raiziss, *Philadelphia Evening Bulletin*, July 16, 1945; *Philadelphia Inquirer*, July 17, 1945; *New York Times*, July 17, 1945.

14. "Toxicity is Cut in Sulfanilamide," *New York Times*, January 25, 1940; "Magic Bullets Aid in Bacterial War," *New York Times*, April 4, 1940; *American Men of Science*, 7th ed. (Lancaster, Pa.: Science Press, 1944), p. 1437.

15. C. F. Schmidt, "Alfred Newton Richards, 1876–1966," *Annals of Internal Medicine* sup. 8, 71 (1969):15–32.

16. A. N. Richards and O. H. Plant, "Urine Formation in the Perfused Kidney. The Influence of Alterations in Renal Blood Pressure on the Amount and Composition of Urine," *American Journal of Physiology* 59(1922):144–90; A. N. Richards and O. H. Plant, "Urine Formation in the Perfused Kidney. The Influence of Adrenaline on the Volume of the Perfused Kidney," *American Journal of Physiology* 71 (1922) 191–202.

17. C. F. Schmidt, "Alfred Newton Richards," p. 20; A. N. Richards and H. H. Dale, "The Vasodilator Action of Histamine and Some Other Substances," *Journal of Physiology* 52(1918):110–65.

18. C. F. Schmidt, "Alfred Newton Richards," p. 21; A. R. Cushny, *The Secretion of Urine* (London: Longmans, Green, 1926).

19. C. F. Schmidt, "Alfred Newton Richards," p. 22.

20. J. T. Wearn, *The Physiologist* 23(1980):1–4.

21. A. N. Richards, "Process of Urine Formation," The Croonian Lecture, *Proceedings of the Royal Society* Ser. B. 126 (1938):398–32.

22. J. T. Wearn and A. N. Richards, "Observations on the Composition of Glomerular Urine with Particular Reference to the Problem of Readsorption in Renal Tubules, *American Journal of Physiology* 71(1924):209–27.

23. S. S. Leopold and C. S. Leopold, "Bronchial Asthma and Allied Allergic Disorders. Preliminary report of a study under controlled conditions of environment, temperature, and humidity," *Journal of the American Medical Association* 84(1925):731–34; D. W. Presser, Penn Engineers (writeup of the work of Charles Leopold. Charles S. Leopold was a pioneer and expert in heating, ventilating, and air conditioning. Among the installations he engineered were the air conditioning of the Pentagon, the United States Senate, the House of Representatives Office Building, the New York Stock Exchange, Convention Hall, Philadelphia, Madison Square Garden, Gimbel Brothers Stores, New York and Philadelphia, Saks Fifth Ave., and the special exhaust system for the Atomic Energy Commission, Los Alamos, N. M.) *New York Herald Tribune*, November 26, 1960.

24. B. C. Hirst, "Memoir of Dr. Edmund Brown Piper," *Transactions and Studies of the College of Physicians of Philadelphia* 4th ser., 3 (1935–1936):xi–xv; personal papers in possession of his daughter Mrs. Donaldson Cresswell, now in the Historical Collections of the College of Physicians of Philadelphia.

25. E. B. Piper, "The Treatment of Puerperal Sepsis by Use of Mercurochrome Intravenously, With a Report of Animal Experimentation in the Chemical Disinfection of Blood," *American Journal of Obstetrics and Gynecology* 4 (1922):532–43: E. B. Piper, "Blood Stream Infection Treated With Mercurochrome 220 Intravenously," *American Journal of Obstetrics and Gynecology* 9 (1924):17–21 (discussion 107–110); E. B. Piper, "A Summary of the Present Status of the Intravenous Use of Mercurochrome," *American Journal of Obstetrics and Gynecology* 10,(1925):371–74.

26. E. B. Piper, "A New Axis Traction Forceps," *American Journal of Obstetrics and Gynecology* 24(1932):625–28; E. B. Piper and C. Bachman, "The Prevention of Fetal Injuries." *Journal of the American Medical Association* 92(1929):217–21.

27. Personal conversation with T. Grier Miller at The Philadelphia Medical Club Meeting.

13

SCIENCE AND PRACTICE: THE NEXT PHASE

Not only is there a certain art in knowing a thing, but also a certain art in teaching it.

Cicero

CARL F. SCHMIDT

Carl F. Schmidt helped A. N. Richards observe the glomerular blood flow of the frog kidney but was forced to stop when the bright arc lights that the research required gave him eye strain. In search of activity, he visited the Office of the China Medical Board in New York City in 1921. The Chinese wanted specialists to investigate the pharmacological activity of and therapeutic possibilities in the many drugs in the Chinese pharmacopeia. The Chinese were also seeking fellows trained in pharmacology, chemistry, and physiology to teach Western methods to their own doctors and medical students. Intrigued, Schmidt signed up.[1]

He arrived in Peking just after the Peking Union Medical School was organized. Charles Read was head of pharmacology there. He welcomed Schmidt because he had little training in pharmacology and needed help with the teaching. He steered Schmidt toward some native drugs—a volatile oil, a diuretic, and a nerve tonic among them—that seemed as though they should have active properties. But Schmidt came up with only negative results, as he did for a number of other drugs. He was discouraged, thinking that none of the Chinese drugs had any activity.[2]

At this time K. K. Chen returned to China, supported by a Boxer fellowship. Schmidt met him, and they discussed their collaboration.

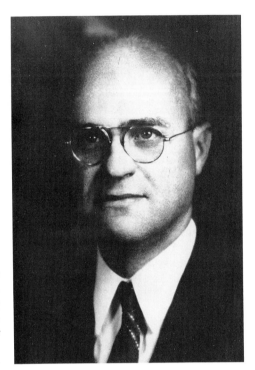

Carl F. Schmidt, Professor of Pharmacology, who brought ephedrine to the United States and was a pioneer in the study of the cerebral circulation. (Archives of the University of Pennsylvania.)

Shortly thereafter, Chen visited his family in central China. While at his home, he told them that he intended to apply modern techniques to explain the chemistry and pharmacology of the ancient native drugs. He also told them about Schmidt's frustrating results. An uncle pointed him to ma huang. Chen obtained some and took it to Schmidt.[3]

Meanwhile, Chen and Schmidt tested other drugs unsuccessfully. One day, after a class experiment, Chen suggested that they test the ma huang on the dog used by the students, which was in sufficiently good condition for a trial. He rushed home for the sample, and on his return, the two placed some of the oily powder in a beaker of hot water. After letting it sit for a few minutes, they drew some of the yellow supernatant fluid into a syringe and injected it into the dog's vein.[4] The dog's blood pressure rose at once—the first promising result from any drug they had tested. They were so surprised that they wondered whether the syringe had been contaminated with epinephrine. But no epinephrine had been used that day; besides, that drug is short-acting, and the dog's blood pressure stayed high for five minutes.[5]

Chen tried to extract the active principle from the crude sample of ma huang. A few days later, he made a white powder which, when injected into the dog, produced the same rise in blood pressure. He learned in the scientific literature that, in 1884, Nagai had discovered a similar substance, determined its structure, and named it ephedrine, after the plant from which he extracted it (*Ephedra vulgaris helviticus*). Others had shown that it causes the pupils to dilate and the blood pressure to rise from vasoconstriction and, in fact, Japanese doctors used it for eye diseases. But there was no complete investigation of its effects.[6]

When Schmidt returned to the United States, he brought 500 grams of ephedrine with him. He gave it to T. Grier Miller, a gastroenterologist, who tested it in the hospital's medical clinic. Miller and his associates found that it was useful for treating nasal congestion, asthma, serum sickness, hives, and low blood pressure.[7]

ISAAC STARR

Isaac Starr might well be the most distinguished clinical scientist Richards trained. Starr graduated from Penn's medical school and interned at Massachusetts General Hospital. He returned to Penn and joined Richards's group investigating the mechanisms by which the kidney formed urine. But he wanted to study other physiological problems. He told Richards, who was supportive—and unusual in encouraging his protégés to pursue their own ideas.[8]

Starr decided to focus on the heart. At the time, the heart was often conceived of as a dynamo whose pumping action could be explained by the small currents produced by its conduction system. Starr, however, saw it as a pump and directed his approach accordingly.[9]

About this time, Richards arranged to have members of the pharmacology department work on the medical wards so that the residents could learn about the pharmacological action of the drugs they administered to patients. Starr and Joseph Heymans assisted Richards, and in 1928 they were both appointed assistant professors of clinical pharmacology, probably the first use of this academic title.[10] Starr liked the work, and the interaction was successful. One result was a course in

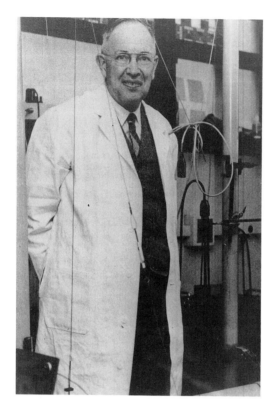

Isaac Starr, Professor of Research Medicine. Pioneer in investigating the fluid mechanics of the circulation and organizer with A. N. Richards of the first course in clinical pharmacology in the United States. (Copied from Scope.)

clinical pharmacology for medical students, headed by Starr and Richards. Starr evidently had some personal magnetism. In 1933 he received an endowed chair, which funded everything except salaries for research assistants; but he soon learned that both ward residents and fellows in pharmacology and physiology were glad to work with him for no pay.[11]

In his first clinical studies, Starr measured cardiac output by a procedure using ethyl iodide; it was laborious and required needle sticks. Since Starr did not like to be stuck with needles himself, he refrained from sticking subjects and patients unless absolutely necessary. He also realized that invasive procedures altered the measurements because of the patient's anxiety and discomfort.[12]

Starr had these problems in mind when he participated in a program on cardiac-output methods given by the American Physiological Society in the early 1930s. Another participant was Yandell Henderson, who reminisced about experiments "on the mass movement of the circulation" some thirty years earlier. Henderson had noticed that, when he stood on a spring scale, the pointer tip moved in time with his heartbeat.[13] To study the phenomenon, he rigged a suspended bed to pick up the resonance frequency and a recorder that amplified it some one hundred times. He simplified the instrument, which he took on the Douglas-Haldane expedition up Pikes Peak in 1913 to measure heart output at high altitudes. Henderson's ballistocardiograph was ingenious but too heavy, and the amplification distorted the record of the heart's action.[14]

Starr was stimulated. Back at Penn, he was helped by Detlev Bronk, head of the Eldridge Reeves Johnson Foundation for Medical Physics, who made available his machine shop and its head machinist, A. R. Rawson. Starr's first instrument resembled Henderson's in design but was lighter and used an optical recording system. It had such a low natural frequency that patients had to hold their breath when the measurements were taken. It was a technique that trained subjects could do much better than many patients. Starr modified the design. He opposed the motion of the bed by a stiff spring so that the frequency would be considerably higher than the heart rate. The problem of respiratory interference was solved, and patients were not required to hold their breath.[15]

Starr used the instrument to measure cardiac output of normal subjects and of patients, some suffering from cardiac diseases. After several years, he realized that it measured not output but cardiac force, which was even more important.[16] He then applied Newton's laws in postmortem studies to analyze his ballistocardiograph, correlating the device's tracings with output of blood from the heart. He attached large syringes into a cadaver's aorta and forced blood into the circulation by striking the syringe plungers with a mallet suspended as a pendulum from the ceiling. This arrangement enabled him to control both the volume of blood ejected and the force of the ejection. The results, made in collaboration with Orville Horwitz and Truman G. Schnabel Jr., were made over a period of ten years and were the first accurate physical measurements of cardiac output.[17]

Combining these data with those obtained from studies on normal subjects and patients, Starr began to understand in detail what the wiggles of the ballistocardiogram tracings really meant: the instantaneous changes of force produced by the cardiac muscle. When the ventricles of the heart contracted during the systole cycle, the rate at which blood ejected into the pulmonary artery and aorta changed— slower at first, rising, then falling at the end of the contraction. Since the ballistocardiogram is a continuous measurement (the upstroke of the wiggly curve), the rate of change of ejected blood can be estimated at each instance of systole.

Thus the ballistocardiogram measures noninvasively the heart's ability to accelerate blood, an element of cardiac function not assessed by any clinical test (the history, physical, EKG, blood pressure, X rays, or even such special studies as cardiac catheterization and visualization of the coronary arteries). Starr realized that patients, even those with heart disease, who accelerated blood rapidly, had large, functional cardiac reserves and the best prognosis. His machine can also detect when the heart chambers do not contract simultaneously.[18]

HENRY CUTHBERT BAZETT

Henry Cuthbert Bazett succeeded Edward Reichert as chairman of physiology; Reichert had held the position for thirty-one years, and Bazett served for twenty-nine years. Under Bazett, and in part because of him, the department was one of the most distinguished in the world.[19]

Bazett was born in England and served in the Royal Army Medical Corps during World War I. He was fearless. He insisted on serving as the first subject in any experiments involving human beings. During one experiment, a catheter placed in the right side of his heart became detached and slipped into his circulation; it had to be removed surgically. He was a subject so often that a colleague quipped that he should write a book called The Physiology of H. Cuthbert Bazett. During World War II, the Canadian Air Force Command issued an order preventing him from flying G-test missions with the most daring of its pilots.[20]

Although Bazett worked on many scientific problems throughout his career, his primary interest was the mechanism by which the body controls its temperature. He identified the venae comites as significant and figured out the arrangement of receptors, blood flow, and thermal gradients. He went on to describe how the body, in cold temperatures, prevents peripheral heat loss and warms the venous blood shunted from its surface, so that the temperature of the peripheral venous blood is kept in equilibrium with that of the central venous circulation. In warm environments or during exercise, he postulated, the temperature of the venous blood deep in the body rises, increasing the blood temperature as a whole. Thermal regulators in the pons respond by producing peripheral vasodilatation and sweating; local control of peripheral capillary flow and sweating is regulated by gradients near receptors in the skin.[21]

This concept of temperature regulation in humans has proved to be essentially correct. Even if it had been proven otherwise, Bazett would not have been disturbed. He boldly stated his hypotheses, openly

H. Cuthbert Bazett, Professor of Physiology, serving as an experimental guinea pig. (Lysle Peterson.)

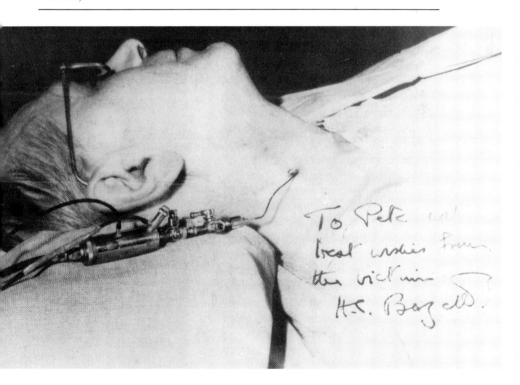

discussed differences of opinion with his colleagues, and took those differences as stimulation to further work.

In addition, he always encouraged science at both fundamental and applied levels. The Johnson Foundation for Medical Physics stems, in part, from his realization that methods were needed to study body function in humans. At the time of his death (he died suddenly at sea while traveling to an international physiology congress), he had just been elected president of the American Physiological Society. At professional meetings he was seen more often discussing research problems with younger scientists and former students than hobnobbing with the scientifically and politically elite.[22]

He was not known as an excellent teacher of medical undergraduates, because his lectures tended to be too advanced for the students, and he customarily presented too many details before he established his main idea. Even so, he recognized and backed brightness. In one class, he asked Herndon B. Lehr, then a first-year medical student, to discuss current theories of congestive heart failure. Lehr, who had studied engineering at Georgia Tech, said that he disdained the physiological theories; he proceeded to put forth a logical, mechanical approach. Bazett was impressed with the forthrightness and ingenuity of Lehr's answer. Before long, he invited the student to work as a physiology assistant. Lehr eventually became chief of plastic surgery at the Hospital of the University of Pennsylvania.[23]

BALDUIN LUCKÉ

Balduin Lucké, a pathologist interested in physiology, succeeded E. B. Krumbhaar as head of pathology in 1948. Lucké was a Hessian who came to the United States as a youth. He received his medical degree from the Medico-Chirurgical College of Philadelphia and served a residency at Philadelphia General Hospital. He joined the Penn staff in 1914.[24]

He made his first important scientific contribution during World War I. He was serving in the medical corps at Camp Zachary Taylor when the influenza pandemic of 1918 broke out. Among its victims were thousands of soldiers. Lucké examined histological and bacteriological specimens from hundreds of autopsies and concluded that death was due to such secondary invaders as pneumococci, staphylococci, and streptococci, rather than to *H. influenzae*, as was widely thought.

On his return to Penn, Lucké studied the changes in cell permeability produced by injury and the changes in electrolyte concentration. In the early 1930s, he began studying tumors of frogs. His sudden shift of interest occurred by chance. A. N. Richards was using frogs in his experiments and one day noticed a sizeable nodule on the renal cortex of a leopard frog. After satisfying himself that it was not a hematoma or a cyst, he asked Lucké to have a look. Lucké found through microscopic examination that it was a carcinoma. He examined its biological properties and found that it could be transferred by freeze-dried dessicated homogenates of the tumor. The tumor was also transferable from one frog to another by extracts free of living cell. In addition, the tumors did not metastasize at low temperatures but did so when the temperature was raised. Lucké's observations suggested a new approach to cancer research. The "Lucké carcinoma" (after decades, still one of the few "name" tumors) was the first carcinoma induced by a virus. Lucké and

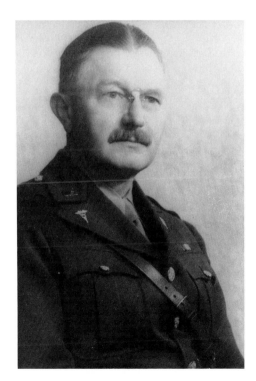

Balduin Lucké, Professor of Pathology. First to demonstrate cancer can be transferred from animal to animal by a filterable virus. During World War II he described the pathology of lower nephron nephrosis and infectious hepatitis. (Historical Collections of the College of Physicians of Philadelphia.)

Hans Schlumberger went on to investigate tumors found in other cold-blooded animals.[25]

During World War II, Lucké served as deputy director of the Army Institute of Pathology, where he made further discoveries. He investigated epidemic hepatitis in the pathological specimens from many service hospitals. After describing the pathological changes seen in "acute catarrhal jaundice" and "idiopathic acute yellow atrophy," he concluded that these were not different diseases, as had been thought, but extreme forms of the same condition. He also described the renal changes associated with the "crush syndrome" and named it the "lower nephron nephrosis." He received the Legion of Merit for his brilliant work. In return, he so valued his military associations that, according to his wishes, he was given a military funeral.[26]

EUGENE M. LANDIS

Eugene M. Landis was still a medical student when he made an essential discovery about the physiology of blood circulation.[27] Three hundred years before his work, William Harvey discovered that blood is pumped from the left side of the heart into the arteries and returns to the right side through the veins. His discovery led him to reason that a network of vessels invisible to the eye must connect the smallest visible arterioles and venules. Antony van Leeuwenhoek and Marcello Malphigi studied the anatomy of this capillary network.

This question remained: was fluid excreted from the vascular bed or passed back and forth by diffusion? Scientists could not understand the diffusion of gases or the transudation of fluids between tissues and the intravascular space until they knew something about blood pressure within the capillaries. In 1733 Stephen Hales made the first measurement of capillary blood pressure, but it was inadequate. Danish scientists tried to measure it in 1925, but technical difficulties stopped them.

Landis was working in the physiology laboratories when Professor Merkel Jacobs pointed out that micromanipulators and micro-injection methods newly developed by Robert Chambers at Cornell might help overcome the difficulties the Danes faced.[28] Landis used the mesentery of a frog for his first experiments. He observed that injection of dye

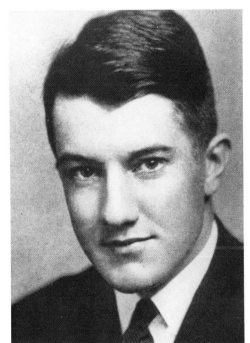

Eugene M. Landis, physiologist, who while a medical student at the University of Pennsylvania was the first to measure accurately the capillary blood pressure. Subsequently he served as Professor of Physiology at the University of Virginia and Harvard Medical Schools. (Historical Collections of the College of Physicians of Philadelphia.)

solutions was variable and realized that, for meaningful results, the capillary blood pressure had to be measured over the entire period of the injection. He proceeded to hold a micropipette in the same position in the lumen for enough time to adjust the pressure within the pipette until it exactly balanced the capillary blood pressure, with no net flow of liquid in either direction. Landis was then able to determine how fluid moves by filtration and absorption through the capillary wall.[29]

Landis received his medical degree in 1926, the same year that his classic paper on his research was published in the *American Journal of Physiology*. He continued at Penn until 1939. During that time, he continued his work on capillaries by studying peripheral circulation with John Gibbon and Hugh Montgomery. Their work led to the development of the suction boot for treating ischemic limbs.

Landis left Penn to head the Department of Medicine at the University of Virginia medical school and then became the George Higgenson Professor of Physiology at the Harvard University Medical School. He helped organize and direct several scientific societies and was given the first Distinguished Graduate Award from Penn's medical school, when the honor was established in 1984.

R. TAIT McKENZIE

R. Tait McKenzie was the first person in America to hold the title of professor of physical education. He also was a pioneer in sports medicine and physical rehabilitation and a remarkable sculptor.[30]

McKenzie was a Canadian who loved his Scottish ancestry so much that, when he died, his heart was buried in Scotland, according to his wishes. He early had an inkling that one could mix professions; his first schooling came from a blacksmith who had become a teacher. While in medical school at McGill University, he was an assistant in the gymnasium. From the outset he wanted to be a great athlete, but his body seemed too frail. With persistent work, however, he became a gymnast champion and football player.[31]

He was appointed medical director of physical training at McGill, a post created just for him. He took the bold step of requiring medical examinations for students entering Canadian colleges. In 1896 he extended his work to teaching and dissecting in the medical school's anatomy department. About 1900 he became interested in modeling human faces in clay.[32]

Through the efforts of J. William White, who had heard him lecture, McKenzie came to Penn in 1904. He instituted compulsory medical examinations for matriculating Penn students. The physical exams turned up many cases of hallux valgus and Morton's toe, foot deformities that restricted the physical activities of those who had them. He was also concerned about the deformities left by infantile paralysis and scoliosis and developed programs to strengthen individuals who had had these diseases. He also wrote extensively on preventing tuberculosis through diet, exercise, and proper living conditions. His motto was "An eager mind in a lithe body" (*mens fervida in corpore lacertoso*).[33]

In 1915 McKenzie volunteered for the Canadian army fighting in Europe. He was assigned to Aldershot Hospital and applied for the course it gave in physical education. One of the texts was his book *Exercise in Education and Medicine*. One day McKenzie was amused when his young instructor asked him if the McKenzie who wrote the book was any relation of his.

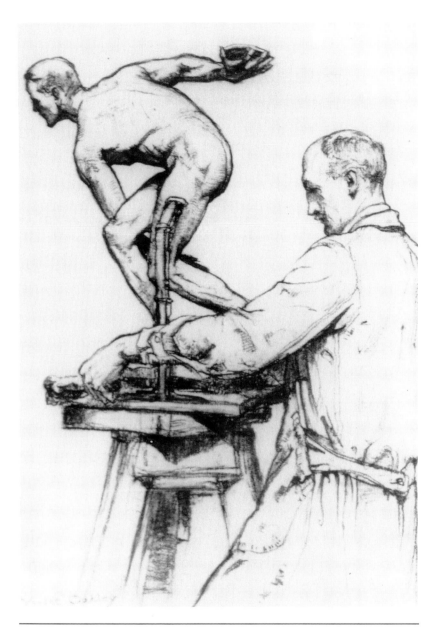

R. Tait McKenzie, Professor of Physical Education and Physical Medicine and Rehabilitation. (Historical Collections of the College of Physicians of Philadelphia.)

In time McKenzie helped establish reconstruction depots for wounded and disabled soldiers, convalescent camps which helped restore their patients to useful lives. He headed the depot at Heaton Park Camp in Manchester and wrote *Reclaiming the Maimed* and a handbook of physical therapy from his experiences.[34]

As a sculptor, McKenzie constantly observed the bodies of athletes performing such activities as running, jumping, and pole vaulting. Their forms led him to idealize the perfect athlete's body in such bronze statues as "The Sprinter" and "The Modern Discus Thrower." The war, in a sense, was the antithesis of both sides of his life's work: It destroyed the bodies of the athletes he had tried so hard to build (as a professor) and to depict (as an artist). Even so he idealized what he felt was the spirit of the unsung heroes of the battlefield in such statues as "Over the Top" (the Canadian national war memorial), "The Home Coming" (Cambridge, England), "The Victor" (Woodbury, N. J.), and "Captain Guy Drummond," created for the soldier's mother.[35]

McKenzie's art had other themes as well. "The Youthful Franklin" (at Penn), "The Call" (a Scottish war memorial in Edinburgh), and a statue of General James Wolf (in Greenwich Park, near London) depict not merely heroes but moments of first resolve, when victory, though distant, is already felt as palpable, like the first spring-like day after a harsh winter.[36]

McKenzie graced the medical world with his work. For Penn he executed panels of Nathaniel Chapman and Samuel Jackson and medallions of Crawford Long (the alumnus who first used anesthesia), Francis Kenlock Huger, Class of 1797 (who made an unsuccessful attempt to rescue General Lafayette from Olmutz prison), among others. He made medallions for organizations to bestow as awards, including one of Joseph Leidy for the American Society of Anatomists. He also made the Mary Ellis Bell prize medal, which Penn's medical school awards for student research each spring. He intended to push this subject further. Just prior to his death, he remarked to a friend that he hoped for another commission for a statue honoring medical research; he intended to portray a youthful, enthusiastic investigator with the inscription *Nondum, O mors* ("Not yet, O death").[37]

McKenzie was a charming gentleman with a sense of humor that could be grim but never caustic or demeaning. Yet he always quarreled with the medical profession's choice of the caduceus as its symbol. He pointed out that the two-snaked caduceus is the staff of Hermes, or

Mercury, the god of commerce, bankers, usurers, and cattle thieves. The true symbol, he insisted, was a single snake coiled around a wooden club, the staff of Aesculapius, the god of medicine.[38]

PHYSICAL MEDICINE AND REHABILITATION

When the Agnew Wing opened in 1897, it contained a "room for the development of muscle power" equipped with apparatus for mechanical massage, gymnastics, applying super-heated air as well as mechanical massage and passive and Swedish movements.[39] These facilities were under the direction of Anna S. Kite. In 1911 a Physical Laboratory was established in addition to the orthopedic gymnasium. The new facility contained baths, equipment for administering dry heat, and appliances for hydrotherapeutic measures. At this time R. Tait McKenzie was appointed professor of physical therapy and Josef B. Nylin, a Swedish physician, was appointed chief of the laboratory. McKenzie gradually phased out his work in physical medicine in the mid 1920s and retired in 1930.[40] Josef Nylin continued as chief of the clinic of physical medicine and rehabilitation until his death in 1945.[41] In 1947 George Morris Piersol was made the first professor of physical medicine and rehabilitation at the University Hospital. William J. Erdman succeeded Piersol as chairman of the department in 1952.[42]

MERKEL JACOBS

Merkel Jacobs came from an academic family; one of his ancestors founded Gettysburg College.[43] The family were adventurous outdoors as well, and Jacobs took treks to the remote wilderness. During one expedition in 1907, when Jacobs was still a graduate student, Edward Heacock, a fellow student in the party, drowned after his canoe overturned in a rushing mountain stream. On another trip that year, a rock fell on Jacobs's leg, fracturing his femur. Herbert Ives, a medical student with the expedition, set the fracture; but it took seven and a half days for Ives and the others (including Jacobs's father and two brothers) to carry Jacobs to a railroad; he finished the trip strapped to the cowcatcher of a locomotive.[44]

Jacobs earned his Ph.D. from Penn in 1908, studied biology in Berlin, then returned to Penn as an instructor in zoology. In 1923 he was appointed professor of general physiology. He also devoted much scientific effort to the Marine Biological Laboratories at Woods Hole, Massachusetts. He rose through the ranks there to the post of director and then trustee.

At Penn Jacobs helped to teach medical undergraduates, although his main responsibility was the education of graduate students and

Medical professors, 1921. Front row: *Neilason, Abbott, Piersol, Marshall, Pepper, Deaver, Lark, Fussel, Meeker, Griffith, Heisler.* Second row: *Riesman, McFarland, Pancoast, Burr, Gill, Taylor, Richards, Wood, Egbert, Addison, Sweet.* Third row: *Stangel, Thomas, Spiller, Hartsell, Grayson, Sailer, Frazier, Stevens. (David Y. Cooper, photograph saved from trash by H. M. Vars.)*

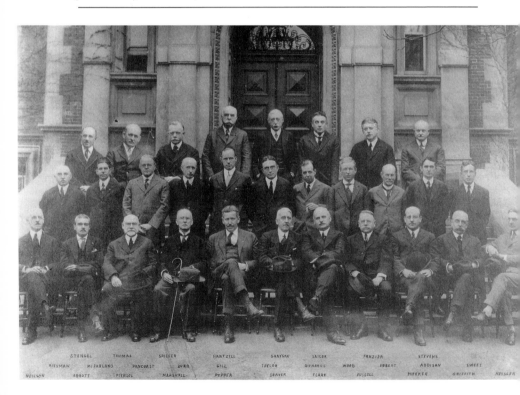

students from other departments. He developed a course in advanced general physiology with David R. Goddard, Lewis V. Heilbrunn, and Rudolph O. A. Hoeber; by many accounts, it was acclaimed as one of the best in the discipline offered anywhere. One of his legacies is the generations of students whom he trained who went on to productive academic careers at Penn and elsewhere.

In 1927 Jacobs was asked to deliver a Harvey Lecture on the subject of the erythrocyte membrane. He had not published any work on that membrane, and in the lecture he cited only one of his papers, a study of the permeability of cells to ammonia gas. In this lecture he displayed his ability to analyze mathematically the physical properties of the diffusion process. He later published a paper called "Diffusion Processes," which was a more detailed presentation of his analysis. A seminal piece for its time, the article was reprinted in 1967 not from historical curiosity but for basic information on processes of cellular diffusion processes; it is still up-to-date, enjoying a remarkable shelf life for a scientific paper.[45]

NOTES

1. Conversation with C. F. Schmidt (February 1983).
2. *Ibid.*
3. *Ibid.*
4. *Ibid.*
5. *Ibid.*
6. Conversation with C. F. Schmidt; K. K. Chen and C. F. Schmidt, "The Action of Ephedrine, The Active Principle of the Chinese Drug Ma Huang," *Journal of Pharmacology and Experimental Therapeutics* 24(1924):339–57.
7. T. G. Miller, "Ephedrine—Its Use in the Treatment of Vascular Hypotension and Bronchial Asthma." *Annals of Clinical Medicine* 4(1926):132–35; T. G. Miller, "A Consideration of the Clinical Value of Epinephrine," *American Journal of Medical Sciences* 170 (1925):157–81; G. Fetterolf and M. B. Sponsler, "Epinephrine Sulphate the Alkaloid of Ma Huang. Effects of Local Application on Nasal Mucous Membranes," Preliminary Report, *Archives of Otolaryngology* 2(1926):713–21.
8. Taped interview with Isaac Starr, by David Y.Cooper (March 1983).
9. *Ibid.*
10. *Ibid.*
11. *Ibid.*
12. *Ibid.*
13. *Ibid.*
14. *Ibid.*
15. *Ibid.*
16. *Ibid.*

17. *Ibid.*

18. Interview with Isaac Starr; I. Starr and A. Nordergraaf, *Ballistocardiography in Cardiovascular Research, Physical Aspects of the Circulation in Health and Disease* (Amsterdam: North Holland, 1967), pp. 82–83, 377–81, 245.

19. A. C. Burton, "Obituary—Henry Cuthbert Bazett," *Lancet* 259 (1950):308–9; L. H. Newbery and O. G. Edholm, "Prof. H. C. Bazett, C.B.E.," *Nature* 166(1950):933.

20. Edholm, "Prof. H. C. Bazett," p. 933.

21. H. C. Bazett, "Theory of Reflex Controls to Explain Regulation of Body Temperature at Rest and During Exercise," *Journal of Applied Physiology* 4(1951):245–61.

22. Personal recollections of David Y. Cooper.

23. Conversations with Dr. H. B. Lehr.

24. E. R. Long and D. T. Rowlands, *The Development of Department of Pathology in the School of Medicine of the University of Pennsylvania* (Philadelphia: Privately printed, 1977); E. R. Long, *A History of Pathology in America* (Springfield, Ill.: Charles C. Thomas, 1962).

25. B. Lucké, "Carcinoma in the Leopard Frog: Its Probable Causation a Virus," *Journal of Experimental Medicine* (1938):457–68; B. Lucké, "Carcinoma of Kidney in Leopard Frog and Significance of Metastasis," *American Journal of Cancer* 34(1938):15–30.

26. Long and Rowlands, pp. 47–49.

27. Letter from Eugene Landis to David Y. Cooper, June 21, 1983; W. O. Fenn, *History of the American Physiological Society: The Third Quarter Century, 1937–1962* (Washington, D.C.: American Physiological Society, 1963), pp. 26–29; A. P. Fishman and D. W. Richards, eds., *Circulation of the Blood: Men and Ideas* (Bethesda, Md.: American Physiological Society, 1962), pp. 355–406.

28. Landis letter, 1983.

29. E. M. Landis, "The Capillary Pressure in Frog Mesentery as Determined by Micro-Injection Methods," *American Journal of Physiology* 75 (1926):548–70; E. M. Landis, "Capillary Pressure and Capillary Permeability," *Physiological Reviews* 14(1934):404–81.

30. E. B. Krumbhaar, "Memoir of Tait McKenzie, M.D.," *Transactions and Studies of the College of Physicians of Philadelphia* 4th ser., 6 (1938–1939):260–61; J. McGill, *The Joy of Effort: A Biography of R. Tait McKenzie* (Ontario: Clay Publishers, 1980); C. Hussey, *Tait McKenzie: A Sculptor of Youth* (Philadelphia: Lippincott, 1930); A. Kozar, *R. Tait McKenzie the Sculptor of Athletes* (Knoxville: Univ. of Tennessee Press, 1975); D. Y. Cooper, "R. Tait McKenzie Athlete, Physical Educator, Artist," *Transactions and Studies of the College of Physicians of Philadelphia* 5th ser., 7 (1985):131–39.

31. Cooper, "Tait McKenzie," p. 132.

32. *Ibid.*, p. 131.

33. McKenzie Papers, Archives of the University of Pennsylvania; Cooper, "Tait McKenzie," pp. 132–33.

34. R. T. McKenzie, *Exercise in Education and Medicine* (Philadelphia: Saunders, 1909, 1915, 1923); R. Tait McKenzie, *Reclaiming the Maimed* (New York: Macmillan, 1918); R. F. Fox, *Physical Remedies for Disabled Soldiers* (London: Balliere, Tindall and Cox, 1917). R. T. McKenzie wrote the ninth chapter entitled "Massage, Passive Movement, Mechanical Treatment and Exercise."

35. Hussey, *Tait McKenzie, Sculptor of Youth:* "Over the Top," p. 58; "The Homecoming," p. 64; "The Victor," p. 68; "Capt. Drummond," p. 60.

36. Hussey, *Tait McKenzie, Sculptor of Youth:* "Gen. James Wolf," pp. 77–80; "The Call," pp. 71–76; "Young Franklin," pp. 50–53.

37. Krumbhaar, "Memoir of Tait McKenzie."

38. R. T. McKenzie, "Notes on some medals and plaquettes relating to medical men and events," *Transactions and Studies of the College of Physicians of Philadelphia*, 4th ser., 3–4 (1935–37):8–13.

39. Program for the Opening of the Agnew Wing at the Hospital of the University of Pennsylvania (Philadelphia: Lippincott, 1897).

40. Annual Report of the Hospital of the University of Pennsylvania, (July 1, 1911–June 30, 1912, p. 128; July 1, 1912–June 30, 1913, p. 15).

41. Annual Report of H.U.P., July 1, 1925–June 30, 1926; July 1, 1930–June 30, 1931.

42. T. G. Miller, "Memoir of George Morris Piersol, 1880–1966," *Transactions and Studies of the College of Physicians of Philadelphia*, 4th ser., 34(1966–1967):159–60.

43. J. R. Brobeck,"Merkel Henry Jacobs, (1884–1970)," *Biographical Memoirs* (American Philosophical Society, 1970), 137–40.

44. H. Palmer, *Mountaineering and Exploration in the Selkirks* (New York: G. P. Putnam's Sons, 1914).

45. M. Jacobs, "Diffusion Processes," *Ergebnisse der Biologie* 12 (1935):2–160; M. H. Jacobs, "The Exchange of Material Between the Erythrocyte and its Surroundings," *The Harvey Lectures* 22(1927):146–64.

14
THE MALONEY CONSTELLATION AND A SEVERE SELF-EXAMINATION

The high prize of life, the crowning fortune of a man is to be born with a bias to some pursuit, which finds him in employment and happiness.

Ralph Waldo Emerson

Alfred Stengel, who became professor of medicine when Edsall resigned in 1911, had a profound, though largely overlooked, effect on academic medicine. He was a builder, like the Peppers, who were his in-laws (he married a cousin of William Pepper, III). He developed a strong clinical department with specialty sections and encouraged research. Medical observers have criticized Stengel for not installing a full-time medical staff in his department, but he made other contributions. He consolidated the hospital services, unified and increased the outpatient traffic, improved the service at Philadelphia General Hospital, brought fourth-year students onto the wards as clinical clerks, and increased the outpatient work of third-year students; and during his term he increased his medical staff from two to eight.[1]

Perhaps most important, Stengel seized the opportunities in the advancing specialization within internal medicine, although the first step was halting enough. In 1919 the Hospital of the University of Pennsylvania established a "cardiac clinic" as part of the medical outpatient service.[2] For nine years it struggled on as the only specialty in medicine. Stengel realized that new sciences and specialties could be fostered by proper housing. He introduced his idea for a new out-

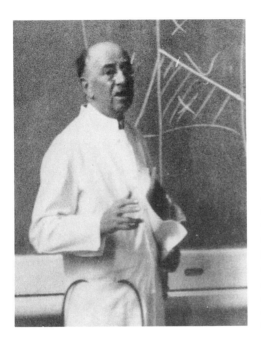

Alfred Stengel, Professor of Medicine, first Vice President in Charge of Medical Affairs. Originator of the Maloney Clinic and, with Eldridge Reeves Johnson, founded the Johnson Foundation. (Photograph Album of Norris Smith, Archives of the University of Pessnylvania.)

patient clinic at a dinner honoring Fred H. Klaer's tenth anniversary as chief of the medical outpatient department in the early 1920s. Stengel outlined his plans for a salaried staff, elaborately equipped research laboratories, X-ray facilities, a comprehensive social-service department, and an efficient clerical force.[3]

Stengel's dream materialized as the Martin Maloney Clinic, completed in 1929 and named for a donor who made a gift of $350,000.[4] At the time the Maloney Clinic was unique. It was not a new hospital or new hospital unit with a single purpose, but a supplementary section of the medical clinic, having multiple functions all connected with the evolving requirements of modern medicine. It housed a medical outpatient department with special sections for cardiovascular disease (headed by Charles C. Wolferth), gastrointestinal disease (headed by T. Grier Miller), allergy (headed by Richard Kern), chest conditions, diabetes, thyroid problems (headed by Edward Rose), and blood diseases (headed by Thomas FitzHugh). It also contained the William Pepper Laboratory of Clinical Medicine, the Eldridge R. Johnson Foundation of Medical Physics, the Department of Physical Therapy, a morgue and autopsy department, a pharmacy, a hospital library, a floor for animal research, twenty-three private rooms, and offices for certain members of the medical staff.[5]

The first three floors of the nine-story building were devoted to the care of ambulatory patients. Organizationally the department was separated into a division for general medical care, which taught medicine to third-year students, and a division for subspecialties, which focused on clinical research, although it offered clinical experience to fourth-year students.[6]

Cardiology, the first of HUP's medical subspecialties, began, primitively enough, when Stengel purchased an early model of an Einthoven electrocardiograph just after World War I. At first Edward Krumbhaar, who was in research medicine at the time, used the instrument. When he transferred to pathology not long afterwards, the device was turned over to Charles Wolferth.[7]

CHARLES C. WOLFERTH

Wolferth was born at Wolferth Station (named for his grandfather) near Clarksboro, New Jersey. His father was a farmer who poked into agricultural research, so his son had early exposure to the importance of new ideas. While at Penn's medical school, he played varsity football but attempted to drop the sport during his fourth year.[8] J. William White, an ardent football fan, asked him why. Wolferth told him that he had slighted his studies for football up to that year but now preferred to concentrate on obtaining a good internship. "Where do you want to intern?" White asked. "Here," Wolferth answered. White told him to play football and promised him the internship. Wolferth served two years as an intern and another year in clinical pathology, then became the hospital's first medical resident, in 1915–16.[9]

Wolferth was a penetrating and logical thinker, a quality which helped him master the experimental approach to clinical science. He also had a vast knowledge of cardiology and of medicine generally. After being mustered out of the Army following World War I, he worked with England's famous heart specialist, Sir Thomas Lewis. When he returned to Penn, Stengel assigned him the task of organizing and directing a heart station at the hospital. Wolferth organized the new

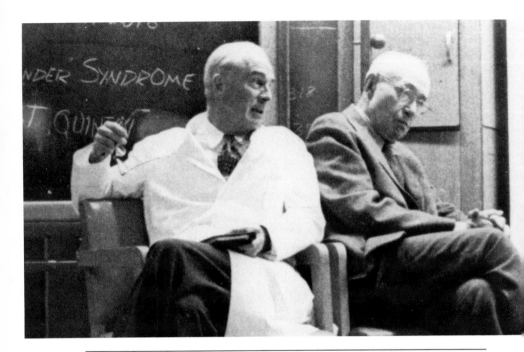

*Charles C. Wolferth (*left*) and Francis C. Wood at a medical seminar. (Scope.)*

clinic on a pattern he learned from Lewis. Shortly after it was started, Edward B. Robinette endowed the clinic.[10]

Personally Wolferth tended to work alone. He attended few national meetings but read scientific journals avidly. He also had a dry sense of humor with which he twitted the peculiarities of his patients, his colleagues, and himself. He was heard to say, "I like my patients to have a lot of bad habits—their prognosis is better." When someone once flattered him, he observed, "It's amazing how an otherwise intelligent, critical person will believe absolutely anything about himself, no matter how fantastic, provided it's complimentary."[11]

Although the staff concentrated on clinical practice, Wolferth encouraged the junior staff to do original work by suggesting stimulating problems that they could examine in the laboratory or the heart clinic. The Robinette Foundation was interested in correlating the heart sounds heard through the stethoscope with the electrocardiograph tracing and the mechanism of cardiac arrythmias. Wolferth himself, along with Francis C. Wood, a young associate, made two pertinent and important discoveries.[12]

One concerned precordial electrocardiogram leads, which improved the ability to diagnose acute myocardial infarction. It also involved the current theories of the cause of angina pectoris. In the early 1930s two theories tried to explain the pain of angina pectoris. One was that it was produced by myocardial ischemia due to disease of the coronary arteries. The other was that anginal pain was caused by distension of the first part of the diseased aorta.

In 1931 one of Wolferth's patients had a spontaneous attack of anginal pain while sitting in the electrocardiographic chair. The attack occurred shortly after a tracing had been taken. A second electrocardiogram recorded during the attack showed changes not present in the first. The change in readings indicated to Wolferth that angina is due to myocardial ischemia. He suggested to Wood that they study electrocardiograms on dogs before, during, and after brief coronary obstruction.[13]

Wood tried clamping the anterior descending and right coronary arteries in turn, using conventional Einthoven limb leads, but found no definite changes in the EKG readings. Pressed for time one day, he clamped all three coronary arteries at once—the anterior descending, the right, and the circumflex. Dramatic changes occurred in leads two and three. Wood later produced the change by clamping the posterior descending artery alone.[14]

What puzzled Wood was that the skin appeared bluish, indicating lack of blood, after either the anterior descending artery or the posterior descending artery was clamped, but the EKG changed only when the latter was occluded. This observation prompted him to put an electrode on the anterior wall of the heart, clamp the anterior vessel, and take the EKG. He found a definite change in that tracing but not in the limb leads.[15]

Since some coronary occlusions in patients do not show up on the EKG, Wolferth suggested that Wood put an electrode on the chest over a patient's heart. That afternoon, an ideal patient entered the office; she had an acute coronary occlusion that produced no diagnostic changes on the EKG. Wood set up the machine as planned. The new lead showed a dramatic change in the S-T segment. It worked simply because it was closer to the damaged region of the heart and could readily detect the disturbed electrical changes. Wolferth and Wood's introduction of the precordial lead significantly extended the diagnostic capabilities of the electrocardiogram. The work also was one of many experiments establishing that heart ischemia caused the pain of angina pectoris.[16]

Wolferth and Wood also collaborated to explain the W.P.W. syndrome. Wolff, Parkinson, and White suggested that the syndrome was due to a functional bundle branch block. Wolferth was skeptical because heart block should have produced different EKG results.[17] He remembered an article by A. F. Stanley Kent, a British physician, who described a structure bridging the atrioventricular groove on the right side of the heart.[18] After some research, Wolferth and Wood published an article that reconciled both the electrocardiographic and the clinical findings of patients with W.P.W. syndrome: the excitatory process was conducted through Kent's bundle as well as through the bundle of His. The present interest in studies of conduction defects originated with this pioneering work.[19]

T. GRIER MILLER

The accomplishments of the gastrointestinal clinic, organized by T. Grier Miller in 1926, include the work of Joseph Stokes and John R. Neefe, who showed that there are two types of viral hepatitis; the studies of Katherine O'Shea Elsom on the effects of vitamin deficiency on the gastrointestinal tract; and a clinic for patients with psychiatric disorders related to intestinal function, the precursor of the hospital's Department of Psychiatry. Miller himself joined with William Osler Abbott to develop the first reliable method of introducing a tube into the jejunum and ileum.[20]

Miller earned his undergraduate degree from the University of North Carolina and entered the textile business. But a philosophy professor, Horace Williams, had encouraged him to be an independent thinker, and Miller found himself out of step with other textile executives. He decided to try medical school for a year and chose Penn for his experiment. The term convinced him that only medicine would "satisfy his curiosities and ambitions." He expected to become a surgeon, and in fact had been helping a surgeon in his hometown of Statesville, North Carolina, during his summer vacations; but Stengel offered him the first

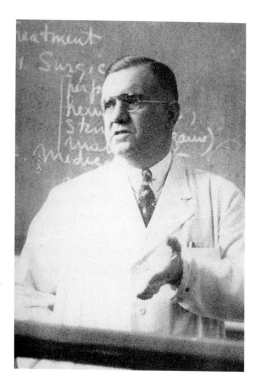

T. Grier Miller lecturing in the Medical Lecture Room. (Photograph Album of Norris Smith, Archives of the University of Pennsylvania.)

medical fellowship granted at the University; it paid $400 a year. Stengel's associate in private practice died at the end of the year, and Miller was given his position; thus he had a private practice while participating in the hospital's clinical activities.[21]

Prior to 1934, gastroenterologists had no reliable technique for passing a tube beyond the duodenum in humans to sample intestinal contents or relieve obstructions. One method, dating from 1919, used an Einhorn's tube; but it was time-consuming, and on those occasions when it was successfully passed into the jejunum and ileum, adequate samples did not always pass through the tube's small lumen.[22]

A chance conversation with Abbott changed clinical procedure. Abbott was the son of Alexander C. Abbott, erstwhile professor of bacteriology and director of the School of Hygiene and Public Health at Penn. His mother was Georgiana Osler, a niece of Sir William Osler, but the younger Abbott made every effort not to trade on his name; in fact, he was called Pete. He specialized in pharmacology.[23] One of his major papers was entitled "Problems of a Professional Guinea Pig."[24]

He had been studying the absorption of electrolytes and foods from the gastrointestinal tract of dogs. In his experiments he used two balloons attached by a cord in order to isolate segments of the bowel at representative levels of the jejunum and ileum. Miller happened to ask how the work was getting along. Abbott complained that he could not control the area of the intestinal tract he intended to isolate because the inflated balloons were pulled down the intestines by the peristaltic waves. Miller saw at once the solution to his own problem. He proposed to Abbott that they hook a balloon to a gastrointestinal tube and have the intestinal peristalsis move the tube to any area of the jejunum or ileum.[25]

The idea seemed reasonable to Abbott. He did not believe in conducting experiments on animals when he could do them in humans, so

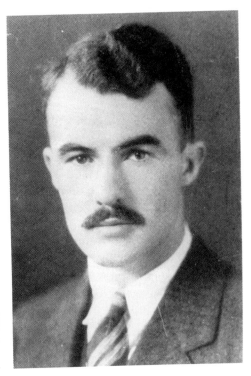

William Osler Abbott. (Historical Collections of the College of Physicians of Philadelphia.)

he built a double-lumen tube with a balloon on the end and immediately tried it in patients. It worked, but to introduce it into clinical use, Abbott and Miller had difficulty finding a manufacturer to make the small tubes. They approached some fifty manufacturers of medical rubber products before they found one to produce their apparatus. The device is still used today for experimental studies as well as for managing intestinal obstructions and for postoperative care of patients who have had serious bowel surgery.[26]

THE GEORGE S. COX INSTITUTE

The George S. Cox Institute was another unit developed through Stengel's efforts.[27] It is a clinical research division of the Department of Medicine and was founded to "find a cure for diabetes mellitus," as a plaque on the eighth floor of the Maloney Clinic states. Institute researchers have produced interesting diabetes work, but one of the most significant studies done there was in another realm: the synthesis of 10-norprogesterone and Maximilian Ehrenstein's discovery that this new steroid exerted its activity even when administered orally—a key step in developing oral contraceptives.

The Cox Institute was opened in 1932 and has had only three directors: Cyril Norman Hugh Long, Francis D. W. Lukens, and Albert Winegrad. Long served for only four years, but in that period made the scientific contributions that determined the remainder of his career.[28]

He was an Englishman who began his research before he became an M.D. He was in organic chemistry when he joined A. V. Hill, a physiology professor at the University of Manchester. Hill was working on the chemical changes involved in muscle contraction, studying the breakdown of glycogen and the formation of lactic acid. He needed a chemist to develop methods for measuring blood levels of these substances in animals and humans during exercise. Long at first was not interested because he had little experience in biology. Furthermore, biochemistry was held in low esteem by pure chemists because it involved extracts of cells, blood, and other body fluids that could not be analyzed with the precise methods of pure chemistry. But Long joined Hill and shortly realized that he enjoyed unraveling the secrets contained in the "biological mess." He published papers with Hill and others on lactic acid formation in exercise and its relation to oxygen consumption.

Hill recommended Long for a position in muscle chemistry at McGill University in Montreal. Long went there and earned his medical degree in 1928 while continuing his research, which he extended to include conditions of anesthesia and diabetes. He was recruited as the Cox Institute's first director and quickly saw the advantages for himself: complete freedom to investigate his own ideas, contact with clinical medicine without direct responsibility for patient care, and association

The early members of the George Cox Foundation. Front row, left to right: *Margaret Gerstley, Edith Fry, Miss Case, Elizabeth Barth, Dorothy Quinn.* Second Row, left to right: *W. C. Whitaker, Maurice Bowie, C. N. H. Long, F. C. Dohan, Russel Richardson, F. D. W. Lukens, Gerald Evans.*

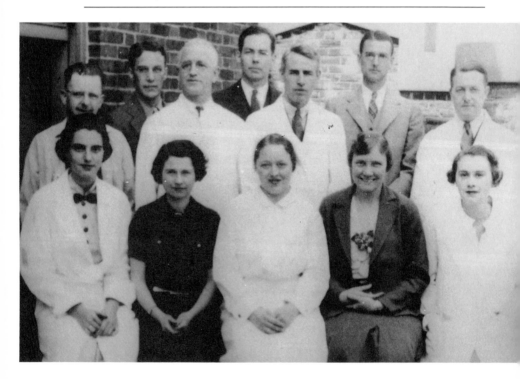

with such innovative scientists as Alfred Newton Richards and Detlev Bronk. The first colleague to join him was Lukens, who was working with Miller in gastroenterology and who would, in a few years, succeed Long as the institute's director.[29]

When Long and Lukens began their work in the Cox Institute, all symptoms of diabetes mellitus were assumed to stem from an underutilization of sugar caused by a lack of insulin. A few years earlier, Bernardo Houssay had discovered that removing the pituitary gland from diabetic dogs ameliorated diabetic symptoms remarkably. Although Long realized that pancreatic dysfunction was the major reason diabetic patients could not utilize sugar, he also knew that removing the cortical portion of the adrenal gland lowered blood sugar and that the adrenal gland atrophied after the pituitary gland was removed.

Long and Lukens started to investigate the role of the adrenal cortex in regulating sugar levels in diabetes. They removed the adrenal gland and pancreas from cats and found that the animals lived eleven days longer than the usual diabetic cat and had lower blood-sugar levels than the controls with only the pancreas removed. The scientists pointed out that the diabetes was ameliorated by the absence of adrenocortical function, not by the lack of medullary or "nervous" function of the adrenal gland, as had been thought. And they observed that body sugar was lowered after the adrenalectomy because other sources of sugar, mainly protein, were reduced.

The adrenalectomy, of course, did not cure diabetes, but Long and Lukens showed that the pituitary and other ductless glands helped produce the clinical picture of diabetes. Long generalized his thesis before the American College of Physicians in 1936, and it remains sound advice today: "The clinical condition that follows hypo- or hyperfunction of an endocrine organ is not merely due to the loss or plethora of that particular internal secretion but is a result of the disturbance of the normal equilibrium of the body."[30]

By 1936, Long had filled the Cox Institute with other collaborators and guests, including the prominent Houssay, whose "office" consisted of a desk at the end of the corridor. Long's reputation, too, had spread, and he was lured to Yale University, where he later rose to be dean of the medical school. He continued his work on the relationship of the pituitary gland to disease, focusing on the relationship of that gland to the hypothalamus. One of his collaborators was John Brobeck, who was recruited to Penn to succeed Bazett as chairman of physiology after Bazett died in 1951.[31]

REORGANIZATION OF THE UNIVERSITY AND MEDICAL SCHOOL

While the clinical work was advancing, the medical school underwent a reexamination as thorough as the original path for medical education set by John Morgan in his *Discourse*. It was precipitated by a change in the top administration of the University. Penn had always been headed by a "provost"; but in the 1920s the trustees created the position of president to govern the University when they tried to lure General Leonard Wood to Pennsylvania. Under this plan the provost would serve as the chief educational officer. General Leonard Wood, however, delayed assuming his duties. After two years of correspondence. the trustees became impatient and Wood resigned (1922). This dilemma was solved by electing Josiah Penniman to serve as president as well as provost. In 1926 the title of president was abolished. Four years later the trustees reestablished the office of president and elected Thomas S. Gates to fill this office.

In 1926 three vice provosts, one responsible for faculty personnel and relations, one in charge of student government, and one in charge of public relations, were created to aid Dr. Penniman in governing the university. In 1928 these duties of the three vice provosts were redefined when vice provosts in charge of undergraduate departments, administration and—a new jurisdiction—of medical departments were created. Because of the enormous responsibilities of the new position, it remained empty for three years. Finally in 1931 Alfred Stengel accepted the position. By that time, the title had been changed to vice president in charge of medical affairs (later health affairs), and he was responsible for the Schools of Dental Medicine, Medicine, Veterinary Medicine, and School of Nursing, the Graduate School of Medicine, the Hospital of the University of Pennsylvania, and the Graduate Hospital. Stengel retained his chairmanship of medicine.[32]

THE RICHARDS-MILLER REPORT

Before Stengel was appointed, Gates commissioned a confidential assessment of the medical school, figuring that such advice would be useful to whoever was chosen as the new vice president for medical affairs. Gates chose Richards and Miller, a basic scientist and a clinician involved in research, for the difficult but important assignment.[33]

Richards and Miller talked to trustees, departmental chairmen, deans, managers and superintendents of the hospitals, directors, and, going outside, leaders in American medical education and science. They concluded:

> Our school embodies one major inconsistency. Our preclinical departments with one exception have become centers of experimental research, and a genuine attempt has been made to give instruction to the student in the spirit of investigation in order that he may cultivate the power of independent thought upon which his future development must rest. In the clinical subjects we think that the instruction is so largely directed at his practical training that the investigative foundation of clinical medicine suffers from relative neglect. . . . Our students in the clinical years do not feel that they are part of an organization which accepts as a major responsibility the enlargement of medical knowledge by modern experimental methods.[34]

The report was never released to the public. Clearly written and as candid and critical as it could be, considering that the authors were passing judgment on their colleagues, it gives a picture of the strengths and weaknesses of a great and proud and sometimes tradition-bound medical school.[35]

Richards and Miller felt that the administrative organization of the school was left too much in the hands of its executive committee, which, they suggested, guided the school laxly and with more regard for the problems of its particular members than for the part that individual activities played in the accomplishments and direction of the school as a whole. They suggested that the hospital replace its nurse supervisors with a male director and that that director and the anticipated vice president for medical affairs reorient the executive committee. They did not give a role to the dean of the medical school. From 1765 the medical faculty had grown in decentralized fashion into departments, and the dean traditionally served as a sort of executive secretary rather than a leader; that model was to be maintained.[36]

The authors were generally enthusiastic about the basic-science departments, which had staffs distinctly larger than is "required for teaching necessities, leaving for each member of the preclinical faculty an impressive fraction of his time for investigative work." They had high praise for anatomy, especially Eliot R. Clark's research on the anatomy of living cells, in which he employed original techniques designed by him and his wife. As a teacher Clark deemphasized the memorization of body parts and their interrelationships, favoring instead fine dissections, accurate observation, and penetrating interpretations. It was a freedom that students did not fully use, Richards and Miller said, but added that Clark underestimated the "wholesomeness" both of some rigid discipline and of the difficult comprehensive examination, distinctive parts of earlier teaching.[37]

Richards and Miller called physiological chemistry one of the best-organized departments, but considered biochemistry too theoretical; it could be made more clinically oriented by choosing chemists more familiar with clinical problems, they advised. They also praised the original research in physiology as well as its laboratory course for first-year students, but felt that the average student was not as interested in it "[as] its intrinsic interest would seem to warrant." They wanted the faculty in both departments to make special efforts to excite students about the field.[38]

The department of bacteriology received the most severe criticism: it had not been reorganized, the faculty were generally unproductive, and students gave the courses neither interest nor respect. Richards and Miller stopped just short of recommending that bacteriology be dropped from the medical curriculum. The severe rebuke was successful. Following their advice, the department was moved to the Medical Laboratories Building and newly equipped for research. Stuart Mudd was appointed chairman and undertook the overdue reforms.[39]

Richards was able to criticize his own department of pharmacology. Its laboratory courses were so rigid and the didactic teaching so excessive that students had little time to think independently, he and Miller stated. They recommended a sort of independent study, in which students would take a subject, design and arrange their own experiments, and carry them through to decisive outcomes.[40]

As for the clinical departments, the physicians noted that Penn had a long-standing reputation for the teaching given to the "intending practitioner of medicine." Even though the clinical faculty often enjoyed nationwide reputations, the authors continued admonishingly, they had not made a fundamental advance in medical science for nearly 30 years.[41]

Richards and Miller had other suggestions. The school should build a new and expanded medical library.[42] It should remember that the Hospital of the University of Pennsylvania "was not primarily established to add to the resources of the city for caring for the sick" but for "instruction and study."[43] It should make the chairman of medicine a full-time post with a salaried staff.[44] It should radically revamp neurology by taking advantage of a recent $200,000 gift for neurological research, plus a proposed merger of the private Orthopaedic Hospital and the Institute for the Study of Neurological Diseases.[45] And it should assemble a faculty of first-rate scientists, clinicians, and teachers at the newly affiliated Children's Hospital of Philadelphia.[46] There was yet more.

Some of Richards and Miller's recommendations have been implemented, some have come to pass, some persist as problems. At the time they were handed up, only a few, chiefly high-placed members of the faculty were privileged to see what had been written; and many of them criticized Richards and Miller for overemphasizing research. It was hardly a criticism that it would have behooved Penn to heed.[47]

NOTES

1. "The Medical Story from Stengel to Wood," *University of Pennsylvania Medical Bulletin* (January 1956); papers of Charles C. Wolferth (hereafter WP), College of Physicians of Philadelphia; Papers of Alfred Stengel (hereafter SP) Archives of the University of Pennsylvania.
2. WP.
3. WP; SP.
4. WP; SP.
5. WP; SP.
7. WP; SP.
8. F. C. Wood, "Memoir of Charles C. Wolferth, 1887–1965," *Transactions and Studies of the College of Physicians of Philadelphia* 4th ser., 34(1967):157–58; T. G. Miller, "Charles C. Wolferth, 1887–1965." *Transactions of the Association of American Physicians* 79(1966):81–83.
9. Wood, "Memoir of Charles C. Wolferth"; Miller, "Charles C. Wolferth, 1887–1965", p. 155.
10. Wood, "Memoir of Charles C. Wolferth," p. 156.
11. *Ibid.*, p. 157.
12. *Ibid.*, p. 156.
13. F. C. Wood and C. C. Wolferth, "Experimental Coronary Occlusion. Inadequacy of the Conventional Leads for Recording Characteristic Action Current Changes in Certain Sections of the Myocardium; An Electrocardiographic Study." *Archives of Internal Medicine* 49 (1933):771–78; F. C. Wood and C. C. Wolferth, "Angina Pectoris. The Clinical and Electrocardiographic Phenomena of the Attack and the Comparison

with the Effects of Experimental Temporary Coronary Occlusion," *Annals of Internal Medicine* 47(1931): 340–65.

14. Conversation with Francis C. Wood.

15. Conversation with Wood.

16. Conversation with Wood.

17. L. Wolff, J. Parkinson, and P. D. White, "Bundle Branch Block with Short P-R Intervals in Healthy Young People Prone to Paroxysmal Tachycardia," *American Heart Journal* 5(1930): 685–704.

18. Conversation with Wood.

19. C. C. Wolferth and F. C. Wood, "The Mechanism of Production of Short P-R Intervals and Prolonged QRS Complexes in Patients with Presumably Undamaged Hearts, Hypothesis of an Accessory Pathway of the Auricular Ventricular Conduction (Bundle of Kent)," *American Heart Journal* 8(1933):297–311.

20. Frank P. Brooks, "T. Grier Miller, 1886–1981." *Transactions and Studies of the College of Physicians of Philadelphia* 5th ser., 4(1982):80–83.

21. *Ibid.*

22. T. Grier Miller and William Osler Abbott, "Intestinal Intubation: A Practical Technique," *American Journal of Medical Sciences* 187(1934):595–99.

23. T. G. Miller, "William Osler Abbott, M. D," *Transactions of the Clinical and Climatological Society* 58 (1946):lxxxiii–lxxxv; W. C. Stadie, "William Osler Abbott." *Transactions and Studies of the College of Physicians of Philadelphia* 4th ser., 12(1944):119–20; Archibald Mallock, "William Osler Abbott (1902–1943)," *Proceedings of the Charaka Club* 11(1947):207–10.

24. W. O. Abbott, "The Problems of a Professional Guinea Pig." *Proceedings of the Charaka Club* 10(1941):249–60.

25. Personal recollections of David Y. Cooper from conversations with David Alexander Cooper, Francis C. Wood, and T. Grier Miller.

26. Miller and Abbott, "Intestinal Intubation."

27. Conversation with Francis C. Wood; conversation with Albert Winegrad.

28. O. L. K. Smith and J. D. Hardy, "Cyril Norman Hugh Long," *Biographical Memoirs of the National Academy of Science* 46(1975):265–309; J. S. Fruton, "Cyril Normal Hugh Long (1901–1970)," *Year Book of the American Physiological Society* (Philadelphia: American Philosophical Society, 1970), pp. 143–45.

29. *Ibid.*

30. C. N. H. Long and F. D. W. Lukens, "Observations on Adrenalectomized Depancreatized Cats," *Science* 79(1934): 569–71; C. N. H. Long, "Recent Studies on the Function of the Adrenal Cortex," *Bulletin of the Johns Hopkins Hospital* 78 (1946):317–21; C. N. H. Long, "Diabetes mellitus in the Light of Our Present Knowledge of Metabolism," *Transactions and Studies of the College of Physicians of Philadelphia* 4th ser., 7 (1939):21–46.

31. J. Brobeck, J. Tepperman, and C. N. H. Long, "Experimental Hypothalamic Hyperphagia in Albino Rat," *Yale Journal of Biology and Medicine* 15 (1943): 831–53; J. Brobeck, J. Tepperman, and C. N. H. Long, "The Effect of Experimental Obesity Upon Carbohydrate Metabolism," *Yale Journal of Biology and Medicine* 15(1943):893–904.

32. E. P. Cheney, *History of the University of Pennsylvania, 1740–1940* (Philadelphia: University of Pennsylvania Press, 1940), pp. 415–16, 420; G. W. Corner, *Two Centuries of Medicine* (Philadelphia: Lippincott, 1965), pp. 262–63.

33. Corner, *Two Centuries of Medicine*, pp. 291–93.

34. A. N. Richards and T. Grier Miller, *Survey of Medical Affairs, University of Pennsylvania*, pp. a–c, (hereafter RMR, for Richards–Miller Report).

35. Corner, p. 292.

36. RMR, pp. b–c.

37. RMR, pp. 1–3.

38. RMR, p. 4.

39. RMR, p. 7.

40. RMR, p. 13.

41. RMR, pp. 14–15.

42. RMR, pp. 10–11.

43. RMR, p. 17.

44. RMR, p. 18.

45. RMR, pp. 24–31.

46. RMR, pp. 62–65.

47. RMR. pp. 80–81.

15
MEDICAL PHYSICS

Imagination is more important than knowledge.

Alfred Einstein

The Eldridge Reeves Johnson Foundation for Medical Physics was the first department in the United States devoted to applying the laws of physics to biological and medical problems. As Stengel announced at the dedication ceremonies, it was charged with studying light and optics relating to sunlight, radium emanation, mercury and quartz-lamp rays, infrared rays, and X-rays; heat in diseases and treatment; sound and instrumental methods for improving hearing (it would also investigate the reproduction and physical effects of sounds); physical measurements in the human body, including heart action, blood flow, stomach and intestine movements, and air distribution; photographic and cinematographic study of body processes and conditions; and electricity in the diagnosis and treatment of disease.[1]

The foundation started with a $600,000 endowment from Eldridge R. Johnson, founder of the Victor Talking Machine Company and Stengel's patient; he gave another $200,000 to add a floor to the projected Maloney Clinic. The foundation opened in 1929 with Detlev W. Bronk as its director.[2]

DETLEV W. BRONK

Bronk taught physics at Penn for a year after graduating from Swarthmore College, then departed for the University of Michigan, where he began studying the physics of living organisms. To broaden his background, he earned a degree in physiology. He studied infrared spectroscopy in physics and the regulation of respiration in physiology.

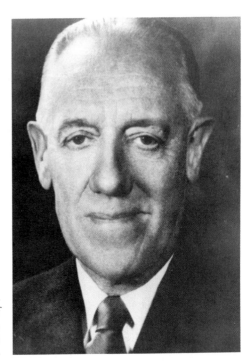

Detlev W. Bronk, first Director of the Johnson Foundation. (Archives of the University of Pennsylvania.)

Henry Cuthbert Bazett, who wanted assistance with his studies on temperature regulation by the central nervous system, brought Bronk back to the Philadelphia area. Bronk took a position in Bazett's laboratory, directing the research of graduate students and also teaching at Swarthmore.[3]

After a few years, Bronk, feeling he was not making sufficient scientific progress, took a fellowship under E. D. Adrian at Cambridge University in England. Adrian was working on nerve conduction. Bronk developed a technique for destroying most of the fibers of a nerve bundle while leaving a sufficient number intact to measure motor activity. He also developed an electrode consisting of a small needle with an insulated wire connected to an amplifier. The needle's sharp tip measured the electrical events in a small number of motor fibers without requiring the fibers to be cut. The instrument later became the electromyograph.[4] Bronk then went to London to study heat generation during muscle activity with A. V. Hill. Bronk's biophysical studies started him in the design and construction of electric instruments to make accurate physical measurements of biological systems—just the background he needed for the new foundation, which he returned to Penn to head.[5]

He assembled a group of associates, most of whom moved elsewhere after finishing a project or two and a few of whom followed him during his later peregrinations. One of their most important projects at Penn provided the basis for our present understanding of the regulation of blood pressure. Bronk and others investigated receptors for detecting changes in blood pressure, the central control centers, the properties of the efferent neuronal systems controlling heart rate, and the diameter of blood vessels. They also investigated the mediation of synaptic transmission. They discovered the important property of trans-synaptic excitation and the prolonged effect of previous activity. In 1937 Penn created a neurological institute to connect the biophysicists and neurological researchers.[6]

Bronk was frequently courted by other research institutions but turned them down until he accepted a post as professor of physiology at Cornell University's medical school in 1940; he took many of his most creative researchers with him. It was revealed later that funding for the Johnson Foundation was in jeopardy and Bronk did not appreciate the unsettledness. But they returned to Penn a year later. Cornell, they felt, was not hospitable to biophysics as an independent discipline and intellectual enterprise. He felt that he and his staff were looked on as mere technical specialists who were supposed to build instruments for the medical faculty, teach them how to use the devices, and repair them when they broke down.[7]

Meanwhile, Penn had resolved the budgetary problems that drove Bronk away. Alfred Newton Richards was not only in charge of medical research at Penn, but he directed the national effort in medical research through the Federal Office of Scientific Research and Development, created by Vannevar Bush. Richards obtained funds to study high-altitude physiology and the nocturnal visual acuity of pilots, and he knew that Bronk had been an aviator in World War I. So the Johnson Foundation, now that most of its major people had returned, collaborated with the Departments of Medicine, Pharmacology, and Physiology to study, among other things, the oxygenation of blood at high altitudes; some of the hemoglobin saturation curves used today resulted from their work.[8]

Ever restless, Bronk left Penn for good in 1948, when he accepted the presidency of Johns Hopkins University. Later he headed the Rockefeller Institute, which he renamed Rockefeller University.[9]

RAGNAR GRANIT AND HALDAN KEFFER HARTLINE

Ragnar Granit, a Finn who had received his M.D. degree from Helsinki University, worked with Adrian in England and was Bronk's first appointment to the Johnson Foundation.[10] He left in 1931, shortly after Haldan Keffer Hartline arrived. Both of them were pioneers in visual physiology and they quoted each other's work freely, but they never worked together. Nonetheless, they are linked forever as sharing the Nobel Prize in Medicine or Physiology. They were the first individuals associated with Penn to win a Nobel Prize, but they were not at the University when they won it.

At Penn Granit investigated the retinal action potential of the eyes of vertebrates, discovered some sixty-five years earlier. He found that the complex time course of the retina's response to light comprised three components. He advanced the theory that the visual responses are molded by an interplay of excitation and inhibition, and his representation of the interplay of the factors forms the basis of the interpretation of the electroretinogram. To explain the relationship between receptor excitation and the generation of nervous activity, he originated the concept of the generator potential, a mechanism that converted the logarithmic signal of the stimulus to a linear output in the neuron.[11]

Scientists at the time also could not explain the change in the retina's sensitivity in adapting to light or to darkness. The prevailing view attributed the changes to the bleaching and regeneration of the visual pigment (visual purple or rhodopsin). Using microelectrodes Granit concluded that neural factors determine the changes. Time proved him correct; the retina adapts to light by using the less light-sensitive cones as detectors, while in darkness its cones are activated.[12]

Later Granit used his microelectrodes to analyze the mechanism underlying color vision. His work provided the first direct evidence that specific cones are sensitive to the three regions of the spectrum representing the three primary colors on which color vision is based.[13]

Hartline began research on the phototropic reactions of land isopods while still an undergraduate at Lafayette College.[14] He received his M.D. from Johns Hopkins. He reportedly graduated last in his class and was given his degree only by promising never to practice medicine. He had an impish sense of humor and a mistrust of the medical and scientific "establishment." When his professor in gynecology asked what a woman with a grapefruit-sized mass in her abdomen was suffering from, Hartline answered, "I suppose she swallowed a grapefruit."[15]

Equally independent in his approach to science, Hartline planned his own experiments and built unique equipment, which he used along with antique instruments scrounged from any source. They were connected by tangles of wire and cables covered with black tape and strung throughout his disheveled laboratory. He draped sheets of tin foil and black cloth over optical parts of the equipment to prevent leaks of light. One collaborator described the scene as "a slightly disorganized but extremely fertile chaos."[16]

At Hopkins Hartline recorded the action potentials of the retinas of living animals and showed that it was feasible to study electrical events in the eye and relate them to the visual processes in humans. At the Johnson Foundation he and Clarence Graham, a physiology graduate from Temple University, developed a method to dissect out and record the output from a single optic nerve fiber of the horseshoe crab. At Woods Hole in the summer of 1931, they made the historic dissection, the earliest record of single-unit activity in the visual system. It enabled them to show that neural impulses in the optic nerve are related to the logarithm of the intensity of the quality of light to which the visual cell is exposed. Their work also demonstrated that the impulses transmitted by the optic nerve are essentially identical and that the intensity of the light incident on the photoreceptor is coded in terms of the frequency of discharge, rather than the shape or amplitude of the signal.

Hartline also showed that the activity of individual fibers differs markedly—some discharge steadily in response to a constant light stimulus, others are activated only by the onset and cessation of illumination, still others discharge when the light is off—but that the response of the whole nerve results from the combined activity of the fibers. He also found a high sensitivity to moving light patterns. He postulated that the processing of visual information begins in the retina with the specialized activity of the ganglia there.

Hartline mapped the retina in detail and determined that a retinal ganglion can receive excitatory and inhibitory influences over many convergent pathways from many photoreceptors. The optic nerve arising from the ganglion is simply the common pathway that carries the impulses, which result from the interaction of impulses from many receptors. As he put it, "Individual nerve cells act independently. It is the integrated action of all units of the visual system that gives rise to vision."[17]

PHILIP W. DAVIES AND FRANK BRINK JR.

Until the early 1940s, medical scientists and clinicians could not easily measure oxygen tension in animal tissues.[18] Oxygen content of blood and plasma could be measured fairly accurately, but tension could merely be estimated by injecting a small bubble of gas and allowing it to equilibrate with the gases in the surrounding tissues, then withdrawing it and analyzing its gas content—a slow, technically difficult technique that permitted only intermittent measurements. The obstacle hindered studies of metabolic and blood gas.

Work that originated in the Johnson Foundation formed the basis of the polarograph used today to measure oxygen tension in biological systems. Bronk involved a graduate student, Frank Brink Jr., in polarographic methods. Brink had learned as an undergraduate at the Pennsylvania State University that oxygen could be measured electrolytically by a dropping mercury electrode. He also was aware that the same process occurred at platinum surfaces. He proposed constructing a respirometer in which a nerve is placed in a closed space containing a known amount of an oxygenated solution and measuring the oxygen consumed with a platinum wire sealed in a glass container.[19]

At this point Bronk packed and left for Cornell. Brink accompanied him and, with Philip W. Davies, a foundation fellow, built such a respirometer. In their first experiments they were unable to record any current because they allowed too much time to elapse after closing the chamber.

They returned to Penn with Bronk and refined their oxygen electrodes. Davies, who later left Penn for Johns Hopkins, where he remained, concentrated on studies of the brains of cats. Brink, who followed Bronk to Hopkins and then to the Rockefeller Institute, focused on peripheral nerves. They covered the electrodes with a collodion membrane to reduce the problem of "electrode aging," which had made long-term measurements in blood particularly difficult. Brink invented a recessed electrode, which eliminated the effects of change in the oxygen diffusion coefficient of the medium and allowed the electrode to be moved from place to place so that wider areas could be evaluated.[20]

Others quickly began using the oxygen electrode. Britton Chance used it to measure oxygen consumption of tissue slices and mitochondria. Hugh Montgomery, chief of the Peripheral Vascular Clinic, was the first to use it clinically to measure the oxygen tension in ischemic limbs. He also used it to explore the extent of gangrenous tissue in patients requiring amputation and to assess the effects of physical procedures and drugs on peripheral oxygen tension. John Sayen and Orville Horwitz used it in their pioneer studies on dog hearts to measure changes in oxygen tension in regions around experimental coronary infarcts. Elsewhere, too, the oxygen electrode was increasingly used until polarographic techniques almost totally replaced their rivals.[21]

JOHN C. LILLY

John C. Lilly developed two of the first electronic devices that continuously measured physiological parameters in human subjects.[22] He grew up in Minnesota and was led to medicine after his eighteen-year-old brother, whose liver had been lacerated in a riding accident, died on the operating table. On the advice of Will Mayo of the Mayo Clinic, Lilly attended Dartmouth's two-year medical program, then transferred to Penn, where he received his M.D. in 1941.

As a medical student and also a member of the Johnson Foundation, Lilly developed a manometer to measure blood pressure and arterial pulse curves electronically. In the 1930s physiologists had made manometers with metallic diaphragms or membranes, but the diaphragms were inconvenient; they had to be fixed rigidly with respect to the recording device. Lilly used the diaphragm as the movable plate of an electrical capacitance electrode. As the diaphragm moved, variations in capacitance were measured by a radio-frequency circuit, amplified, and displayed on an oscilloscope or a strip-chart recorder, essentially the principle of the radio microphone.[23]

Lilly's device was useful in aviation research during World War II, as was a meter he made to measure the percent of nitrogen in respired gases. Lilly used a vacuum system to pull gases through a tube. A high electrical voltage applied to a hollow electrode caused the flowing gas to emit light in the manner of a neon sign so that it could be measured photoelectrically. The device gave continuous and accurate recordings and was used to study nitrogen concentrations in the gas delivery systems of pilots and others who breathe oxygen at high altitude. Later Julius Comroe and Ward Fowler used the meter to measure changes in dead space during the respiratory cycle. They also used it to compare the degree of respiratory mixing in normal subjects to that in subjects with respiratory diseases.[24]

After World War II, Lilly turned to neurological research. In the late 1940s he developed a 25-channel television-like display device to measure brain activity. He left Penn in 1953 for the National Institutes of Health. He became interested in the physiology and life habits of dolphins, studies of which gained him international attention.

GLENN MILLIKAN

Glenn Millikan invented an oximeter with which he measured the amount of oxidized and reduced myoglobin in muscle without removing the muscles from the animal.[25] This in vivo technique enabled him to calculate the metabolic activity of muscles and estimate their oxygen supply under physiological conditions. His thinking pioneered the development of difference spectroscopy, a type of spectral analysis that could be applied to turbid solutions.

His oximeter cleverly uses the spectral properties of oxidized and reduced hemoglobin, the properties of red and green gelatin filters, and the response characteristics of Weston photocells to tungsten light. The subject's ear lobe is fitted comfortably in a trough between a small tungsten light source and a colorimeter fitted with two small photocells. One photocell reflects the amount of tissue and blood in the optical path, the other reflects the degree of oxygenation of blood.[26]

Although Millikan felt that the instrument would be widely applied clinically, its most important uses have been in physiology and biochemistry. Even before he came to Penn, he met Britton Chance and showed him an early version of his idea. Chance realized that the approach could be used to measure oxidation reduction in respiratory pigments of mitochondria, which he was studying then. But the concentration of pigments in mitochondria are so small that Chance had to improve the optics and sensitivity of the instrument. He substituted a grating or prism monochrometer for the filters, which enabled him to obtain many wave lengths of monochromatic light. He ultimately developed the dual-wavelength spectrophotometer, later modified into a split-beam device, so that scientists could scan wide ranges of the spectrum rather than being restricted to reaction rates at one wavelength.

Coincidentally Millikan, Chance, Davies and Brink, and Lilly all published papers on their respective inventions in the same issue of *Review of Scientific Instruments*—surely one of the most significant issues of that journal. Millikan, whose father was the physicist Robert A. Millikan, was an inveterate designer. He liked to hike and camp in the wilderness but also enjoyed the comforts of home, so he made a shower bath that folded into the trunk of his car so that he could bathe during expeditions. His career was cut short when he was killed in a mountain-climbing accident.[27]

RAYMOND E. ZIRKLE

Raymond Zirkle was one of the early scientists who investigated what parts of the cell X-ray irradiation damaged. While at the Johnson Foundation he developed methods that allowed him to study these processes and found that radiosensitivity was altered by changes in pH within the cell.[28]

LESLIE A. CHAMBERS

The use of ultrasound to disrupt cells, make emulsions, and cleanse surfaces is an important technique in use in science, dentistry, and industry today. Leslie A. Chambers and his collaborators did much in the mid-1930s while he was a member of the Johnson Foundation to explore the use of this method for disrupting the cell walls of bacteria and viruses and forming emulsions.[29]

THOMAS F. ANDERSON

Thomas F. Anderson, one of the early electron microscopists in America, provided an important experimental base for much of the information required to discover the double helical structure of DNA. Anderson was born in Manotowoc, Wisconsin.[30] His father organized and built a power and light company, which consisted of a dam and an electric generator; he also organized a company that sold electrical appliances to subscribers and repaired the instruments. Thus the son grew up in a technical world, and he enhanced his knowledge of science at the California Institute of Technology and later by studies in Europe. Anderson was studying at the University of Wisconsin when he was offered a fellowship by the National Science Foundation to explore the biological and medical uses of an electron microscope, the nation's first, at the RCA facility in Camden. He was skeptical initially because so little had been written about the microscope, but his doubts were quickly dispelled after he arrived and worked with it.[31]

Since the endeavor was new, Anderson worked under the guidance of a committee headed by Penn bacteriologist Stuart Mudd. Mudd and David Lackman had already published excellent pictures taken with the new machine that showed bacterial chains of streptococci held together by their cell walls. Within weeks Anderson and Harry Morton took electron micrographs of *Corynebacterium diphtheriae* grown in potassium tellurite and showed that tellurite crystals had developed inside the bacteria.[32]

Anderson pushed on. With Wendel Stanley he obtained the first electron micrographs of several plant viruses, directly confirming the dimensions that had been estimated from suspensions containing 10^{10} viral particles per milliliter. These studies helped persuade a doubting scientific community that DNA and RNA were large polymers. He and Salvatore Luria examined phage through the electron microscope. Virologists had thought that there was only one type of phage, but the micrographs showed several different morphologies, indicating many phage families.[33]

When Anderson's fellowship expired, Bronk brought him to the Johnson Foundation. Anderson and L. A. Chambers worked with the first commercial model of the RCA electron microscope, applying themselves at first to the structure of *Rickettsia*. But Anderson soon returned to phage, which was rapidly becoming an exciting subject.[34]

As more phages were discovered, it was obvious that each phage carried an increasingly elaborate set of instructions to the host bacterium for assembling the daughter particles. With various collaborators, Anderson showed that 37 percent of T2 phage was DNA, then that the DNA of the phage was contained mostly in the head of the virus and released by osmotic shock. This discovery was made in two steps. First,

Anderson discovered that T4 phage would not adsorb to the host bacterium unless it was activated by an aromatic amino acid; the amino acid frees the phage's long tail fibers so that the connectors on their tips can attach to the surface of the host.

Second, he devised an experiment to test osmotic pressure. When the pressure is lowered rapidly, water passes into the phage faster than sodium chloride passes out; the increased pressure ruptures the viral membrane. When the pressure is lowered slowly, sodium chloride escapes as rapidly as the water enters, and the cells do not rupture. The high viscosity of the suspension solution in which the phage particles are ruptured suggested to Anderson that DNA is released into the solution. He confirmed his supposition when he saw that the solution contained DNA; by contrast, the heads sedimented by centrifugation contain only protein. Since the phage "ghosts" were not infectious, it was evident that infection requires DNA.[35]

Anderson also answered the question of whether the phages attach to the bacterium by their heads or tails. Electron micrographs of air-dried specimens were inconclusive, seeming to show both ways. Anderson developed methods to eliminate surface tension when the sections were being prepared. Through improved micrographs he demonstrated that phage attach by their tails.[36]

The work of Anderson and others did not totally dispel the skepticism of some scientists that DNA is a string of genetic material directing an organism's development or that it is a two-dimensional structure which transfers three-dimensional information. In 1952 Hershey and Chase improved on the experiments of Anderson and his colleagues by using double-labeling radioisotope techniques. They finally convinced the skeptics that DNA is the material that transfers genetic information. Two years later, James Watson and Francis Crick further clarified the genetic mechanism when they resolved the double helical structure of DNA.

Anderson was on the threshold of discovering the role of DNA in phage genetics, but he stated later that he was not prepared to advance any further than he had at the time. He stayed at Penn until 1958. By then his old RCA microscope was outdated, but the Johnson Foundation could not afford to buy him a modern one. The Institute of Cancer Research at the Fox Chase Cancer Center in Philadelphia lured him away with a new, more powerful instrument.[37]

NOTES

1. "Big Gift for Medical Education, Eldridge R. Johnson Contributes $800,000 to Endow Foundation for Research in Medical Physics. Fund Now Reaching the $10,000,000 Mark," *Pennsylvania Gazette* 26 (October 27, 1927); A. N. Richards and T. G. Miller, Survey of Medical Affairs, University of Pennsylvania, Prepared for President Gates and Submitted to Him on March 5, 1931, pp. 45–46; D. Y. Cooper, "The Johnson Foundation for Medical Physics and Biophysics," *Transactions and Studies of the College of Physicians of Philadelphia* 5th ser., 6(1984):113–24.

2. Cooper, "Johnson Foundation," pp. 114–16.

3. F. R. Brink, Jr., "Detlev W. Bronk," *Biographical Memoirs of the National Academy of Sciences* (Washington, D.C.: National Academy of Sciences, 1979) vol. 50, pp. 3–87; Britton Chance, "Detlev W. Bronk (1897–1975)" *Year Book of the American Philosophical Society* (1978):54–66.

4. Chance, "Detlev W. Bronk," p. 56.

5. Chance, pp. 56–57.

6. Brink, pp. 8–18.

7. Chance, p. 62; Brink, pp. 27–28.

8. Brink, pp. 30–33.

9. Chance, p. 62.

10. F. Ratliff, "Nobel Prize: Three Named for Medicine-Physiology Award," *Science* 158(1962):468–73.

11. R. Granit, *Receptor and Sensory Perception* (New York: Yale University Press, 1955), pp. 11–28.

12. *Ibid.*, pp. 143–50.

13. *Ibid.*, pp. 134–42.

14. H. K. Hartline, "A Quantitative and Descriptive Study of the Electrical Response to Illumination of the Arthropod Eye," *American Journal of Physiology* 83(1928):466–83; H. Keffer Hartline, "The Dark Adaptation of the Eye of the Limulus, as Manifested by its Electrical Response to Illumination," *Journal of Cellular and Comparative Physiology* 1(1930):379–89; H. Keffer Hartline and C. H. Graham, "Nerve Impulses from Single Receptors in the Eye," *Journal of Cellular and Comparative Physiology* 1(1932):277–95.

15. Obituary of Keffer Hartline being prepared by F. Ratliff; L. A. Riggs, "Recollections of Early Laboratory Experiments on Vision," in *Foundations of Sensory Science*, ed. William Dawson and J. M. Enock (New York, Heidelberg: Springer Verlag, 1984), pp. 195–97; conversation with Louis Flexner, a classmate of Keffer Hartline at the Johns Hopkins Medical School.

16. Experience visiting and working in the Johnson Foundation.

17. H. K. Hartline, "The Neural Mechanism of Vision," *Harvey Lectures* XXXVI(1942):39–68.

18. Letter to David Y. Cooper from Frank Brink, Jr., describing work on the oxygen electrode and some of his experiences in the Johnson Foundation.

19. J. H. Comroe, *Retrospectroscope* (Menlo Park, Calif.: Von Gehr Press, 1977), pp. 20, 102; P. W. Davies and F. Brink, Jr., "Microelectrodes for Measuring Local Oxygen Tension in Animal Tissue," *Review of Scientific Instruments* (1942): 524–33; C. M. Connelly, D. W. Bronk, and Frank Brink, Jr., "A Sensitive Respirometer for the Measurement of Rapid Changes in Metabolism of Oxygen," *Review of Scientific Instruments* 24(1953):683–95; Comment in L. Brown and J. H. Comroe, Jr., "Blood pO_2

Derived from Measurements of O_2 Physically Dissolved in Blood." in *Methods in Medical Research*, ed. J. H. Comroe, Jr. (Chicago: Year Book Press, 1950), pp. 169–77.

20. Letter from Frank Brink to David Y. Cooper, February 17, 1984; Letter from Philip Davies to David Y. Cooper, June 15, 1984.

21. J. J. Sayen, W. F. Sheldon, O. Horwitz, H. F. Zinsser, and J. Meade, Jr., "Studies of Coronary Disease in Experimental Animals II. Polarographic determination of local oxygen availibility in the dog's left ventricle during coronary occlusion and pure oxygen breathing," *Journal of Clinical Investigation* 30 (1951):932–40.

22. J. C. Lilly, *The Scientist* (Philadelphia: Lippincott, 1978), pp. 45, 69–73, 76–77.

23. J. C. Lilly, "The Capacitance Diaphragm Manometer," *Review of Scientific Instruments* 13(1942): 34–37.

24. J. C. Lilly, "Mixing of Gases Within the Respiratory System with a New Type of Nitrogen Meter," *American Journal of Physiology* 161(1950):342–51

25. E. H. Wood, "Oximetry," in *Medical Physics*, vol. 2, ed. O. Gasser (Chicago: Year Book Press, 1950), pp. 664-80; K. Matthes, "Untersuchungen uber die Sauerstoffsattigung des menschlichen Artierenblutes," *Archiv für Experimentellen Pathologie und Pharmakologie* 179(1935): 698–711.

26. G. A. Millikan, "The Oximeter, an Instrument for Measuring Continuously the Oxygen Saturation of Arterial Blood in Man," *Review of Scientific Instruments* 3(1942): 434–44; E. H. Wood, "Oximetry"; K. Matthes, "Untersuchungen uber die Sauerstoffsattigung," p. 698.

27. Personal conversation with Thomas Redman.

28. R. E. Zirkle, "Modification of Radiosensitivity by Means of Readily Penetrating Acids and Bases," *Radiology* 35 (1936):230–37; R. E. Zirkle, "Biological Effects of Alpha Particles and their Relation to the Effects of Neutrons," *Occasional Publications of the American Association for the Advancement of Science*, 4 (1937):220–24; R. E. Zirkle, P. C. Abersold, and E. R. Dempster, "The Relation of Biological Effectiveness of Fast Neutrons and X-Rays Upon Different Organisms," *American Journal of Cancer* 29(1937):535–62.

29. L. A. Chambers, "Sound Waves, A New Tool for Food Manufacturers," *Food Industries* (New York: McGraw Hill, 1938); collected papers of the Johnson Foundation, vol. 2, 1936; L. A. Chambers and A. J. Weil, "Immunological Properties of a Sonic Extract of Pneumococcus," *Proceedings of the Society of Biology and Medicine* 38(1938):924–27; W. Henle, G. Henle, and L. A. Chambers, "Studies on the Antigen Structure of Some Mamalian Spermatozoa," *Journal of Experimental Medicine* 68(1938): 335–52.

30. T. F. Anderson, "Some Personal Memories of Research," *Annual Review of Microbiology* 29(1975):1–17; T. F. Anderson, "Reflections on Phage," *Annual Review of Genetics* 15(1981):405–17.

31. W. M. Stanley and T. F. Anderson, "A Study of Purified Viruses with the Electron Microscope," *Journal of Biological Chemistry* 139 (1941):325–38; T. F. Anderson and W. M. Stanley, "A Study by Means of the Electron Microscope of the Reaction Between Mosaic Virus and Antiserum," *Journal of Biological Chemistry* 139 (1941):339–41.

32. H. E. Morton and T. F. Anderson, "Electron Microscopic Study of Biological Reactions I. Reduction of Potassium Tellurite by *Corynebacterium diphtheriae*," *Proceedings of the Society of Experimental Biology and Medicine* 46(1941):272–76.

33. Stanley and Anderson, "A Study of Purified Viruses."

34. Anderson, "Personal Memories," pp. 8–10.

35. G. S. Stent, *Molecular Biology of Bacterial Viruses* (San Francisco: W. H. Freeman, 1963), pp. 110–15; F. H. Portugal and J. S. Cohen, *A Century of DNA—A History of the Discovery of the Structure and Function of the Genetic Substance* (Cambridge, Mass.: MIT Press, 1977), pp. 180–83.

36. Anderson, "Reflections on Phage," pp. 409–10.

37. Anderson, "Personal memoirs," pp. 13–14.

16

DISCOVERIES THAT TURNED INTO HOUSEHOLD NAMES

Restlessness is discontent and discontent is the first necessity of progress. Show me a thoroughly satisfied man and I will show you a failure.

Thomas A. Edison

ELIOT R. CLARK

The Department of Anatomy, which had deteriorated when George A. Piersol fell into a long illness, rebounded under his successor, Eliot R. Clark.[1] A Johns Hopkins medical graduate, Clark chaired anatomy departments at two institutions before coming to Penn in 1927. He had the opportunity to plan and design the anatomy facilities in the new Anatomy-Chemistry Building, completed in 1929. He arranged for all of the anatomy courses to be taught in the same semester, so that the faculty had long stretches of time for research.[2]

Clark also brought a new attitude toward his subject. He was more interested in the morphology of living cells than that of dead ones. Early in his career, he figured that fixation processes in preparing microscope slides destroyed many of the normal structural relationships within tissue. His first in vivo study was an examination of the thin, transparent tissues of the tail fins of amphibian larvae.[3] He observed the cells, nerves, connective tissue, and blood flowing through the tiny vessels. Eventually Clark decided to study higher animals in the same way.[4]

Clark soon found that the observation of normal living tissue in normal higher animals under the high-power microscope was not a simple procedure, for he could find no tissues that were sufficiently transparent for microscopic study. It was clear that before he could extend these studies to warm-blooded animals a number of difficult technical problems would have to be solved. His first step was the construction of a chamber with a uniform depth, sufficiently thin for use under high-power, oil-immersion microscope objectives. Next he had to develop techniques to implant and maintain the observation chamber in rabbit ears. The two most difficult problems encountered were pressure necrosis and infection, complications that altered normal tissue function and caused extrusion of the chamber from the rabbit's ear.

The first successful chamber that permitted an area of tissue to grow while being observed under the microscope was reported in the *Anatomical Record* in 1928 (work done while Clark was still at the University of Georgia Medical School). This early chamber had a thin transparent observation area made of Kodaloid (celluloid) that was connected by small holes to a deeper cavity through which a thin strip of tissue containing the central artery of the rabbit's ear could be placed and not be damaged by pressure.

The bay chamber, the most successful of the chambers for general use, was an improvement over the early designs. Next Clark devised the round table chamber was developed to improve observation with high power oil-immersion lenses of the tissue growth processes.

To observe tissues that had already formed, Clark developed a chamber that he called the "preformed tissue chamber." With this visualization device, the normal behavior of cells, blood vessels, nerves, and connective tissue and their response to physical and chemical stimuli could be observed for prolonged periods of time. The last chambers that Eliot Clark developed were the "combination chambers," designed to observe the function of preformed tissues as well as growth of new tissue simultaneously.

OSCAR V. BATSON

A student of Eliot Clark at the University of Missouri, Oscar Batson was, unlike his teacher, a classical anatomist who used modern tech-

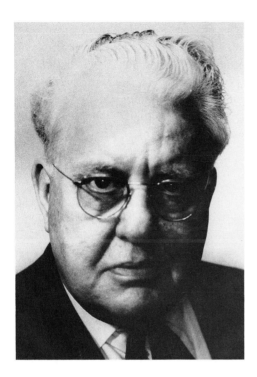

Oscar V. Batson, Professor of Anatomy in the Graduate School. Discoverer of the function of the vertebral veins. (Historical Collections of the College of Physicians of Philadelphia.)

niques to demonstrate anatomical structures, especially by combining X rays with anatomical dissection techniques.[5]

In the 1920s otologists frequently ligated the jugular vein to prevent the spread of infection from mastoiditis. An otologist himself, Batson was puzzled about how the blood left the brain when the main drainage channels were blocked. He investigated the problem by making preparations in which he injected plastic material into the venous system and corroded away the tissue with alkali. The extensive network of veins demonstrated by the cast that was left convinced him of the importance of the vertebral veins in drainage of blood from the head and neck.

Batson used similar procedures to investigate the extent of the venous system in the spinal column. When he had injected radio-opaque material into the dorsal vein of the penis (which is connected to the vertebral veins by the pelvic venous plexus), he found that the material rapidly filled the vertebral veins, or bone veins, of the spine and then flowed into the cranial veins. The architecture of the injected veins, paralleling the distribution pattern of metastases, explained how tumors spread to the spine and skull from the pelvis and thorax.[6] Batson's studies also explained how the venous system functioned when the air way is cut off during such straining actions as lifting, defecation, and parturition.

Batson was a large man with a huge head and long, wavy, white hair. He customarily wore a black suit, black shoes, and a black string bow tie, giving him the appearance of a cross between an undertaker and an evangelist. He was all business and rather abrupt, unless a student's question interested him, in which case he would discuss it in great detail. He was a histrionic lecturer. He used a large elephant's thigh bone to demonstrate the strength required to support the animal's great weight. Straining as if he were lifting a 500-pound barbell, Batson raised the bone just a few millimeters from the desk top. Students examining the structure afterwards found it was only a light replica made of papier-mâché.[7]

STUART MUDD AND EARL FLOSDORF

When the medical school pulled bacteriology from the School of Hygiene and elevated the course into a department in 1931, it hired Stuart Mudd to organize it. Mudd not only developed a strong department but also made his own contributions. One was administrative: he helped intro-duce electron microscopy into bacteriology.[8] Another was scientific: he and Earl Flosdorf developed a freeze-drying process for preserving serum and bacteria.[9]

Since the end of the nineteenth century, it had been known that dried serum was stable over prolonged periods; various methods of dessication were available, but all had flaws, especially for making individual sterile doses suitable for patient use.[10]

By the late 1920s, measles and the secondary infections that all too frequently followed were treated by serum, but only after an epidemic was well under way. The serum was drawn from patients convalescing from the disease; but since measles appeared in epidemics every two to three years, no serum was available for the early cases. Even if patients convalescing from the previous epidemic were found, their titers were so low that their serum was useless. Mudd looked no farther than an early case of measles in his own family for the idea of permanently preserving convalescent serum.[11]

To help him with the research, he brought Earl Flosdorf, who had a degree in high-vacuum physics, to Penn and collaborated with Borner of Graduate Hospital, who was improving the Wassermann test.[12] They developed aseptic techniques that maintained sterility throughout the freeze-drying process; they devised a system of automatically regulating temperature, so that it could be kept constant in the containers; they improved the vacuum system, thereby shortening the freeze-drying process; and they simplified the seal without losing the vacuum.[13]

They tested their apparatus with lyophilized guinea-pig complement, which is unstable and hard to preserve. They made a series of small, individual containers which could be individually sealed without disturbing the vacuum.[14] Their work was simplified by the genius of James D. Graham, the medical school's glassblower, who was so adept at his craft that he could fashion instruments without drawings or blueprints—especially useful since most biological scientists do not have the engineering skills to make the mechanical drawings required by a toolmaker. His legacy includes an improved McCloud gauge, which he reduced from 36 inches to 10 inches and made safer by constructing it of heavier glass; his enhancements are used in the Stokes-McCloud gauges sold today.[15]

The instrument proved reliable.[16] Although Mudd was more interested in lyophilization for medical purposes, Flosdorf explored its possibilities for food; he preserved orange juice, coffee, and a complete Christmas dinner that he carried to England and ate with his son who was in school there. Later he used the process to preserve tissue, even a whole fetus. When aneurysms were first treated by aortic grafts, human aortas were harvested from the morgue and preserved by the process.[17]

Except for improved refrigeration and modern design, the lyophilizer of today differs little from Mudd and Flosdorf's original version. Its popularity spread, and it is a widely used technique in biology, chemistry, pharmaceuticals, and physics as well as in food processing.[18]

GEORGE L. WEINSTEIN AND MAXIMILIAN EHRENSTEIN

The development of oral contraceptives is usually attributed to Gregory Pincus and John Rock, but Penn scientists made two fundamental and

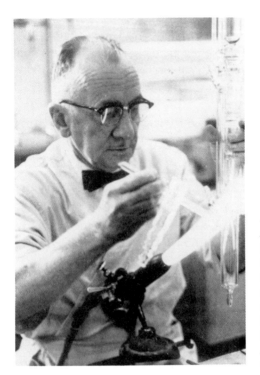

James D. Graham, Glassblower for the School of Medicine of the University of Pennsylvania. Skilled craftsman whose ingenuity designed many of the instruments that made the discoveries described here possible. (Copied from a photograph belonging to his son James D. Graham, Jr.)

independent discoveries that made "the pill" possible. The story starts at the University of Rochester, where George Corner (who later would write a history of Penn's medical school) discovered progesterone in 1928; with W. M. Allen, he developed an assay method to quantify and standardize progestational activity in extracts from ovarian follicles, pituitaries, and urine.[19]

The story moves to Penn with A. W. Makepeace. He worked in Corner's laboratory and learned the technology for physiological studies of female hormones. At Penn, he joined George L. Weinstein and Maurice Friedman in studying the physiology and endocrinology of rabbits. The researchers raised the question of why pregnancy prevents ovulation.

They reasoned, from their own work as well as studies by others, that the presence of a functioning corpus luteum must interfere with physiological processes that take place during ovulation. They investigated the block by injecting extracts of either sow corpora or progesterone prepared from stigmasterol into female rabbits after mating. Both preparations inhibited ovulation. Since the tissue concentration of progesterone was equal to that existing during pregnancy, the scientists implicated progesterone as the blocking hormone.[20] In 1937 they deduced that the progesterone did not act directly; subsequently it was learned that it inhibits the pituitary's release of gonadotropin.[21]

Weinstein, a resident in gynecology, was eager to pursue the research but was only rebuffed by an ordinarily perceptive mentor. The industrious postdoctoral fellow approached A. N. Richards and sought his help in obtaining a grant to continue the work. But Richards had not been impressed by the research and, in one of the few mistakes he ever made, advised Weinstein to finish his residency and go into private practice.[22]

The second crucial Penn contribution to "the pill" was made in the early 1940 s by Maximilian Ehrenstein, an organic chemist in the George S. Cox Foundation, based in the Department of Medicine.[23] He was synthesizing derivatives of steroid hormones from the aglycone strophanthidin in order to track the physiological changes in various substituents of the steroid molecule.[24] In one series of experiments, he removed the angular methyl group attached to carbon-10 of the molecule. The resulting compound was 10-norprogesterone. He sent a sample of this new substance for assay to Allen, who had moved to St. Louis University. (Ehrenstein, very choosy in picking consultants, had the highest regard for those trained under George W. Corner.) Allen administered the material to rabbits and found that its progestational activity was equivalent to that of the natural progesterone. Moreover, it could be administered orally, unlike the natural substance. (Later, the Hungarian chemist Carl Djerassi showed that oral administration actually depended on the absence of the angular methyl group.)[25]

Ehrenstein published a paper describing his synthesis of 10-norprogesterone in 1944.[26] Just then, the pharmaceutical firm financing his work notified him that it was withdrawing its support because his studies had not been productive. Thus both avenues of the medical school's basic work on oral contraceptives closed before Penn realized the scientific, not to mention commercial, value of the work done within its walls.[27]

JOHN H. GIBBON, JR.

John H. Gibbon, Jr., and his wife, Mary, developed the heart-lung machine, and Penn was a major, but not the only, site of their work.[28] Gibbon stepped into medicine reluctantly; he would have preferred to be a poet or painter if he could have made a living at it. He became intrigued by research during his internship at Pennsylvania Hospital. There he assisted Joseph Heymans in double-blind studies on the effects of diets containing sodium or potassium chloride on the blood pressure of hypertensive patients. Gibbon grew excited when he saw the sort of information that controlled experiments could yield.

He became a research fellow in the laboratory of Edward Churchill at the Harvard University Medical School. His first project was to measure the pulmonary artery pressure in cats with closed and open arteriovenous fistulae. He found that pulmonary blood flow increased

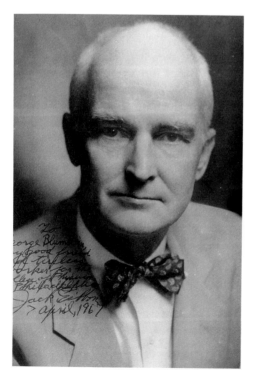

John H. Gibbon, developer of the heart-lung machine. While at the University of Pennsylvania in the 1930s he worked with Eugene Landis on the peripheral circulation and in the Harrison Department of Research Surgery where he tested early models of his heart-lung machine. (Historical Collections of the College of Physicians of Philadelphia.)

markedly when the fistula was opened, but pulmonary artery pressure changed little.[29]

The laboratory group—which included Mary Hopkinson, a technician whom Gibbon married—moved from Boston City Hospital to Massachusetts General Hospital. An unsuccessful operation there in 1931 gave Gibbon his first inkling of developing a heart-lung machine. Churchill tried to remove a pulmonary embolus in a patient. The embolus was so difficult to diagnose and the surgical procedure so uncertain (the standard procedure at the time had been performed 142 times worldwide, and only nine patients had survived) that the operation was held off until the patient was practically moribund.

Churchill opened the artery, removed the clot, and closed the vessel in six and a half minutes, but it was still too late. He and Gibbon stood by, helplessly, watching the patient's veins distend and her blood darken. Observing this tragedy, Gibbon found himself thinking that he could have helped her if only there were some way of taking out the blue venous blood, removing carbon dioxide, adding O_2, and then putting the blood back into the arterial system.[30]

Gibbon finished his residency in 1931 and came to Penn to work in Eugene Landis's physiology laboratory. For three and a half years, he, Landis, and Hugh Montgomery studied the effect of temperature and tissue pressure on the flow of fluids through the capillary wall. During this time Gibbon began to conceptualize an extracorporeal blood circuit that could temporarily take over cardiorespiratory functions. With Landis's encouragement, he asked Churchill for a one-year fellowship (with Mary as his assistant) to start his project. Churchill agreed, although he had little enthusiasm for the idea.

The problem of pumping the blood from the venous to the arterial side of the circulatory system was the simplest part of the task to solve. The larger problem was obtaining suitable gas exchange. They tried many methods, but all of them produced foaming, hemolysis, or the forming of vasoconstrictor substances. Finally, after consulting with a professor of steam engineering at Harvard, the Gibbons designed a vertical revolving cylinder which spread the blood in a thin film, increasing the gas exchange without excessive drawbacks.[31]

Cats, including strays when the laboratory supply ran low, were used in the early experiments because they were of appropriate size. The Gibbons' first machine was a Rube Goldberg apparatus of metal, glass, water baths, electric motors, and other parts—unimpressive in appearance but it worked. To test it, the Gibbons gradually closed the pulmonary blood before removing blood for oxygenation. With each successful partial bypass, they further constricted the artery until it was closed completely and the cat's pulmonary function was supplied solely by the machine.[32]

The researchers returned to Penn in 1933 and set up a laboratory in the Harrison Department of Surgical Research. The department's director, I. S. Ravdin, was determined to invigorate the area of surgical research started by J. William White, and he allotted funds to the Gibbons.[33] For the next six and a half years, they built improved models of the machine, affectionately called Queen Mary I and II. They also performed studies demonstrating that prolonged cardiopulmonary bypass did not damage the internal organs of animals that survived.[34]

John Gibbon joined the Army Medical Corps during World War II, and after four years of service, he and his wife moved to Jefferson Medical College, where they improved their machine and built larger ones with greater pumping and gas-exchanging capacities. But their budget was meager, especially since they needed an engineer to design the device and a machinist to build it. At a friend's suggestion, they approached Thomas J. Watson, the founder and chairman of I.B.M. Watson was so impressed with their work that he provided engineering expertise and paid for constructing the machine. Later John Gibbon would say that Watson and Eugene Landis, who championed his idea of an extracorporeal circuit when it was merely an idea, were the only colleagues to encourage his far-fetched plan.[35]

The Gibbons had one more obstacle to overcome: maintaining adequate gas exchange for human beings. T. Lane Stokes and John Flick, two residents studying under John Gibbon's direction, solved the problem. They found that oxygenation could be increased eight-fold by creating turbulence in the blood film. They oxygenated the blood without producing foam by flowing the substance over a vertical screen of stainless steel.[36] I.B.M. improved the design of the system, and on May 6, 1953, the machine was first used on a twelve-year-old patient who had a large atrioventricular septal defect. It opened a new era in surgery, an era that it continues to help expand.[37]

ELDRIDGE L. ELIASON

Eldridge L. Eliason was appointed John Rhea Barton Professor of Surgery on the basis of his clinical abilities, but he was a good friend to basic scientists. Otto Rosenthal, a biochemist in surgical research, was conducting studies with the Warburg respirometer and frequently needed fresh tissue, both normal and cancerous, from patients.[38] Most of the surgeons supplied his request but left the specimens, uniced, on the radiator; or they neglected to inform him that the specimens were available. According to Rosenthal, Eliason was unfailingly cooperative and even deferential. He called when the tissue was ready, and it was iced when Rosenthal picked it up in the operating room. Rosenthal always thanked him, and Eliason would reply deferentially, "I hope this is what you want."[39]

Eliason was born on Maryland's eastern shore, went to Yale University as an undergraduate, and entered Penn through a mistake. He was set on entering Jefferson Medical College, and upon arriving in Philadelphia, asked a streetcar conductor how to get to "the medical school." The conductor said, "I go right past it," and dropped Eliason at 36th Street. Eliason made his way to Medical Hall (now Logan Hall) and found the admissions office. Dean John Marshall happened to be standing there and recognized Eliason from a gymnastics meet held at Philadelphia's Academy of Music a few years earlier. Marshall addressed Eliason by name and gave him a card to fill out. When he saw it had the Penn name, Eliason said that he had come to the wrong place. Marshall answered, "No, Mr. Eliason, you have come to the right place." Already impressed by Marshall recognizing him, Eliason elected to attend Penn.[40]

He turned out to be bold but not brash. During a clinic, Eliason rolled a patient's bed over the foot of the eminent J. William White, who bellowed, "What the hell are you doing?" Eliason, although scared, rapidly replied, "Your foot should not have been there, Dr. White." White liked his spunk and later offered him a position on his surgical service.[41]

Eliason had not previously considered surgery as a career, but he went on to train some of the best clinical surgeons in Philadelphia history, including William Erb, L. Kraeer Ferguson, Julian Johnson, and Lloyd Stevens; one resident, Robert Brown, became Surgeon General of the Navy. He backed his nurses and taught them and, after the tension of a tough operation, would pat the scrub nurse on the shoulder and say (in the patronly manner of his day), "Child, you did a grand job." He was the only member of the faculty ever to become an honorary member of the Nurses Assocation.[42]

Aphorisms spilled out of him: "A good surgeon is a good doctor who can cut. . . . Don't cut until you know what it isn't. . . . If the clinical and laboratory findings don't agree, do 'em again. . . . Keep the chemistry up and the belly down. . . . Do a rectal examination, and in 50 percent of the cases, you won't need a consultant. . . . Give me a dependable boy, and you can keep the brilliant ones. . . . Treat the patient, not the film."[43]

I. S. RAVDIN

The medical school's overall leader and commanding figure after World War II through its bicentennial in 1965 was I. S. Ravdin.[44] He was born in Evansville, Indiana; his father and grandfather had been physicians. He earned his bachelor's degree from Indiana University and his medical degree from Penn in 1918. His first significant paper concerned the status of blood transfusion; he collaborated with Elizabeth Glenn, whom he would later marry. Although the paper was simply a review article, the researchers gained an appreciation that blood transfusion could serve a nutritional role by supplying the body with protein. When Ravdin realized, in further research, that only so many calories could be administered to a patient, he crusaded for programs which built up a patient's protein reserves preoperatively and began postoperative oral feeding as soon as possible. His work laid the foundation for the development of total parenteral nutrition, which was developed by his students and colleagues.[45]

In the 1920s he extended his laboratory work to include the biochemistry and physiology of bile and the mechanism of gallstone formation. He became known as an expert on liver physiology and disease, and in the early 1930s he was asked by Merck Chemical Company to evaluate the safety of divinyl ether as an anesthetic agent. This compound had been synthesized by Merck, but the wife of one of the company's top executives died following anesthesia with it. Ravdin assembled an interdisciplinary group of top Penn scientists, including Balduin Lucké in pathology, Samuel Goldschmidt in physiology, and (later) Harry Vars in biochemistry, to determine whether the substance was toxic to the liver. They demonstrated that glycogen did not protect the liver from toxins and anoxemia. They found that protein was necessary for cellular repair and that, if there was insufficient protein in the liver, that organ drew on the total body protein to fulfill its requirements.[46]

Ravdin began his administrative climb in 1928 when he was appointed the first J. William White Professor of Surgical Research.[47] Later he was appointed the John Rhea Barton Professor of Surgery and, still later, Penn's vice president for medical affairs.

Ravdin could be charming, cunning, or ruthless by turns, but he was always honest with himself and with his colleagues. He was also known for accurately assessing the capabilities of others and picking the right people for jobs. He was not afraid to surround himself with people who were better than he or who did not like him if they happened to be the best for a task.[48]

His personality is best revealed by anecdote. When Julian Johnson had to bide time before becoming Eliason's resident, he signed on for Frazier's thyroid service. But he was so lackadaisical about it that Frazier, annoyed, was going to turn him down. Ravdin advised Johnson to apply for a residency to Harvard or Yale and ask Frazier for a letter of recommendation. Johnson did so and was accepted at Yale almost by return mail—such a rapid response that Frazier was convinced that Johnson was worthy of a spot with him.[49]

Ravdin headed the 20th General Hospital, a Penn-staffed facility, during World War II. His administrative skills were needed from the moment the staff arrived in India. It was monsoon season, and the roads to the hospital compound were a quagmire; trucks became mired up to their axles. Coolies were trying to make the road passable by bringing rocks from a nearby stream bed, but they were carrying the stones in pans on their heads. Ravdin knew it would take years to make a road in this manner. He went to the stream bed, where G.I.s were digging up the stones. He told them that they would probably get malaria but that they would never make it to the hospital because of the bad roads; and even if they reached the hospital, they could receive no treatment because supplies would never get through. The G.I.s asked him how much stone he needed. Ravdin told them 200 truckloads. The soldiers said they could move the stone but had no trucks. Ravdin asked where trucks were located. They pointed him to a motor pool. Ravdin went there and convinced the commander to lend him twenty trucks. Then he drove one truck back to his unit, loaded it with men who could drive trucks, and returned to the motor pool and borrowed the trucks he needed. Within a few days he had his road, long before regular military channels would have built it.[50]

Ravdin's tactics were not always obvious to his unit. When the 20th General received its first shipment of building materials, he allocated

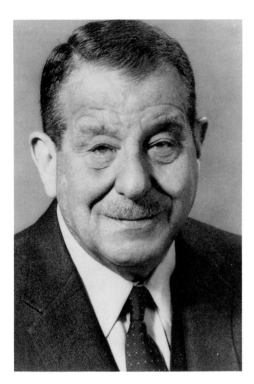

I. S. Ravdin, John Rhea Barton Professor of Surgery, Director of Harrison Department of Surgical Research, Vice President of Medical Affairs. (Archives of the University of Pennsylvania.)

the small allotment to constructing a smart, waterproof building to treat the top brass rather than to replace the bamboo huts (or "basies") used by regular patients and staff. The staff was livid. But shortly a high-ranking officer came for treatment. Ravdin was so courteous and the facility so pleasant that, when he was about to be discharged, he asked Ravdin if the doctor had any needs. Ravdin then took him by jeep past the huts and tents and asked for speedy delivery of building supplies. Not long thereafter, he had his request.[51]

His talent was hardly wasted in civilian life. Under Ravdin the Department of Surgery was always active. He spurred residents to hurry up by threatening to administer "grasshopper suppositories." He had a good clinical touch. When his gallbladder became inflamed, he could have had any eminent surgeon operate on him—for instance, his friend Allen O. Whipple, professor of surgery at Columbia, who had been called in as a consultant, or Eliason. Instead, Ravdin chose the young

Jonathan Rhoads because he had trained Rhoads and because Rhoads was the surgeon he recommended to others.[52]

Ravdin had the graces of the old paternalism. He entered one patient's room to find the crepe all but hung; the patient had been told he had a large mass on his kidney, most likely malignant, and the family was already in mourning. Ravdin asked a resident for the X ray. He held it up to the window so that the patient could see it. He pointed to the mass and told the patient, "This is a cyst on your kidney. It is not malignant. Dr. Murphy and I will remove it in the morning at 8:00, and you are going to be all right." The tumor proved to be a cyst. Ravdin's first comment on seeing the lesion was, "It is better to be a lucky surgeon than a good one." In the dressing room later, he told the residents gathered around, "Even if it had been malignant, I was going to tell him it was benign. What purpose would it have served to depress him with impending doom when there was little else that could be done at the moment."[53]

NOTES

1. R. G. Williams, "Memoir of Eliot Round Clark," *Transactions and Studies of the College of Physicians of Philadelphia* 4th ser., 32(1964–65):82–84.

2. E. R. Clark, "Department of Anatomy University of Pennsylvania School of Medicine," *Methods and Problems of Medical Education* 17th ser. (New York: Rockefeller Foundation, 1930).

3. Williams, "Memoir of Clark."

4. E. R. Clark, H. T. Kirby-Smith, R. O. Rex, and R. G. Williams, "Recent Modifications in the Method of Studying Living Cells and Tissues in Transparent Chambers Inserted into Rabbits' Ears," *Anatomical Record* 47(1930):187–211.

5. Paul Nemir, "Memoir of Oscar Batson," *Transactions and Studies of the College of Physicians of Philadelphia* 5th ser., 2 (1980):67–70.

6. O. V. Batson, "The Function of the Vertebral Veins and their Role in the Spread of Metastases," *Annals of Surgery* 112(1940):138–49.

7. Personal remembrance as a student in Batson's class, David Y. Cooper.

8. E. R. Long, "Memoir of Stuart Mudd, 1893–1975," *Transactions and Studies of the College of Physicians of Philadelphia* 4th ser., 43(1975–76):435–46.

9. S. Mudd and T. F. Anderson, "Demonstration by Electron Microscope of the Combination of Antibodies with Flagella and Somatic Antigen," *Journal of Immunology* 42(1941):251–66; K. Knaysi and S. Mudd, "The Internal Structure of Certain Bacteria as Revealed by the Electron Microscope," *Journal of Bacteriology* 45(1943):349–59; S. Mudd and T. F. Anderson, "Selective 'Staining' for Electron Micrography. The Effects of Heavy Metal Salts on Individual Bacterial Cells," *Journal of Experimental Medicine* 76(1942):103–8; S. Mudd, K. Polevitzky, and T. F. Anderson, "Bacterial Morphology as Shown by the Electron Microscope IV. Structural Differentiation Within the Bacterial

Protoplasm," *Archives of Pathology* 34(1942):199–207; S. Mudd, K. Polevitzky, and T. F. Anderson, "Bacterial Morphology as Shown by the Electron Microscope V. *Treponema pallidum, T. macrodentium and T. microdentium," Journal of Bacteriology* 46(1943):15–24.

10. E. W. Flosdorf, and S. W. Mudd, "Procedure and Apparatus for Preservation in 'Lyophil' Form of Serum and Other Biological Substances," *Journal of Immunology* 29(1935):389–425.

11. Conversation with Harry Morton.

12. Conversation with Harry Morton.

13. Conversation with Harry Morton.

14. Conversation with Harry Morton.

15. Many personal conversations with J. D. Graham; Obituary, J. D. Graham, *Philadelphia Inquirer,* September, 6, 1974; "University Glass Blower," *Pennsylvania Gazette* 41 (1943):293(cover photograph of J. D. Graham); "He Puffs to Help Doctors to Save Lives," *Philadelphia Evening Bulletin,* April 10, 1939; E. William, "He Puffs for Science." *Philadelphia Inquirer,* March 12, 1950; Jimmy Graham Birthday Party, Excerpt from Scholander's memoirs.

16. Taped conversation with Harry Morton.

17. Conversation with Harry Morton.

18. Flosdorf and Mudd, "Procedure and Apparatus."

19. K. S. Davis, "The Story of the Pill," *American Heritage* 29(1978):80–91.

20. Conversation with George L. Weinstein.

21. A. W. Makepeace, G. L. Weinstein, and M. H. Friedman, "The Effect of Progestin and Progesterone on Ovulation in the Rabbit," *American Journal of Physiology* 119(1937):512–16.

22. Conversation with George L. Weinstein.

23. Personal conversation with Maximilian Ehrenstein.

24. C. Djerassi, "Steroid and Oral Contraceptives, The Chemical Developments which Led to the Currently Employed Steroid Contraceptive Agents is Reviewed," *Science* 151(1966):1055–61.

25. *Ibid.*

26. M. Ehrenstein, *Journal of Organic Chemistry* 9(1944): 435; W. M. Allen and M. Ehrenstein, *Science* 100 (1944): 251–252.

27. Personal conversation with Maximilian Ehrenstein.

28. J. E. Rhoads, "Memoir of John Heysham Gibbon, Jr., 1903–1973," *Transactions and Studies of the College of Physicians of Philadelphia* 4th ser., 41(1973–74):194–97; "Memorial Service for John Heysham Gibbon Jr.," *Transactions and Studies of the College of Physicians of Philadelphia* 4th ser., 41(1973–74):176–97.

29. "Contemporaries, J. H. Gibbon,Jr.," *Modern Medicine* 38 (1970):18–21; J. H. Gibbon,"Medicine's Living History, John H. Gibbon, Jr.," *Medical World News* (November, 1972):46–53; Mrs. J. H. Gibbon, "Personal Recollections of the Early Years of the Development of the Heart Lung Machine," *Journal of Extra-Corporeal Technology* 10(1978):77–88; H. B. Schumacker, Jr., "John H. Gibbon, Jr. The Heart Lung Machine and Progress in Cardiovascular Surgery," *Transactions and Studies of the College of Physicians of Philadelphia* 5th ser., 6 (1984):249–63; H. B. Schumacker, Jr., "John Heysham Gibbon, Jr.," *Biographical Memoirs of the National Academy of Sciences* (Washington, D.C.: National Academy of Sciences Press, 1982), pp. 213–47.

30. Conversation with Francis Wood.

31. *Medical World News,* "Medicine's Living History, John H. Gibbon, Jr.," p. 51; *Modern Medicine,* "Contemporaries, John H. Gibbon, Jr.," pp. 18–19.

32. *Modern Medicine,* p. 18; *Medical World News,* p. 51.

33. Harrison Department of Surgical Research, Ravdin Papers.

34. J. H. Gibbon, Jr. "Artificial Maintenance of Circulation During Experimental Occlusion of Pulmonary Artery," *Surgery, Gynecology, and Obstetrics* 69 (1939):1583–94.

35. Schumacker, "John Heysham Gibbon," pp. 223–33; *Medical World News*, pp. 51–52.

36. *Medical World News*, p. 50.

37. *Medical World News*, p. 52.

38. E. P. Pendergrass, "Memoir of Eldridge L. Eliason," *Transactions and Studies of the College of Physicians of Philadelphia* 4th ser., 18(1951):136–39.

39. Experience of David Y. Cooper as a collaborator of Otto Rosenthal.

40. Pendergrass, "Eldridge L. Eliason," p. 136..

41. *Ibid.*, p. 137.

42. *Ibid.*, p. 138.

43. *Ibid.*, pp. 137–38.

44. B. Roberts, "Memoir of I. S. Ravdin, 1894–1972," *Transactions and Studies of the College of Physicians of Philadelphia* 4th ser., 41(1973–74):237–41; J. E. Rhoads, "I. S. Ravdin, 1894–1972." *Medical Affairs, University of Pennsylvania* (Fall, 1972).

45. I. S. Ravdin, E. Thorogood, C. Riegel et al., "The Prevention of Liver Damage and the Facilitation of Repair in the Liver by Diet," *Journal of the American Medical Association* 121(1943):322–24; S. Goldschmidt, I. S. Ravdin, and B. Lucké, "Anesthesia and Liver Damage I. The Protective Action of Oxygen Against the Necrotizing Effect of Certain Anesthetics on the Liver," *Journal of Pharmacology and Experimental Therapeutics* 64(1938):111–29; I. S. Ravdin, H. M. Vars, and S. Goldschmidt, "Anesthesia and Liver Damage II. The Effect of Anesthesia on the Blood Sugar, the Liver Glycogen, and Liver Fat," *Journal of Pharmacology and Experimental Therapeutics* 59(1937):1–14; S. Goldschmidt, I. S. Ravdin, and B. Lucké, "The Effect of Oxygen in the Prevention of Liver Necrosis by Volatile Anesthetics," *American Journal of Medical Sciences* 189(1935):155–56.

46. *Ibid.*

47. R. H. Ivy, "Personal Recollections of Holders of the John Rhea Barton Professorship of Surgery at the University of Pennsylvania School of Medicine," *Transactions and Studies of the College of Physicians of Philadelphia* 4th ser., 42 (1975):239–62.

48. Personal experience of David Y. Cooper on I. S. Ravdin's surgical service.

49. Conversation with Julian Johnson.

50. Conversation with Francis Wood.

51. *Ibid.*

52. Conversations with Jonathan E. Rhoads and Francis Wood; also heard many times while on the surgical service by David Y. Cooper.

53. Episode witnessed by David Y. Cooper while serving as resident on Ravdin's surgical service.

17

RESEARCH DURING WORLD WAR II AND AFTERWARDS

The greatest and noblest pleasure which we have in the world is to discover new truths and the next is to shake off old prejudices.

Frederick the Great of Prussia

A. N. RICHARDS AND THE WAR EFFORT

As unprepared as the United States was, in December of 1941, to enter World War II, it had begun to prepare for the eventuality of war. President Franklin D. Roosevelt asked A. N. Richards to head the Committee on Medical Research, an advisory group to the Office of Scientific Research and Development, directed by Vannevar Bush. Richards's task was difficult.[1] Medical research was not particularly extensive, and there was no precedent for planning and coordinating research nationwide.[2]

Richards appointed his committee, which included the Assistant Surgeon General of the United States and the director of the National Institutes of Health. The committee determined that any war effort would require research in shock, surgical infection, tropical diseases, war neuroses, blood procurement and transfusion, and the development of plasma expanders.[3]

Richards's greatest contribution as chairman of the committee was his effective effort to put penicillin into mass production in time to treat the war casualties expected in the invasion of Europe and the war in the Pacific. Alexander Fleming had discovered penicillin in 1929 and in a paper that year suggested that "it might be an efficient antiseptic."

President Truman congratulating ten key scientists for their wartime work in the Office of Scientific Research and Development, January 20, 1947. Seated, left to right: James B. Conant, President of Harvard University; the President; Alfred N. Richards, Vice President, University of Pennsylvania. Standing: Lewis H. Weed, Chairman, Division of Sciences, National Research Council; Vannevar Bush, Chairman, new Army-Navy Joint Research and Development Board; Frank B. Jewett, President, National Academy of Sciences; J. C. Hunsaker, Massachusetts Institute of Technology; Roger Adams, University of Illinois; A Baird Hastings, Harvard University. All those present, as well as Karl T. Compton, President of the Massachusetts Institute of Technology; A. R. Doley, Columbia University; and Richard C. Tolman, California Institute of Technology, received a letter of thanks from President Truman. We are indebted to the Truman Library, Independence, Mo., for this illustration. Another picture of the same group appeared on the cover of Science, *January 31, 1947, and in many newspapers about this time.* (Annals of Internal Medicine 71, Supplement 8 [1969].)

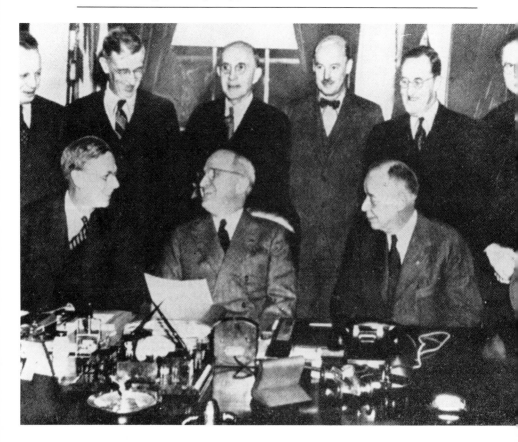

Development was slow until the war, and even then most drug companies were not interested in the cooperation that testing of the drug would require; one firm feared that the penicillin mold would contaminate its vats. By March 1942, there was enough penicillin to treat one test case; by June, 10 more; and by February of 1943, ninety more. The military began using the drug in April. By the time Japan surrendered, September 2, 1945, more than 650 billion units a month were being produced.[4]

CHRISTIAN J. LAMBERTSEN AND THE INSTITUTE FOR ENVIRONMENTAL MEDICINE

In recent decades, one of Penn's most successful and unusual research units has been its Institute of Environmental Medicine; it owes its origin to other aspects of the war effort. In 1941 the Division of Medical Sciences of the National Research Council organized a committee on aviation medicine. The committee pointed out the need for research on masks to deliver oxygen at high altitude, on methods to improve night vision, and on the gravitational effects of altitude on the body.

Penn landed a contract for $90,000—the largest given by the council—to build two high-altitude chambers in the basement of the John Morgan Building. There, an interdisciplinary group from medical physics, pharmacology, physiology, and research medicine developed instruments to measure physiological function under flight conditions and studied such topics as oxygen breathing at high altitudes, night blindness, and the psychological effects of combat during flight.[5]

After the war, those chambers were given to Christian J. Lambertsen, who founded the first institute in the United States dedicated to studying human physiology when exposed to oxygen and inert gas mixtures in high-pressure environments.

Lambertsen made his own significant contributions to the war effort, even as a medical student. A lean, muscular, and large-boned individual, Lambertsen had no buoyancy as a swimmer unless he kicked continuously, a tiresome chore.[6] Yet he enjoyed swimming underwater so much that, early on, he tried to make a breathing unit so that he could remain submerged for prolonged periods of time. Putting together parts used in rebreathing circuits of anesthesia machines, he made his first successful self-contained diving unit in 1939. He used physiological principles that designers of diving equipment had not used before and understood the physiology of respiration, even though he was a year away from entering Penn's medical school.[7]

In medical school, Lambertsen continued to refine his device—a "self-contained underwater breathing apparatus," eventually familiar as scuba—and found a champion in Henry Bazett. Bazett called friends on the National Research Council and in 1941 traveled with Lambertsen to Washington to offer the device to the United States Navy. Much to their surprise, naval authorities seemed fully satisfied with their hose-to-helmet diving techniques. They dismissed both Lambertsen's device and his idea that underwater teams could swim under submarine nets and clamp explosives to the hulls of ships.[8]

Lambertsen was referred to the Office of Strategic Services, a branch of the army, which accepted his ideas. Only Dean William Pepper knew about his student wartime activity, helping the OSS establish a secret operational underwater force.[9]

As a civilian at Penn after the war, the navy called him back from the laboratory to train its surface frogmen to become divers. In memorable maneuvers in the Caribbean, Lambertsen, with a navy associate, made the first exit from and reentry into a submerged submarine that was under way. He then piloted a one-man midget submarine in the first landing onto (and subsequent takeoff from) the deck of a large submarine cruising underwater. These demonstrations firmly established the concepts he had formulated as a student and marked the beginning of modern underwater demolition teams and sea air and land teams. During his research, he had what he later called the "good fortune" of twice being saved after he became unconscious on the sea floor.[10]

For years, Lambertsen continued to improve his diving units, eventually overcoming two persistent problems, that of residual air in the rebreathing circuit and that of oxygen toxicity. In the late 1940s he converted the high-altitude chambers into a positive-pressure-thermal laboratory by reversing the doors and locks and installing pressurizing equipment. He made the first quantitative studies in humans of the effects of high oxygen pressures on gas transport, respiratory control, and the acid-base internal environment of the brain.[11]

Lambertsen favored using humans in his respiratory experiments. "If sensible," he said, "make yourself the first subject." His guiding philosophy was to "make the experimental conditions produce large physiological changes, so that definitive measurement is practical." By increasing the severity of stresses and thereby magnifying the effects of adaptations or disruptions, he turned pressure itself, temperature, gas density, high partial pressures of gases, narcotic drugs, and physical work into controllable forces, even though the effects they produce are not readily detectable under normal conditions of the sea-level laboratory.[12]

In 1965 his laboratory, redesigned by himself, was established as the Institute for Environmental Medicine. Over the past two decades, it has undertaken a series of multidisciplinary predictive studies, correlating measurements of the effects of oxygen and environmental stresses upon specific neural, sensory, cognitive, pulmonary, cardiovascular, hematologic, endocrinal, and other functions. Lambertsen adapted the fundamental pharmacologic principle of "dose-response" to the quantitative study of human physiological tolerance, thereby improving the predictive capability of the research. Among the significant results was his finding that disruptive neurologic effects of rapid compressions were due to hydrostatic pressure rather than to the gases breathed. Lambertsen and his associates also discovered a means for markedly increasing oxygen tolerance. In addition, they uncovered a new, incapacitating, and potentially lethal occupational gas-embolic disease of divers. They identified the mechanism that causes it and devised a method to prevent it completely.

JULIUS COMROE AND ROBERT D. DRIPPS

Julius Comroe headed the graduate department of pharmacology and physiology, and that department largely made pulmonary physiology practical for physicians. Comroe's book on respiratory physiology was the first complete summary of the pulmonary function tests and their interpretations.[13]

He came to Penn in 1936. He first worked under the direction of Carl Schmidt, who was studying the relationship between cerebral blood flow and respiration. Failing to find a way to measure blood flow, Schmidt began examining the connection between respiration and the carotid sinus and body.[14] Comroe extended this work with Robert Dripps, who joined the group in 1938.

Comroe and Dripps found that lobeline, nicotine, and relatively small decreases in oxygen tension directly activated the carotid body, which, in turn, directly increased respiration in the respiratory center. Small changes in carbon-dioxide tension had the same effect.[15]

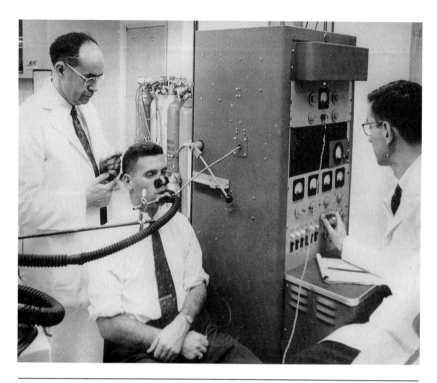

Julius Comroe and Robert Forster using the mass spectrograph. (Nadine Landis.)

Using buffered solutions of the gas in varying strengths, Comroe located the respiratory center in the forma reticularis and showed that only the bicarbonate radical and carbon dioxide stimulated respiration. The main regulatory factor, he established, was bicarbonate concentration. He, Dripps, and Schmidt concluded that decreased oxygen tension, lobeline, and nicotine only reflexively stimulated respiration through their action on the carotid body, dispelling the misconception that carbon dioxide was involved. That gas, they suggested, controlled respiration. Whether it or pH is the actual regulator has not yet been settled.

Extended their collaboration, Comroe and Dripps defined the effects of prolonged breathing of 100 percent oxygen. Breathing oxygen of more than 50 percent for longer than 12 hours, they found, created thoracic pain when patients breathed deeply; it also created difficulties in breathing and a decrease in vital capacity. In other studies they found that arterial gas tensions usually considered normal were, in fact, too low. And by measuring the percent of saturation of hemoglobin in subjects, they concluded that the degree of arterial saturation could not be estimated reliably by looking at the skin and mucous membranes of the mouth, as was the customary clinical practice.[16]

Dripps and Comroe also revised techniques of artificial respiration. They happened to have patients who suffered respiratory arrest, one for two and a half hours, the other for seven hours, and were able to gather the first quantitative information on artificial respiration in unconscious human subjects. They concluded that a satisfactory technique must not only oxygenate the blood but also eliminate excess carbon dioxide—so that rhythmic chest movements were required.[17]

Dripps recommended the mouth-to-mouth method as a last resort.[18] Army officials, interested in ways to combat nerve-gas poisoning, felt that the technique would spread disease in contaminated environments; in addition, disproportionate sizes between rescuer and victim might damage the victim's lung. But these objections were overcome when David Y. Cooper and Richard J. Johns hooked together two gas masks with a tube and made an efficient respirator.[19]

Comroe went on to a career as an essayist. His regular pieces in the *American Review of Respiratory Diseases* dealt with the origin of scientific discoveries as well as the philosophy of science; they were collected in the book *Retrospectroscope*, the title of his column.[20]

Dripps became Penn's first long-term anesthesiologist. His and Comroe's work, as well as research by Schmidt and I. S. Ravdin, made clinicians aware that many medical and surgical complications originated as asphyxia. Penn's first physician-anesthesiologist was Ivan B. Taylor, who arrived in 1938 and left in 1941. He was succeeded by Philip Gleason, who stayed less than a year before he joined the Army and served at the 20th General Hospital. Dripps succeeded him and held the position for twenty-three years, during which time he built the Department of Anesthesiology into one of the finest anywhere.[21]

Dripps's most important clinical contribution was the follow-up study, made with Leroy Vandam, of 10,098 patients who had received spinal anesthesia at the Hospital of the University of Pennsylvania.

Prior to this study, patients feared that spinal anesthesia produced permanent neurological damage. Dripps and his associates demonstrated not one instance of such damage. Some patients had temporary causalgias of the thighs and back. A larger number had headaches and auditory and ocular difficulties, dubbed "spinal headache," but the investigators traced the problem to the leakage of spinal fluid from the hole made by the needle in the dura. A smaller needle reduced the incidence of the syndrome.

Dripps also helped introduce such nonexplosive anesthetics as halothane. And he measured cerebral blood flow by radioactive krypton in anesthetized normal subjects.[22]

ROBERT E. FORSTER II

Robert E. Forster II replaced John Brobeck as the chairman of physiology. He had been in Julius Comroe's Department of Physiology and Pharmacology in the Graduate School and remained at Penn when the two departments were combined. While working with Comroe he mastered the new infrared meter for measuring carbon monoxide and their recently obtained mass spectrometer for measuring helium. With these methods, he, with Fowler and Bates, modified Krog's method of measuring the difusion coefficient and devised a rapid and clinically useful single breath technique for measuring diffusion capacity. Forster is one of ten Pennsylvania professors to serve as president of the American Physiological Society.[23]

GEORGE LUDWIG AND THE CLINICAL USE OF ULTRASOUND

Penn contributed to echo techniques, or ultrasound, to study the biological structures of tissue long before the 1960s, when ultrasound became a fashionable subject for clinical medicine. In the early 1940s, Leslie Chambers, based in the Johnson Foundation for Medical Physics, experimented with ultrasound to disintegrate bacteria and other cells. George D. Ludwig, working at the Naval Medical Research Institute, joined with Francis Struthers, an institute employee, to produce two of the first four papers on the topic.[24]

Their focus on "sonar" techniques was prompted by Charles K. Kirby, then a surgical resident at Penn. Kirby felt that reflected ultrasound might help detect gallstones lodged in the common duct. Surgeons never knew precisely where to open the common duct and search for stones and were never sure, after the operation, that they had removed all of the stones. One device, a probe with a microphone on its end, had been made. It amplified the sounds when the metal probe hit the gallstones; with experience, a surgeon could distinguish the sound produced by a common duct stone. But it was not as definitive as desired.

Ludwig and Struthers first had to determine whether the amount of reflected energy was sufficient to be detected by sonar. The energy is measured indirectly by an "impedance mismatch," for instance between bone and gas. They measured the impedance of various tissues, gallstones, and metal objects and found the reflected energy well above the minimum that the available equipment needed. But the mismatch between bone and gas was so great, they learned, that it interfered with the measurement of the less intensely reflected sounds.[25] Air produced the most difficulty. Unless the abdomen was opened or all gas otherwise removed from the gastrointestinal tract, the researchers felt that ultrasound was not a good detection device. But they pointed out that it might help locate foreign objects and solid tumors.

After his naval service, Ludwig started a surgical residency at the Massachusetts General Hospital, then returned to Penn and shifted to medicine with a joint appointment in the Department of Medicine and the Johnson Foundation for Medical Physics. He worked at Penn for fifteen years but shifted his research interest from ultrasound to the biochemistry of genetic diseases and the production of carbon monoxide associated with hemoglobin breakdown.

Research in ultrasound was taken up by others. Rudolph Hoeber, a Penn biologist, invited Herman Schwann to give a seminar on ultrasound effects on red blood cells.[26] Schwann was studying the broader effect of electromagnetic waves on body tissues. He had observed that microwaves caused severe burns. His studies led to the standardization of radar waves and defined safe exposure levels, which have been important ever since microwave ovens became commonplace.

As a result of the seminar, Schwann was offered a joint appointment in the Department of Physical Medicine and the Department of Medicine. (He later took an appointment in Penn's Moore School of Electrical

Engineering.) For a decade he carried out extensive and systematic studies of the interaction of ultrasound with tissues. Then he extended it to cardiac diagnosis. Claude Joyner, John Reid, and James Bond, under Schwann's direction, made the first echocardiographic records of mitral valve disease and helped improve the design of equipment to make such records.[27]

SEYMOUR KETY AND THE CEREBRAL CIRCULATION

Carl Schmidt, who had been unable to find the relationship between blood flow and respiration, joined with Paul Dumke to make the first accurate measurements of the quantity of blood required to supply the brain. They were able to direct all of the brain's blood flow into a simple device, a bubble flow meter. They also found a correlation between blood flow and blood pressure and demonstrated an intrinsic response to a number of drugs, anoxia, and carbon dioxide. Their results were published in 1943.[28]

The Dumke-Schmidt paper drew Seymour Kety, a Penn graduate, back to his medical alma mater. Kety had been working in the laboratory of Joseph Aub, in Boston, and was impressed by the numerous homeostatic mechanisms that are evoked to preserve the cerebral circulation. Kety's work concentrated on applying the Fick principle—a way to measure pulmonary blood flow—to cardiac output. The Fick principle dated back to 1870 and involved measuring the amount of oxygen taken up in the lung in a given period of time, the oxygen content of the pulmonary artery flowing into the lung and that of the pulmonary vein flowing out. Kety read the Dumke-Schmidt paper and realized that the principle could be applied to measure cerebral blood flow, and he returned to Penn to work with Schmidt on it.[29]

Others about the same time were applying the Fick principle to measure blood flow in the kidney and in the liver. These organs excrete a foreign substance at a constant rate that can be measured independently. The brain does not selectively remove or specifically secrete any foreign substance that can be accurately measured. It does, however, absorb by physical solution inert gases which reach it through arterial blood. If the rate at which the brain takes up inert gas depends upon the characteristics of physical solubility rather than mental activity, then, Kety knew, he could calculate a value for part of the Fick equation.[30]

Kety began studies to determine the solubility of nitrous oxide in the brain. He quickly found that it had the same solubility in blood and brain, in living brain tissue and dead, and was not altered by mental activity or disease states. His experiments showed that after 10 minutes the brain was in equilibrium with the venous blood that drained from it, so samples of that blood would give him the number he needed.[31]

But what about measuring the brain arterio-oxygen difference? Initially the difference is large, but it progressively decreases until equilibrium. Kety devised an equation to calculate the varying difference. He also conducted experiments to show that blood draining from the brain was not significantly contaminated by blood from such extracer-

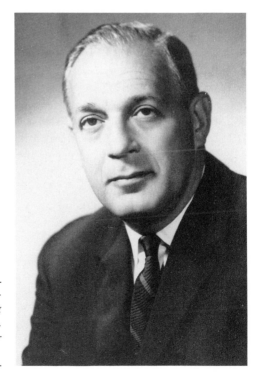

Seymour Kety, who devised the nitrous oxide method for measuring cerebral blood flow in humans. (Photo given to author by Seymour Kety.)

ebral regions as the face and scalp. Kety's results also tallied with values established with the bubble flow meter. In 1948 Kety and Schmidt published the first accurate values for cerebral blood flow, oxygen consumption, glucose metabolism, and cerebrovascular resistance in humans.[32]

In physiology the new method was first used to measure the effect of altering oxygen and carbon dioxide concentrations on the cerebral circulation. These measurements confirmed the classical observations that carbon dioxide is a potent cerebrovascular vasodilator and that low oxygen and carbon dioxide tensions produce cerebral constriction. These studies suggested that cerebral circulation is largely controlled chemically.

Kety's techniques were used to determine the changes wrought by brain tumors, hypertension, diabetes, coma, senility, and many other conditions of cerebral physiology. Kety left Penn in 1949, continuing his innovative research and assuming a distinguished series of administrative posts at the National Institute of Mental Health, Johns Hopkins, and the Mailman Research Center at McLean Hospital in Massachusetts.[33]

The nitrous oxide method was superseded in time by techniques which employed the use of radioactive krypton-85 gas. At the N. I. H., Martin Reivich and Louis Sokoloff measured metabolic rates throughout the brain using a nonmetabolized radioactive agent to determine glucose uptake. Later, at Penn, Reivich applied the method to humans by using positron emission tomography and a suitably labeled deoxyglucose.[34]

NOTES

1. C. F. Schmidt, "Alfred Newton Richards (1876–1966)," *Biographical Memoirs of the National Academy of Sciences*, vol. 42 (New York: Columbia University Press, 1971), p. 301

2. D. Bronk, "Aviation Medicine," *Scientist Against Time* (Boston: Little Brown, 1946), chap. 24, pp. 377–93.

3. Minutes of Richards committee meeting, Richards Papers, Archives of the University of Pennsylvania.

4. A. N. Richards, "Production of Penicillin in the United States," *Nature* 201(1964):441–45; Research, Development, and Production of Penicillin in the United States [Text as submitted to Lady Fleming], unpublished manuscript, Archives of the University of Pennsylvania; Timetable of events leading to Production of Penicillin [Carbon copy of material on American Penicillin Production sent to Lady Fleming, October, 1956], Archives of the University of Pennsylvania.

5. Minutes of the Richards committee meeting, Richards papers, Archives of the University of Pennsylvania.

6. Personal taped interview with Christian J. Lambertsen; Experience working in Christian J. Lambertsen's laboratory, 1949–50.

7. C. J. Lambertsen, Patent Application, Breathing Apparatus, Filed December 16, 1940, No. 2,348,074, May 2, 1944.

8. Conversation with C. J. Lambertsen.

9. Conversation with C. J. Lambertsen.

10. Conversation with C. J. Lambertsen.

11. Conversation with C. J. Lambertsen.

12. C. J. Lambertsen, Patent Application, Breathing Apparatus, Filed January 31, 1945, No. 2,456,130, December 14, 1948; The LARU (Lambertsen Amphibious Respiratory Unit), *A self contained respiratory apparatus for shallow water swimming and diving, and for use in atmospheres containing noxious gases, Instructions for Use and Maintenance. OSS Public Relations Release, The Lambertsen Amphibious Respiratory Unit.* Lambertsen Papers; letter of July 15, 1949, to Chief of Naval Operations, Navy Department, Washington, D.C. from C. J. Lambertsen, "Subject: Current Status of Underwater Operation Program of the U.S. Navy Underwater Demolition Teams"; personal experience of David Y. Cooper working in laboratory of C. J. Lambertsen, 1949–50; C. J. Lambertsen, Schematic Diagram of Flatus II and Description, August 5, 1945. Personal papers of C. J. Lambertsen; Patent application, filed December 14, 1956, Breathing Apparatus [Breath saving unit], No. 2,871,854, February 3, 1959; C. J. Lambertsen, Patent 3,794,021, February 26, 1974. Dual Mode Mixed Gas Breathing Apparatus.

13. J. H. Comroe, Jr., R. E. Forester, A. B. DuBois, W. A. Briscoe, and E. Carlson, *The Lung, Clinical Physiology and Pulmonary Function Tests* (Chicago: Year Book Publishers, 1964; First Edition 1955).

14. Jacque Cattell, ed., *American Men and Women of Science*, 15th edition, vol. 2 (New York: Bowker, 1982), p. 321.

15. C. F. Schmidt, J. H. Comroe, Jr., R. D. Dripps, and P. R. Dumke, "The Function of the Carotid and Aortic Bodies," *American Journal of Medical Sciences* 198 (1939):7; J. H. Comroe and C. F. Schmidt, "Reflexes from the Carotid Body to the Respiratory Center," *American Journal of Medical Sciences* 193(1937):735; J. H. Comroe and R. D. Dripps, "Effects of Direct Chemical Stimulation of the Respiratory Center," *American Journal of Medical Sciences* 201(1941):783; R. D. Dripps and J. H. Comroe, Jr., "The Respiratory and Circulatory Response of Normal Man to Inhalation of 7.6 and 10.4 Per Cent CO_2 with a Comparison of the Maximal Ventilation Produced by Severe Muscular Exercise Inhalation of CO_2 and Maximal Voluntary Hyperventilation," *American Journal of Physiology* 149 (1946):43–51; J. H. Comroe and R. D. Dripps, Jr., "The Oxygen Tension of Arterial Blood and Alveolar Air in Normal Human Subjects," *American Journal of Physiology* 142(1944):700–07.

16. R. D. Dripps and J. H. Comroe, Jr., "The Effect of Inhalation of High and Low Oxygen Concentrations on Respiration, Pulse Rate, Ballistocardiogram and Arterial Oxygen Saturation (Oximeter) of Normal Individuals," *American Journal of Physiology* 149(1947):277–91.

17. J. H. Comroe, Jr. and R. D. Dripps, "Artificial Respiration: A Comparison of the Shafer, Eve and Meltzer-Auer Method in Two Apneic, Asphyctic Patients," *American Journal of Medical Sciences* 210(1945):7.

18. Personal experience of David Y. Cooper attending the lectures of R. D. Dripps.

19. D. Y. Cooper, "Mouth-to-Mouth Artificial Respiration: Influence of Alcohol on Revival of an Old Technique," *Life Sciences* 16(1975):487–500.

20. J. H. Comroe, Jr., *Retrospectroscope* (Menlo Park, Calif.: Von Gehr Press,

1977); J. H. Comroe, Jr., *Exploring the Heart: Discoveries in Heart Disease and High Blood Pressure Research* (New York: W. W. Norton, 1983).

21. "Dr. Dripps is Named V.P. for Health Affairs," *Health Affairs* (Fall 1972):11–12; H. Wollman, "Memoir of Robert Dunning Dripps—1911–1973," *Transactions and Studies of the College of Physicians of Philadelphia* 4th ser., 42 (1974–1975):291–92; J. E. Eckenhoff, *Anesthesia from Colonial Times—A History of Anesthesia at the University of Pennsylvania* (Philadelphia: Lippincott, 1966).

22. R. D. Dripps and L. D. Vandam, "Long-Term Follow-Up of Patients Who Received 10,098 Spinal Anesthetics. Failure to Discover Major Neurological Sequelae," *Journal of the American Medical Association* 156 (1954):1486–91.

23. Comroe, *Retrospectroscope*, pp. 28–29; R. E. Forster, W. S. Fowler, D. V. Bates, and B. Van Lingen, "The Absorption of Carbon Monoxide by the Lung During Breathholding," *Journal of Clinical Investigation* 33(1954):1135–45; Presidents of the American Physiological Society who have worked at Penn include S. Weir Mitchell, Henry C. Bazett, John Brobeck, Julius Comroe, Eugene Landis, Robert F. Pitts, A. C. Burton, John Pappanheimer, Alfred P. Fishman, and R. E. Forster.

24. D. White, G. Clark, and E. White, *Ultra Sound in Biology and Medicine* (Oxford and New York: Pergamon Press, 1982); G. D. Ludwig and F. W. Struthers, "Considerations Underlying the Use of Ultra Sound to Detect Gallstones and Foreign Bodies in Tissue," *Naval Medical Research Institute Project* NM. 004-001 Report No. 4 (June 1949).

25. G. W. Ludwig, "The Velocity of Sound Through Tissues and the Acoustic Impedance of Tissues," *Journal of the Acoustical Society of America* 22(1950):862–66; G. D. Ludwig and F. W. Struthers, "Detection of Gallstones with Ultrasonic Echos," *Electronics* 23(1950): 172–78.

26. Conversation with Herman Schwann.

27. C. and P. Reid, "Applications of Ultra Sound in Cardiovascular Physiology," *Progress in Cardiovascular Diseases* 5(1962–63):482–97; P. G. Thompson, "Medical Applications of Ultra Sound," *Medical Affairs* (Fall, 1971): 8–12.

28. C. F. Schmidt, "The Influence of Cerebral Blood Flow on Respiration I. The Respiratory Response to Changes in Cerebral Blood Flow," *American Journal of Physiology* 84(1928):202–22; C. F. Schmidt and J. P. Hendrix, "The Action of Chemical Substances on Cerebral Vessels," *Proceedings of the Association for Research in Nervous and Mental Diseases* 18(1938):229–76; conversation with C. F. Schmidt.

29. P. R. Dumke and C. F. Schmidt, "Quantitative Measurements of Cerebral Blood Flow in the Macaque Monkey," *American Journal of Physiology* 138 (1943):421–28.

30. S. S. Kety, "The Cerebral Circulation," in *Circulation of the Blood: Men and Ideas*, ed. A. P. Fishman and D. E. Richards (Bethesda, Md.: American Physiological Society, 1964), pp. 703–38; S. S. Kety, "The Metamorphosis of a Psychobiologist, "*Annual Review of Neurological Science* 2(1979):1–15.

31. C. F. Schmidt, S. S. Kety, and H. H. Pennes, "The Gaseous Metabolism of the Brain of the Monkey," *American Journal of Physiology* 143(1945):33–52; S. S. Kety and C. F. Schmidt, "The Determination of Cerebral Blood Flow in Man by the Use of Nitrous Oxide in Low Concentrations," *American Journal of Physiology* 143(1945):53–66.

32. S. S. Kety and C. F. Schmidt, "The Nitrous Oxide Method for the Quantitative Determination of Cerebral Blood Flow in Man: Theory, Procedure and Normal Values," *Journal of Clinical Investigation* 27(1948):476–83; S. S. Kety, "Study of the Cerebral Circulation by Means of Inert Diffusible Tracers," in *Progress in Brain Research*, ed. J. S. Meyer and J. P. Schade [Cerebral Blood Flow], vol. 35 (Amsterdam: Elsevier, 1971), pp. 375–85; C. F. Schmidt, "The Early Days of Indifferent Gas Methods for

Measuring Cerebral Blood Flow," *Journal of Cerebral Blood Flow and Metabolism* 2(1982):1–2.

33. S. S. Kety, "The Metamorphosis of a Psychobiologist," *Annual Review of Neuroscience* 2(1979):1–15.

34. B. A. Bell, "History of the Study of the Cerebral Circulation and the Measurement of Cerebral Blood Flow," *Neurosurgery* 14(1984):238–46.

18

ADVANCES IN PENNSYLVANIA'S PEDIATRIC SERVICE AT THE CHILDREN'S HOSPITAL OF PHILADELPHIA

Like changing leaves the life of man is found
Now green in youth, now withering on the ground.

Alexander Pope

JOSEPH STOKES

Although Joseph Stokes brought modern scientific medicine to The Children's Hospital of Philadelphia, he made his first mark as a clinician. After graduating from Penn's medical school, interning at Massachusetts General Hospital, and completing his residency at Pennsylvania Hospital, he opened a private practice in the Germantown section of Philadelphia in 1923. It was said that he could hear more with a stethoscope than anyone else-and that he could even see through it. He also initiated a novel fee system of contracts for families.[1]

He joined Penn's pediatric service in 1924 and throughout his career devoted his research to preventing viral diseases in children. In 1934 he noted the discovery that active immunity could be produced in animals by an attenuated influenza virus and began studies to produce active immunity in humans. He collected a group of researchers and also brought Werner and Gertrude Henle, the pioneer virologists, to Children's Hospital to conduct the study.[2]

Meanwhile, Stokes shifted his interest to other viral diseases. In 1940 he looked into a vaccine for measles, but it failed because he and his associates could not maintain an attenuated strain of measles virus. Some twenty years later he helped John Enders and Frederick C. Robbins attenuate the rubella virus reliably, and a vaccine was developed.[3]

During World War II Stokes became intrigued by hepatitis when some Army recruits, given passive immunity against mumps by being vaccinated with serum from convalescent patients, acquired viral hepatitis. On the Penn campus Francis D. W. Lukens, professor of medicine and director of the Cox Foundation, almost lost his life when he was

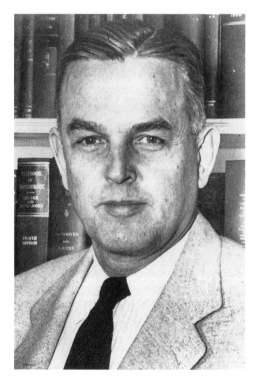

Joseph Stokes, Professor of Pediatrics, specialist in the infectious diseases of children and developer of numerous vaccines for their prevention. (Archives of the University of Pennsylvania.)

given convalescent serum for his severe case of mumps. His mumps was mild, however, compared to the almost fatal case of hepatitis he contracted from the viral contaminated convalescent serum which had been sent to Children's Hospital for evaluation. Subsequently investigators there and elsewhere determined that hepatitis could be transmitted by human serum.[4]

Stokes demonstrated that a mumps virus could be grown in monkeys. Then he, along with John Enders, developed a diagnostic skin test for susceptibility to mumps. They went on to develop a successful mumps vaccine from emulsions of parotid glands of monkeys infected with mumps, but it was not placed on the market because the war ended and no one developed it until later.[5]

After the war Stokes expanded research at Children's Hospital. He brought Seymour Cohen to study genetics and chemotherapeutic agents for cancer and Robert McAllister and Lewis Corielle to develop cancer research. Stokes appointed Alfred M. Bongiovanni to head the endocrinology clinic and laboratory; Bongiovanni and his colleagues helped clarify the endocrinology and pathogenesis of adrenal virilizing hyperplasia.

Stokes also helped organize a full-time pediatric surgical service headed by C. Everett Koop, later the United States surgeon general. Extramurally he organized the Philadelphia Serum Exchange, so that the public could have access to gamma globulin. Jonathan Rhoads, Penn's eminent surgeon and former provost, said, "It's hard to enumerate the accomplishments of Joe Stokes's lifetime, for he worked so much through others."[6]

CHARLES CHAPPEL

No hospital that treats children can do without an isolette, that small, plastic, rectangular chamber with closable ports to admit the arms and hands of attendants who do not interrupt its controlled levels of temperature, humidity, oxygen, and carbon dioxide. Much of the credit for the isolette goes to Charles Chappel. He entered pediatric practice in the early 1930s.[7] After two years of residency at Children's Hospital, he stated, "I saw [only] one baby come out of the premature nursery alive. You can image the heartbreak of those whose baby survived its birth and early life only to succumb to infection."

Chappel studied airborne infections in nurseries and concluded that the attending doctors and nurses were the chief factor in spreading respiratory and intestinal infections among the infant patients. He sketched out, then built, a cardboard model of an incubator for preemies and persuaded a friend, Philo Farnsworth, a television pioneer at Philco, to help him construct it.[8]

In 1937 Chappel brought a primitive isolette to the hospital. It was a closed box with two round ports on one side; to the ports were attached long cloth sleeves closed at the ends with elastic bands. The wooden front could be opened to admit the infant. All of the patient's needs could be supplied by a nurse through the sleeved ports. A filtering system eliminated the danger from infectious bacteria and viruses that contaminated the air of the wards and nurseries.[9]

It was obvious that the device would work after its first clinical trial, but a statistical trial helped interest other pediatricians. Chappel man-

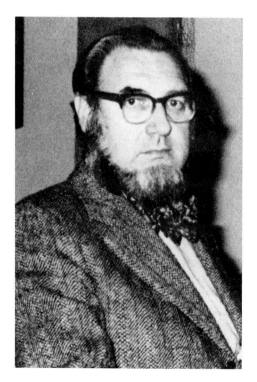

C. Everett Koop, pioneer pediatric surgeon and Surgeon General of the United States. (Scope.)

aged 50 preemies with his incubator, and only one died from infection (others died from congenital defects and other untreatable problems of infancy).

The clear nose cone of World War II bombers gave Chappel the idea of making his incubator from Lucite. It permitted adults to observe the patient better, and it was easier to clean. Chappel left Children's Hospital in 1950 to head clinical research at the Veterans Administration in Washington, D.C., concluding his career at the University of Nebraska medical school.[10]

WERNER AND GERTRUDE HENLEY

Werner and Gertrude Henle left Germany in the 1930s. Werner worked in bacteriology and physiology at Penn, where, under Stuart Mudd and Clarence Gambel, he studied transient sterilization by immunizing female animals against spermatozoa. Henle produced antibodies against the sperm, but they did not prevent pregnancy because they circulated in the plasma rather than in vaginal secretions.

In 1939 Stokes gave the Henles a laboratory for viral research at Children's Hospital. He wanted someone to carry on his work to develop an influenza vaccine. Using the chick allantoic sac as a culture medium, the Henles were able to culture the virus and develop a successful vaccine. When the influenza B virus was discovered, the Henles obtained the strain in order to incorporate it into their vaccine. As they evaluated it, they found that the more the virus was diluted, the more greatly it proliferated in the host. Evidently they were diluting out or inhibiting an inactivating factor. They called this the "interference phenomenon," which brought them early fame.[11]

The Henles discovered the neurotoxic properties of the influenza virus almost by chance. Gertrude Henle was conducting safety tests and wondered whether any neurotropic virus developed in the amniotic fluid used in the vaccine for the flu virus. She injected mice with virus preparations, and all of them died or were near death within twenty four hours. Intravenous and intraperitoneal injection of the virus, they found, produced hepatitis and hepatic damage. They felt that this type of cerebral infection produced the symptoms now described as Reyes syndrome, seen in children during flu epidemics or after severe respi-

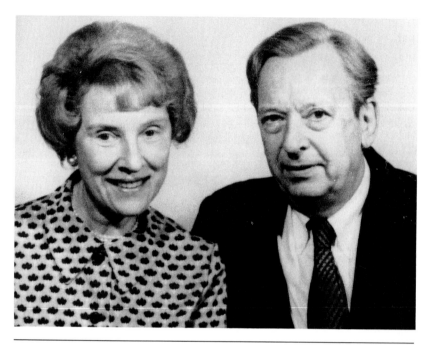

Gertrude and Werner Henle, pioneer virologists. Werner Henle was the first Professor of Virology appointed in the world. (Gertrude Henle.)

ratory infections, especially if they have been treated with large doses of aspirin.[12]

In the 1940s the Henles looked into a mumps vaccine. Although they never obtained optimal attenuation of the virus, they described the epidemiology of the disease. Contrary to popular belief, mumps, they found, was most contagious just prior to the onset of symptoms and during the early days of its clinical manifestation.

The Henles also first traced the link between the Epstein-Barr virus and Burkett's lymphoma. Dennis Burkett, a British surgeon at Makerer University in Uganda, investigated an unusual massive tumor of the jaw that produced grotesque disfigurement and rapid death, most commonly in children between six and eight years old. His studies showed that the lymphoma was infectious and transmitted by mosquitoes.

In 1964 Epstein and Barr suggested that cells cultured from these lymphomas were infected with a virus. It was assumed that the virus particles in the tumor cells were merely passengers, since no species of herpes virus was then suspected of causing tumors in animals. Epstein sent the Henles some viral cells, and the researchers found that the Epstein-Barr virus had the characteristics of a herpes virus. They were convinced that they were dealing with an unknown organism and began to study the link between the virus and Burkett's lymphoma. [13]

Using an immunofluorescence technique that detects the presence of antibodies to a virus, the Henles confirmed that patients with the lymphoma had antibodies to the Epstein-Barr virus. Further investigation found, first, that nearly all healthy African children, not only those with Burkett's lymphoma, had antibodies to the Epstein-Barr virus; and second, that children all over the world had antibodies to the virus, more so in poor or unhygienic conditions. Patients with Burkett's lymphoma turn out to have titers of the virus that are ten times those of healthy individuals.

The Henles happened to find that the Epstein-Barr virus causes infectious mononucleosis. Their technicians were routinely screened, and when one of them came down with infectious mononucleosis, strong titers of antibodies to the virus suddenly appeared in her serum. The Henles confirmed their finding by using the serum collection of James Niederman and Robert W. McCollum of the Yale University medical school. The Yale researchers had collected serum from hundreds of college students as they entered college; if the student developed mononucleosis, they took another serum sample, then yet another after the disease subsided. The samples, which had been stored away, were a perfect source for the Henles to cinch the connection. Their work made it possible to delineate in detail the pathogenesis and epidemiology of infectious mononucleosis.

JOSEPH L. HOLLANDER

Probably no arthritis treatment relieves joint and muscle pain as successfully as steroid injection, a treatment that started at Penn. The idea of steroid therapy occurred to Joseph Hollander about 1950 when he and Steve Horvath were using small thermocouples to study temperatures inside joints, measuring the efficacy of various therapeutic agents. [14] As their work was in progress, cortisone became available;

and they tried it first on a patient with two arthritic knees. They injected one knee with steroid, and it improved; the other did not. The trial suggested that the therapeutic action was local—an important finding since cortisone could be administered orally but only with undesirable side effects. Hollander and his associates carried out an extended study, publishing the results in *Journal of the American Medical Association* in 1951.[15]

Joseph Hollander, Professor of Medicine, rheumatologist, and his chamber for studying the influence of changing climatic condition on arthritis. (Joseph Hollander.)

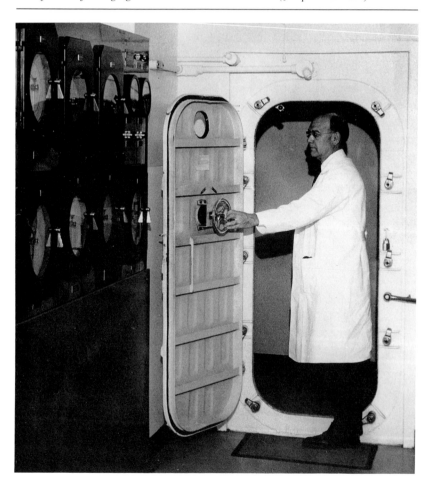

Hollander expected to become an orthopaedic surgeon, but one day he was making rounds with Jesse Nicholson at Children's Hospital when he saw three children sealed in total body casts of plaster; they had juvenile arthritis, and the treatment ankylosed the joints in functional positions. Hollander commented that the casts were a terrible way to treat children. Nicholson replied, "Hollander, when you go off this ward, go to the library and read what's known about arthritis. If you come up with any better treatment, I will try it." Hollander did the library work and realized that arthrology was a field needing advances; he shifted his field to internal medicine.[16]

Hollander also proved the truth in the old saw that patients with arthritis can predict storms. He built a controlled climate chamber in his rehabilitation center and convinced two patients to live in it for a time. Barometric pressure, humidity, air flow, and air ionization were all controlled. Windows permitted the patients to see the weather outside. Throughout the study the environmental conditions were changed without the patients' knowledge in sequences unrelated to the outside weather. The researchers found that lower barometric pressure and higher humidity always made the patients feel worse, their pains increase, and their joints swell.

But Hollander could never show exactly what caused the association of atmospheric changes and pain. Since the pain occurred in areas of scar tissue (amputation stumps or operative scars as well as in inflammatory tissue), he figured that such tissue could not adjust its pressure to atmospheric change as rapidly as did the surrounding normal tissue, and the differences produced the symptoms.[17]

WILLIAM J. RASHKIND

Cardiac catheterization and the heart-lung machine made possible the diagnosis and treatment of congenital heart defects in infants and children, and some important contributions to the field were made by William J. Rashkind at The Children's Hospital of Philadelphia.[18] He and an associate, William Miller, noticed that about 20 percent of children who die of congenital heart disease have a transposition of the great vessels and that most of these patients die in their first six months of life (50 percent in the first month). Although the defect can be corrected, surgery is most definitive when the children are more than six months old. Rashkind developed palliative measures to keep the children alive until the anatomy of their cardiovascular systems had grown sufficiently and would not complicate the surgery.[19]

The standard procedure removed a portion of the atrial septum. Rashkind realized that it would damage the heart less and be simpler if he produced this defect without thoracotomy and general anesthesia. He devised a double-lumen catheter which he threaded into the heart through the femoral vein. The catheter is guided into the left atrium. A balloon at the end of one lumen is inflated, then withdrawn rapidly into the right atrium, thereby tearing the septal wall. The balloon is deflated and the procedure repeated until the filled balloon can be drawn from the left atrium into the right with no resistance.[20]

Rashkind and his colleagues went on to develop a prosthesis to close a patent ductus arteriosus. An early version was a miniature grappling hook made of stainless steel and filled with a cone of medical polyurethane or polyvinyl alcohol foam. The device had an elaborate folding mechanism and a positive release so that it could not release prematurely. But because it failed for more than half of the patients on which it was tried, Rashkind developed a double-disc non-hooked prosthesis. This device made use of the funnel shape of the ductus to anchor it.[21]

NOTES

1. J. E. Rhoads, "Joseph Stokes, Jr. (1896–1972)," *Year Book of the American Philosophical Society* (Philadelphia, American Philosophical Society, 1972), 239–44; A. M. Bongiovanni, "Memoir of Joseph Stokes, Jr. 1896–1972," *Transactions and Studies of the College of Physicians of Philadelphia* 4th ser., 40(1972):147–48; A. C. McGuinness, "Address given on the occasion of a farewell dinner to Dr. Stokes, June 16, 1961," *Journal of Pediatrics* 59(1961):797–807.

2. Rhoads, p. 240; McGuinness, pp. 798–99.

3. Bongiovanni, p. 147.

4. J. F. Enders, L. W. Kane, E. P. Maris, and J. Stokes, Jr., "Immunity in Mumps V. The Correlation of the Presence of Dermal Hypersensitivity and Resistance to Mumps," *Journal of Experimental Medicine* 84 (1946): 341–64.

5. McGuinness. "Address," p. 800.

6. Rhoads, "Joseph Stokes, Jr.," pp. 240, 244.

7. Notes of Charlie Chappel.

8. Notes of Charlie Chappel.

9. Notes of Charlie Chappel.

10. Notes of Charlie Chappel.

11. W. Henle, G. Henle, K. Humler, and F. Lief, "The Changing Aspects of the Serodiagnosis of Viral Infections," *Journal of Pediatrics* 6(1961):827–35.

12. G. Henle and W. Henle, "Studies on the Toxicity of Influenza Viruses I. The

Effect of Intracerebral Injection of Influenza Viruses," *Journal of Experimental Medicine* 84(1946):623–37; W. Henle and G. Henle, "Studies on the Toxicity of Influenza Viruses II. The Effect of Intra-Abdominal and Intravenous Injection of Influenza Viruses," *Journal of Experimental Medicine* 84(1946):639–60.

13. W. Henle, G. Henle, and E. T. Lennette, "The Epstein-Barr Virus," *Scientific American* (July 1979):50–59; W. Henle and G. Henle, *The Association of Epstein-Barr Virus with Nasopharyngeal Carcinoma* (Philadelphia: Children's Hospital of Philadelphia and the School of Medicine, University of Pennsylvania, 1981), p. 1.

14. Personal conversation with Joseph Hollander.

15. J. L. Hollander, E. M. Brown, Jr., R. A. Jessar, and C. Y. Brown, "Hydrocortisone and Cortisone Injected into Arthritic Joints," *Journal of the American Medical Association* 147(1951):1–19.

16. Conversation with Joseph Hollander.

17. J. L. Hollander, and S. Y. Yeostros, "The Effect of Simultaneous Variation of Humidity and Barometric Pressure on Arthritis," *AIBS Bulletin* 13(1963):24–28.

18. Memorial talk of Sidney Friedman for William J. Rashkind.

19. W. J. Rashkind, "Trans-Catheter Treatment of Congenital Heart Disease," *Circulation* 57(1983):711–16.

20. W. J. Rashkind and W. Miller, "Creation of an Atrial Septal Defect Without Thoracotomy," *Journal of the American Medical Association* 196(1966):991–92; W. J. Rashkind and W. Miller, "Transposition of the Great Arteries: Results of Palliation by Balloon Arterioseptostomy in Thirty-one Infants," *Circulation* 38(1968):453–62; W. J. Rashkind, "Balloon Arterioseptostomy Revisited: The First Fifteen Years," *International Journal of Cardiology* 4(1983):369–72.

21. W. J. Rashkind and C. C. Cuaso, "Transcatheter Closure of Patent Ductus Arteriosus," *Pediatric Cardiology* 1(1979):1–3.

19
INTRODUCTION TO THE MODERN ERA

Without freedom of thought there can be no such thing as wisdom, and no such thing as public liberty, without freedom of speech, which is the right of every man, as far as by it he does not hurt and control the right of another and this is the only check it ought to suffer and only bounds it ought to know.

Benjamin Franklin,
Dogwood Papers

As the twentieth century progressed, biochemistry looked increasingly intensively at the cell. Earlier, medical students were taught to focus on the constituents of body fluids and wastes, the chemical and physiologic action of vitamins, the chemistry of proteins, carbohydrates, and lipids, and the body's nutritional requirements. There was virtually no mention of the metabolic processes that were being catalyzed by the enzymes of the cell. Several formidable scientists at Penn helped determine the direction of cell physiology.

DAVID WRIGHT WILSON

Physiological chemistry under the chairmanship of David Wright Wilson was one of Penn's most distinguished departments. Wilson, whom friends called by his middle name, became chairman after World War I and held the post for thirty-two years, presiding over innovative research during the entire period.[1] Wilson earned his Ph.D. from Yale University in 1914. During World War I, he studied the physiological effects of poisonous gases for the army and navy. At the British Research Center for Poisonous Gases at Porton, England, he volunteered to test

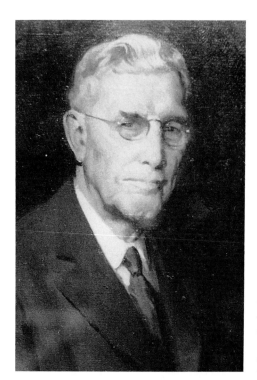

D. Wright Wilson, Benjamin Rush
Professor of Physiological Chem-
istry. (Biographical Memoirs of the
National Academy of Sciences.)

clothing designed to protect soldiers from mustard-gas burns. He was
severely burned by the gas during a test.

SAMUEL GURIN AND CARL BACHMAN—
GONADOTROPIN PURIFICATION

As an academic administrator, Wilson promoted interdisciplinary work.
Carl Bachman, the obstetrician, was an appreciative visitor. He worked
with the biochemist Samuel Gurin in the first purification of a glyco-
protein, gonadotropin. They succeeded because they used urine from
pregnant women whose hormone output was greatest (60 to 80 days after
conception) and because they improved extraction procedures.[2] Bachman later pointed out that collaborative research involved some dozen
members of his and Wilson's departments and produced more than 25

scientific papers in six years. "Whatever benefits Wright and his group may have obtained from their joint activities," Bachman wrote, "there can be little doubt that the rewards for our own group were both substantial and enduring."[3]

SAMUEL GURIN AND THE INTRODUCTION OF RADIOISOTOPES INTO MEDICAL SCIENCE

Wilson was also a visionary scientist. He perceived the importance of isotopes in biochemistry. The stable isotopes of carbon, nitrogen, and oxygen permitted new studies into the complicated metabolic pathways of the body.[4] He worked with Samuel Gurin, among others, to find two sources of the stable isotope ^{13}C, used to investigate the metabolism of carbohydrates. Gurin, long an advisor to Wilson, succeeded him as

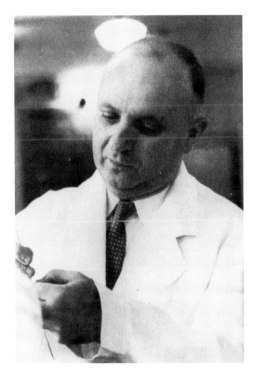

Samuel Gurin, Benjamin Rush Professor of Biological Chemistry, pioneer in the use of stable isotopes and introducer of the radioactive carbon (^{14}C) isotope for metabolic tracer studies. (Scope.)

head of the department. Gurin eventually moved on to become the first non-M.D. dean of Penn's medical school.[5]

In the mid-1940s Gurin and Wilson joined with John M. Buchanan and Warwick Sakami to study the oxidation of fatty acids. They ultimately found that the last group of the fatty acid chain (the methyl terminal two-carbon fragment) is handled differently from the other three two-carbon fragments formed from the alpha or carboxyl end of octanoic acid—the first clue that the fragments had different metabolic origins.[6] Their work also pointed to the now-well-established fact that acetoacetic acid is formed by reaction of acetyl CoA with malonyl CoA.[7]

Gurin and Ross O. Brady discovered that fatty acid synthesis did not occur without carbon dioxide and bicarbonate in the system. They also found that citrate stimulates fatty acid synthesis.[8]

The Penn scientists were so skilled in synthesizing substrates for studies using metabolic tracers that Oak Ridge chose them for the first trial use of ^{14}C carbon in biochemical experiments.[9]

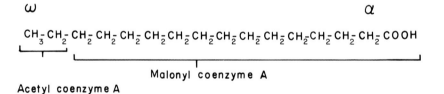

Gurin, Crandall, Buchanan, and Brady demonstrated that there were two kinds of two-carbon units in fatty acids, indicating that the alpha two-carbon fragment had a different origin from the omega fragment. Subsequently Brady and Gurin discovered that fatty acid synthesis did not occur in the absence of CO_2. The latter finding led to the independent discovery by Wakil and Brady that acetyl CoA and malonyl CoA are not formed in the absence of CO_2. F. Lynen's elegant multi-enzyme complex fatty acid synthetase resulted from the realization that the omega two-carbon fragment unit originated from acetyl CoA and the other two-carbon fragments from malonyl CoA.

JOHN M. BUCHANAN AND THE MECHANISM OF PURINE SYNTHESIS

Another important series of studies on the biosynthesis of purine was initiated by John M. Buchanan.[10] He and John Sonne, a second-year medical student, began this work by studying uric acid formation by pigeon liver tissue slices. Since the rates of uric acid synthesis by these liver slices were too slow, they turned to studying uric acid formation in the intact pigeon.[11]

They were joined by Adelaide M. Delluva and Joel Flacks, and the group found the sources of various atoms of the uric acid molecule. Their finding that C atoms 2 and 8 derived from formate led to the discovery of a new class of enzymes, the tetrahydrofolate catalysts, which are important in transferring one-carbon fragments in synthetic reactions.[12]

DALE REX COMAN

Dale Rex Coman studied pathology at Penn after obtaining his medical degree at McGill University. After studying elsewhere, he returned to

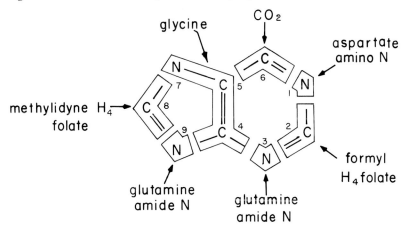

John Buchanan and his collaborators Adelaide Delluva and John Sonne found that the atoms of uric acid were derived from the following precursors: nitrogen 7 and carbon atoms 5 and 4 from glycine; ureide carbon atoms 2 and 8 from folate (formate); nitrogen atoms 3 and 9 from glutamine; carbon 6 from CO_2; nitrogen 1 from aspartate.

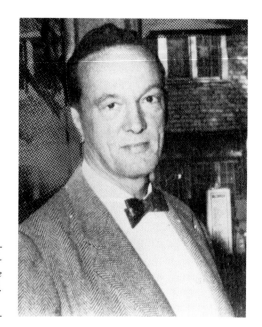

Dale Coman, Professor of Pathology and pioneer in the study of the
mechanism of cancer spread.
(Scope.)

Penn in 1937. In 1944 he wrote a paper on why cancer metastasizes. His finding explained one of the earliest measurable biophysical properties of cancer cells and formed the basis of present work on the structure and chemistry of cell surfaces.[13]

Coman had observed that neoplastic cells, unlike normal cells, tended to wander away from each other. He suspected that their lack of cohesiveness enabled them to spread. His experiments proved his suspicion. He then demonstrated that cancer cells are unable to bind calcium at their surface, a characteristic associated with their decreased adhesiveness. The unusual distribution of metastatic cancer is due not to the type of tissue, or soil for growth, but to the nature of the blood supply to the organ.[14]

LATER WORK OF THE JOHNSON FOUNDATION

When Britton Chance became director of the Johnson Foundation for Medical Physics in 1949, the foundation's emphasis changed from neurophysiology to cell physiology.

Chance, trained as a biologist, holds a doctorate in electrical engineering; thus he has been able to combine the study of biological systems with an understanding of stable, sensitive electronic instruments for making measurements. His work began in the late 1930s when he developed methods to study the kinetics of the changes in color of horseradish peroxidase that occur when peroxide is added. Others had found the changes, the first demonstration of an enzyme-substrate complex, but they could not describe the relationship between the formation of the intermediate compound and the enzyme activity. Chance developed an apparatus using sensitive photocells, filters, and an oscilloscope for following the rapid color changes that occurred when peroxidase changed its oxidation states. With this sensitive photoelectric colorimeter he was able to measure the reaction constants of the various steps that occur during peroxidation; confirming the reaction mechanism postulated by Hugo Theorell.[15]

During World War II, Chance worked at the Massachusetts Institute of Technology. There he invented a small operational amplifier that used subminiature tubes which could be replaced as a single unit, simplifying the construction and repair of complicated electronic equipment. The principle he used subsequently became important in the design of electronic circuits.[16]

After the war, Chance examined the electron transport chain of mitochondria. Studying the cytochromes of this transport system was problematic because the suspensions of mitochondria containing the electron carriers were turbid. He had to overcome the scattering of light and also find a satisfactory wavelength for reference. An oximeter using two wavelengths had been made practical elsewhere. Chance extended it by substituting an end-on photomultiplier tube for the photo cell, two Beckman monochromators for the filters, and adding an optical system with a short light path, which alternately flickered the two wavelengths of light on a single, sample cuvette.[17]

Until Chance developed this spectrophotometer, it could only be surmised thermodynamically that the respiratory chain of mitochondria was an arrangement of the known pyridine nucleotides, flavin, and cytochromes in the order of their relative oxidation reduction potentials. His instrument was sufficiently quick, stable, and sensitive to measure the spectral changes occurring when the intracellular electron carriers became oxidized and reduced. Thus he provided direct experimental evidence that supported the hypothesized sequence of reactions.

Eric Ball, formerly a biochemist at Penn, described the process of capturing biological energy:

> The energy liberated when substrates undergo air oxidation is not liberated in one large burst, as was once thought, but is released in stepwise fashion. At least six separate steps appear to be involved. The process is not unlike the locks of a canal. As each lock is passed in the ascent from a lower to a higher level, a certain amount of energy is expended. Similarly the total energy resulting from the oxidation of foodstuffs is released in small units or parcels, step by step. The amount of free energy released at each step is proportional to the difference in potential of the systems comprising the several steps.[18]

When the advantages of Chance's new spectrophotometers became known, scientists worldwide came to work at the Johnson Foundation for periods ranging from a day to months or longer. The laboratory virtually never closed. Guests or permanent members of the foundation gave so many seminars that they sometimes extended into the evening. And Chance's doors were never closed to visitors; only a black drape hung across the doorway to his laboratory to prevent light from disturbing his optical experiments. His instruments revolutionized biochemistry and biophysics because they permitted accurate kinetic and spectral studies on intact cells and tissues.[19]

ADRENALECTOMY AND SYMPATHECTOMY FOR THE TREATMENT OF MALIGNANT HYPERTENSION

One of the projects that occupied the interests of the departments of cardiology and surgery during the 1950s was the evaluation of the use of adrenalectomy and sympathectomy for the treatment of severe high blood pressure.

Since the organization of the cardiovascular clinic (the Robinette Foundation) by Wolferth there had been a division for the treatment and investigation of hypertension. Early members of the hypertension section were J. Q. Griffiths, August Lindauer, William Jeffers, and

Joseph Hafkenshiel. This small group managed the hypertensive patients who visited the clinics of the Hospital of the University of Pennsylvania, and in addition carried on experimental work on hypertension.

Charles C. Wolferth's interest in hypertension intensified in the late 1940s when his wife developed a severe case of this disease. The evaluation of adrenalectomy for treating hypertension at the University Hospital originated when he discussed with his colleagues what treatment they would recommend.[20]

The idea of removing adrenal tissue originated with the clinical observation that an individual who develops Addison's disease becomes hypotensive, suggesting that adrenal cortical secretions are essential to the abnormal vascular activity of hypertensive patients. Based on this observation Wolferth and his colleagues raised the question whether decreasing adrenal cortical function by removal of most of the adrenal tissue would lower the blood presure of severely hypertensive patients. Before the adrenalectomy project had advanced beyond the planning stage, the favorable result of the treatment of a young woman with diabetes and hypertension by total adrenalectomy was reported by Green, Nelson, and Dodds. The patient's blood pressure remained lowered, and it was possible to control the adrenal insufficiency by administering adrenocortical extracts. This success stimulated the group in the Robinette Foundation to investigate further whether removal of adrenal tissue should be considered for the treatment of essential hypertension.[21]

The goal of the first studies planned was to determine whether it was possible to reduce adrenal function enough to lower blood pressure without producing adrenal insufficiency.[22]

The first patient included in these studies was Wolferth's wife. Actually she had had a partial adrenalectomy before the work at the Hospital of the University of Pennsylvania began. Since Wolferth had been unable to persuade any of the surgeons at the hospital to operate upon his wife, he went to Temple and persuaded George Rosemond to perform the first stage of a bilateral adrenalectomy. Her second adrenal was removed at the Hospital of the University of Pennsylvania by Harold Zintel. Mrs. Wolferth's hypertension was not arrested by this treatment.[23]

The original report of the use of adrenalectomy was given by Wolferth at the Clinical and Climatological Society. It described the clinical course of six patients who had had 90 percent of their adrenal tissue removed. The report revealed that there was striking improvement which lasted for six months in one patient with advanced hypertension, the death of one patient seven days after operation, and some improvement in four patients. Adrenalectomy of 90 percent produced no adrenal insufficiency and these cases required no replacement therapy. This early partial success led to further exploration of adrenalectomy as a treatment for hypertension.

In order to see whether the response would be improved by simultaneously reducing the sympathetic nerve activity, Wolferth examined the response of blood pressure to 90 percent adrenalectomy combined with a limited sympathectomy (a modified Adson procedure). The study of 125 patients followed for three to seven years after being treated by the combined procedure showed that adrenalectomy and sympathectomy compared with sympathectomy alone had higher incidence of good blood pressure response, more improvement of the electrocardiogram tracings, greater decrease in heart size, a decreased postoperative morbidity, and a longer period of survival. The operative mortality was 5 percent higher in those patients who underwent the combined adrenalectomy and sympathectomy.[24]

Similar results were found when the results of total adrenalectomy and Adson sympathectomy were compared with the limited procedure. The summary of the treatment of hypertension by all of these procedures was published in 1958 in a paper by Balkemore, Zintel, Jeffers, Sellars, Sutnick, and Lindauer. These authors concluded that, although the mortality of the more drastic procedure was higher (5 percent) as compared with thorocolumbar sympathectomy alone (0.9 percent), there was a greater improvement in blood pressure, electrocardiographic picture, heart size, and occular fundal changes in patients treated by combined adrenalectomy and sympathectomy. All of the patients who survived the operative procedure had significantly reduced attacks of severe headaches, angina pectoris, and cardiac failure.

This project, which lasted through the early 1950s, had a wide influence on the activities of the Department of Medicine and Surgery. Not only were many members of these departments involved in the management of the patients after surgery as well as their long term care, but several investigators also carried out important studies on these patients that led to advances in the knowledge of the physiology of the circulation and the biological chemistry of the adrenal gland.[25]

SEYMOUR S. COHEN

Seymour Cohen applied phage techniques to characterize the viral-infected cell both metabolically and chemically. At first, however, he had a false start. When World War II ended, he tried working on viruses with the experimental pathologist Dale Coman but soon learned that biochemical studies were not suited to examine viral-infected tissue cultures.[26]

Cohen went to Thomas Anderson, the electron microscopist, who gave him a brief practical course in phage techniques. In his first paper, coauthored with Anderson in 1946, he noted that bacteria infected with phage respired normally but stopped multiplying; that is, the metabolism required to maintain the bacteria's life was not altered, but phage interfered with some step in the reproductive process. Cohen won a Guggenheim Fellowship, which allowed him to work at the Pasteur Institute in Paris.[27] There he told Jacques Monod that he wanted to know more about bacterial metabolism so that he could study the shifts in nucleic acid metabolism that occur after phage infection. Monod introduced him to the use of various strains of *E. coli*. On returning to Penn, Cohen taught a course on the biochemistry of nucleic acids. His work showing that viral proteins and nucleic acids were made de novo attracted the attention of other scientists, because it demonstrated that the same building blocks serve for viral growth as well as for the infected cell; it was, therefore, evident that different synthetic processes were involved in the formation of viral and cell proteins and nucleic acids. Support for the study of the biochemistry of viruses grew quickly.[28]

In 1951 Cohen collaborated with George R. Wyatt, an analytical biochemist, who had used a hydrolytic procedure to discover that plant DNA contained 5-methylcytosine. When he and Cohen applied the procedure to viruses, they saw new spots on the chromatograms. They eventually learned that the material was an unknown phage pyrimidine, 5-hydroxymethylcytosine (HMC), which completely replaced cytosine in the phage's DNA. The next year, they obtained a unique bacterium that required thymine; when infected with phage, it began to make both thymine and HMC, demonstrating that a virus could induce an acquired function in bacteria that it did not possess before infection. Cohen later satisfied himself that the experiment represented de novo enzyme induction.[29]

Cohen also found that, in the absence of thymine, the bacterium lost its ability to multiply and died out, reminiscent of the effects of antifolic acid agents. Others had developed the chemotherapeutic agent 5-fluorouracil and asked Cohen to examine its biochemical mechanism. Cohen and his associates demonstrated that the agent killed bacterial cells by inhibiting the formation of thymidine. Subsequent work by Cohen and others has led to an interest in arabinose nucleotides as chemotherapeutic agents.[30]

THE COMAN REPORT

In 1956 Penn President Gaylord P. Harnwell instituted a University-wide academic study. Dale Coman, who by then had succeeded Balduin

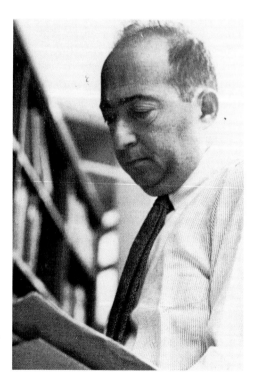

Seymour Cohen, pioneer in the studies of the biochemistry of phage. (Scope.)

Lucke as chairman of pathology, was chosen to head the committee studying the state of the medical school. In the opening pages of the final report, Coman felt obliged to apologize for the list of shortcomings, as if they suggested that medicine at Penn "has more faults than virtues." He warned that "nothing could be farther from the truth. It is one of the finest institutions of its kind in the world. Perhaps it is because of this proximity to excellence that a few major problems confronting the institution are so glaringly evident and the cause of such great concern to the faculty."[31]

The problems were hardly minimal: a shortage of funds for a first-rate clinical and preclinical faculty; a need to renovate and expand facilities; a need for an endowment to reduce reliance on outside funds (Coman and his committee worried that departments may suffer financial chaos when a recipient of large grants retires); difficult relations between the medical school and the hospital; a problematic relationship between the school and the Graduate School of Medicine; inconsistent policies to finance the various clinical departments; and a "crazy-quilt pattern" of compensating hospital residents. The committee also complained that some departments—neurology, obstetrics and gynecology, ophthalmology, and otorhinology—were substandard in organization and original research.[32]

Most of the problems proved to be cyclical. New chairmen reinvigorated the lackluster departments, and a new generation of clinicians and medical scientists made them shine. Compensation of residents was regularized; the graduate school was sold off. Facilities have more than doubled since that report, and construction continues, the latest being a new building for clinical research, which opened in 1989. And many of the problems—the struggle for funds, for space, for new management structures—are perennial. Not that they can be ignored simply because they are ever-present, but important research is clearly capable of thriving in an encouraging atmosphere that, at times, may fall to having a mere "proximity" to excellence.

For 225 years the scientists and clinicians persisted, rarely working under perfectly utopian conditions. They made their discoveries nonetheless, for what was more important than mythical utopian conditions was that they were free to think, to pursue their ideas without the restrictions of a rigid academic discipline. No doubt the next 225 years of Penn's history will turn up its share of undeterrable discoverers.

NOTES

1. E. G. Ball and J. M. Buchanan, "D. Wright Wilson, 1889–1965," *Biographical Memoirs of the National Academy of Sciences,* vol. 43 (New York: Columbia University Press, 1973), pp. 261–84.

2. S. Gurin, C. Bachman, and D. W. Wilson, "The Gonadotrophic Hormone of Urine of Pregnancy I. A Simple Method for Extraction and Purification," *Journal of Biological Chemistry* 128(1939):525–36.

3. Letter from Carl Bachman to D. Wright Wilson.

4. Ball and Buchanan, "Memoir, D. Wright Wilson," pp. 270–73.

5. Life sketch of Samuel Gurin, by Roscoe O. Brady, sent to D. Y. Cooper.

6. J. M. Buchanan, "A Backward Glance," in *Comprehensive Biochemistry*, ed. A. Neuberger, L. M. Van Deenen, and G. Semenza, vol. 36 (Amsterdam: Elsiever, 1986), pp. 9–12; conversation with Samuel Gurin; letter from Sidney Weinhouse to David Y. Cooper (February 18,1985).

7. J. M. Buchanan, W. Sakami, S. Gurin, and D. W. Wilson, "A Study of the Intermediates of Acetate and Acetoacetate Oxidation with Isotopic Carbon," *Journal of Biological Chemistry* 159 (1945):695–709; Buchanan, "A Backward Glance," pp. 9–12; J. M. Buchanan, W. Sakami, and S. Gurin, "A Study of the Mechanism of Fatty Acid Oxidation with Isotopic Acetoacetate," *Journal of Biological Chemistry* 169(1947):411–18; J. M. Buchanan, W. Sakami, S. Gurin, and D. W. Wilson, "Intermediates in the Biological Oxidation of Isotopic Acetate," *Journal of Biological Chemistry* 169(1947):403–09.

8. R. O. Brady and S. Gurin, "The Biosynthesis of Radioactive Fatty Acids and Cholesterol," *Journal of Biological Chemistry* 186(1950):461–69; R. O. Brady and S. Gurin, "The Biosynthesis of Fatty Acids in Cell-Free Systems," reprinted from *Major Metabolic Fuels*, Brookhaven Symposia in Biology No. 5, BNL 206(C-15) (Upton, N.Y.:1952), pp. 162–75; R. O. Brady and S. Gurin, "Biosynthesis of Fatty Acids by Cell-Free or Water Soluble Enzyme Systems," *Journal of Biological Chemistry* 199(1952):421–32.

9. Conversation with Samuel Gurin, 1984.

10. J. M. Buchanan, "A Backward Glance," pp. 22–28; Joseph Fruton, *Molecules of Life: Essays in the History of Biochemistry* (New York: John Wiley, 1973), pp. 428–29.

11. J. C. Sonne, J. M. Buchanan, and A. M. Delluva, "Biological Precursors of Uric Acid Carbons," *Journal of Biological Chemistry* 166(1946):395–96; J. C. Sonne, J. M. Buchanan, and A. M. Delluva, "Biological Precursors of Uric Acid I. The Role of Lactate, Acetate, and Fumarate in the Synthesis of the Ureide Group of Uric Acid," *Journal of Biological Chemistry* 173(1948):69–79; J. M. Buchanan and J. C. Sonne, "The Utilization of Formate in Uric Acid Synthesis," *Journal of Biological Chemistry* 166 (1946):781; J. M. Buchanan, "Biosynthesis of Purine Nucleotide, in *The Nucleic Acids*, ed. E. Chragaff and J. N. Davidson, vol. 3 (New York: Academic Press,1955), pp. 303–22; J. M. Buchanan, J. C. Sonne, and A. M. Delluva, "Biological Precursors of Uric Acid II. The Role of Lactate, Glycine, and Carbon Dioxide as precursors of the Carbon Chain and Nitrogen 7 of Uric Acid," *Journal of Biological Chemistry* 173(1948):81–98.

12. Letter from Dale Coman to David Y. Cooper detailing how he became interested in his experiments in cancer research. Letter not dated, but was received in the spring of 1984.; E. R. Long and D. T. Rowlands, *The Development of the Department of*

Pathology in the School of Medicine of the University of Pennsylvania (Philadelphia: Privately printed, 1977), pp. 50–53.

13. D. R. Coman, "Decreased Mutual Adhesiveness, A Property of Cells from Squamous Cell Carcinomas," *Cancer Research* 4 (1944):625–29.

14. B. Chance, "The Accelerated Flow Method for Rapid Reactions, Part I," *Journal of the Franklin Institute* 229 (1940):455–76; B. Chance, "The Properties of the Enzyme Substrate Compound of Horse Radish Peroxidase," *Science* 109(1949):204–08; B. C. Saunders, A. G. Holmes-Siedel, and B. P. Stark, *Peroxidase* (Washington, D.C.: Butterworth, 1964), pp. 91–100.

15. B. Chance, J. N. Thurston, and P. L. Richman, "Some Designs and Applications for Packaged Amplifiers Using Subminature Tubes," *Review of Scientific Instruments* 18(1948):610–16.

16. J. S. Fruton, *Molecules of Life*, pp. 387–88, 359–86; E. G. Ball, "Oxidative Mechanisms in Animal Tissue," in *A Symposium on Respiratory Enzymes* (Madison: University of Wisconsin Press, 1942), pp. 160–62.

17. B. Chance and G. R. Williams, "The Respiratory Chain and Oxidative Phosphorylation," in *Advances in Enzymology*, ed. F. F. Nord (New York: Interscience, 1956), pp. 65–134.

18. B. Chance, "Techniques for the Assay of Respiratory Enzymes," in *Methods in Enzymology*, vol. 4, ed. Sidney P. Colowick and N. O. Kaplan (New York: Academic Press, 1957), pp. 273–322; B. Chance, "A Sensitive Spectrophotometry I. The Accelerated Stop-Flow Method for Measurement of the Reaction Kinetics and Spectra of Unstable Compounds in the Visible Region of the Spectrum," *Review of Scientific Instruments* 22(1951):619–38; Chia-Chih Yang and V. Legllais, "A Rapid and Sensitive Recording Spectrophotometer for the Visible and Ultraviolet Region. I. Description and Performance," *Review of Scientific Instruments* 25(1954): 801–7; Chia-Chih Yang, "A Rapid and Sensitive Recording Spectrophotometer for the Visible and the Ultraviolet Region II. Electronic Circuit," *Review of Scientific Instruments* 25(1954):807–13.

19. Personal experience of David Y. Cooper while working with Ronald Estabrook in the Johnson Foundation on Cytochrome P-450.

20. Observations and experiences of David Y. Cooper on the medical service as junior intern and intern, as well as resident on the surgical service.

21. Zintel note describing his part in the adrenalectomy study (sent to D.Y.C., to be published).

22. Zintel note; personal experience of David Y Cooper on the medical and surgical services.

23. Experience of D.Y.C on the medical and surgical services.

24. F. D. W. Lukens, C. C. Wolferth, and (by Invitation) W. A. Jeffers, H. A. Zintel, and J.Hafkenshiel, "Observations on Subtotal Adrenalectomy in Hypertension," *Transactions of the Clinical and Climatological Society* 62 (1951):229–36.

25. H. A. Zintel, A. M. Sellers, W. A. Jeffers, J. A. Mackie, J. H. Hafkenshiel, and M. A. Lindauer, "A Three to Seven Year Postoperative Evaluation of 76 Patients with Severe Hypertension Treated by Thoracolumbar Sympathectomy," *Surgery, Gynecology, and Obstetrics* 101(1955): 48–54; W. S. Blakemore, H. A. Zintel, W. A. Jeffers, A. M. Sellers, A. I. Sutnick, and M. A. Lindauer, "A Comparison of Thoracolumbar Sympathectomy and Adrenalectomy with Adson Sympathectomy in the Treatment of Severe Arterial Hypertension," *Surgery* 43 (1958):102–13.

26. The adrenals removed at adrenalectomy were studied to determine what steroids are produced by human adrenals which at that time was not fully known. It was this study of human adrenals that led eventually to the discovery of the function of cyto-

chrome P-450 as the terminal oxidase for microsomal mixed function oxidase catalyzed oxidations.

27. S. Cohen, Personal communication, letter dated March 29, 1983.

28. Cohen Letter.

29. Cohen Letter.

30. S. S. Cohen, J. G. Flaks, H. D. Barner, M. R. Loeb, and J. Lichtenstein, "The Mode of Action of 5-Fluorouracil and its Derivatives," *Proceedings of the National Academy of Sciences* 44 (1958):1004–12; S. S. Cohen and H. D. Barner, "The Conversion of 5-Methyl Deoxycytidine to Thymidine in Vitro and in Vivo," *Journal of Biological Chemistry* (1958): 631–42.

31. Willets Survey, Report of Dale R. Coman's Committee, Archives of the University of Pennsylvania.

DEPARTMENT HEADS

Leaders of the University of Pennsylvania School of Medicine

DEANS

DATE	NAME
1805	Benjamin Rush[a]
1808	Philip Syng Physick
1809	John Syng Dorsey
1813	John Redman Coxe
1814	Philip Syng Physick
1815	Nathaniel Chapman
1815	Thomas Chalkley James
1816	Caspar Wistar
1817	Nathaniel Chapman
1819–1822	John Redman Coxe
1822–1852	William Edmonds Horner
1852–1856	Joseph Carson
1856–1877	Robert E. Rogers
1877–1888	Joseph Leidy
1888–1892	James Tyson
1892–1902	John Marshall
1902–1909	Charles Harrison Frazier
1909–1912	Allen J. Smith
1912–1945	William Pepper III
1945–1948	Isaac Starr
1948–1962	John McK. Mitchell
1962–1969	Samuel Gurin
1969–1973	Alfred Gellhorn
1974–1988	Edward Stemmler (acting, 1974–1975)
1988–1989	Arthur K. Asbury (acting)
1989–	William N. Kelley

[a] Until the turn of the eighteenth century, the school was a loosely associated group of lecturers with almost no central administrative organization. Early "deans" rotated in office; they chiefly admitted classes, arranged for examinations, and awarded degrees.

HEADS OF DEPARTMENTS AND DIVISIONS

Into the 20th century, there was usually only one "professor" in a specialty, and he chaired the department. The following lists reflect that professor, then, as professorships expanded in number, the chairman or division chief. The departments or divisions are listed by their current titles, except Hygiene and Public Health, which no longer exists; changes in title are noted.

When the University of Pennsylvania opened its doors in 1753, it was called the Academy of Philadelphia. In 1755 it became the College of Philadelphia and in 1779 the University of the State of Pennsylvania. It received its current name in 1791.

Anatomy

DATE	NAME
1765–1779	William Shippen
1779–1791	William Shippen
1792–1808	William Shippen[a]
1808–1818	Caspar Wistar
1818–1818	John Syng Dorsey[b]
1818–1831	Philip Syng Physick
1831–1853	William Edmonds Horner
1853–1891	Joseph Leidy
1891–1921	George Arthur Piersol
1922–1926	John C. Heisler (Acting)
1926–1947	Eliot Round Clark
1947–1951	William F. Windle
1951–1967	Louis B. Flexner
1967–1976	James M. Sprague
1977–	Frank Pepe

[a] William Shippen was professor of anatomy, surgery and midwifery at first. In 1805, when Philip Syng Physick was given the chair of surgery, the department name was changed to anatomy and midwifery. In 1810 Thomas Chalkley James was appointed professor of midwifery, and at that time the title of this chair was changed to anatomy.

[b] John Syng Dorsey assumed the chair of anatomy May, 1818. He, however, died suddenly November 10, 1818.

Anesthesiology

DATE	NAME
1938–1941	Ivan B. Taylor
1941–1942	Philip Gleason
1942–1972	Robert Dunning Dripps[a]
1972–1987	Harry Wollman
1987–1988	Norig Ellison (acting)
1988–	David E. Longnecker

[a] In 1966 anesthesiology gained departmental status. Prior to that, it had been a division of surgery.

Biochemistry and Biophysics

DATE	NAME
1769–1781	Benjamin Rush
1783–1789	Benjamin Rush[a]
1789–1791	James Hutchinson
1789–1791	Caspar Wistar
1792–1793	James Hutchinson[b]
1794–1794	Joseph Carson[c]
1795–1809	James Woodhouse
1809–1818	John Redman Coxe
1818–1847	Robert Hare
1847–1852	James Blyth Rogers
1852–1877	Robert Empie Rogers
1877–1897	Theodore G. Wormley (?)
1897–1910	John Marshall[d]
1910–1922	Alonzo E. Taylor
1922–1954	D. Wright Wilson
1954–1962	Samuel Gurin[e]
1964–1971	Howard Rasmussen
1971–1975	James Ferguson
1975–1976	Takashi Yonetani (acting)[f]
1976–1977	Harold Bright (acting)
1977–1983	David Trentham
1983–	Franz Matschinsky

[a] When the College's charter was abrogated in 1777, Rush did not take his chair in chemistry in the University of the State of Pennsylvania until 1783. For six years there was no professor of chemistry in the University.

[b] James Hutchinson accepted the chair of chemistry in the university in 1789, and since he was drawing classes larger than Wistar in 1792 when the schools united, he continued in this position.

[c] Carson never lectured in chemistry as he died October 24, 1794.

[d] In 1908 the name of the department was changed to physiological chemistry and toxicology. When the Benjamin Rush chair was established in 1910, John Marshall was given the chair of chemistry and toxicology and his chair was demoted to second rank. John Marshall vacated the chair in 1921, and it was discontinued in 1923.

[e] Appointed as professor of biological chemistry.

[f] Biophysics was combined with biochemistry in 1975, and the department name changed to the Department of Biochemistry and Biophysics.

Dermatology[a]

DATE	NAME
1875–1910	Louis A. Duhring[b]
1910–1921	Milton Bixby Hartzell
1921–1924	Frederick D. Weidman (acting)
1924–1945	John H. Stokes
1945–1965	Donald Pillsbury
1965–1980	Walter B. Shelley
1980–1982	Margaret Gray Wood (acting)
1982–	Gerald Lazarus

[a] Originally the department was named the Department of Diseases of the Skin (1875). The name was changed to Department of Dermatology in 1903 and to the Department of Dermatology and Syphilology in 1923. It was changed back to the Department of Dermatology in 1951.

[b] In 1875 Louis Duhring became Professor of Diseases of the Skin at the Hospital of the University of Pennsylvania. He was elected Professor of Clinical Dermatology of the Skin in the Medical School in 1883.

Human Genetics[a]

DATE	NAME
1965–1971	Rupert E. Billingham[a]
1971–1972	Willys K. Silvers (acting)
1972–1980	William J. Mellman
1980–1981	Willys K. Silvers (acting)
1981–1988	Roy J. Schmickel
1988–	Willys K. Silvers (acting)

[a] Medical genetics was the department's original name, changed to human genetics in 1973.

The Henry Phipps Institute for the Study, Treatment, and Prevention of Tuberculosis was founded in 1903. After tuberculosis was conquered in the 1950s, the institute shifted its interest to other community diseases, and its name was changed to the Henry Phipps Institute for Research in Community Disease. In 1965 that thrust was ended, and the institute's endowment was assigned to the Department of Human Genetics. Directors of the Phipps Institute:

1903–1910	Lawrence Flick
1910–1913	Paul Lewis
1913–1923	Charles J. Hatfield
1923–1932	Eugene L. Opie
1932–1955	Esmond R. Long
1955–1965	Theodore H. Ingalls

Medicine

DATE	NAME
1765–1779	John Morgan[a]
1783–1789	John Morgan[a]
1780–1784	Thomas Bond[b]
1789–1791	Benjamin Rush
1789–1791	Adam Kuhn
1792–1797	Adam Kuhn[c]
1805–1813	Benjamin Rush[d]
1813–1815	Benjamin Smith Barton
1815–1850	Nathanial Chapman[e]

[a] John Morgan retained the chair of the theory and practice of physic (medicine) until his death in October 17, 1789. He never returned to teaching, however, after he entered the service of the Continental Army in 1775. From the minutes of the Trustees' meeting of March 13, 1789, "Morgan Professor of Theory and Practice of Physic not being present within the state, the Trustees considered him as reinstated and permitted to continue in his office until his return home when he is to be waited upon by the committee in like manner as the other professors have been, in order to know whether it belies his intention to resume the exercise of his post heretofore." Benjamin Rush was chosen to fill this chair October 24, 1789.

[b] When the University of the State of Pennsylvania was formed, Thomas Bond (then 69) filled in and taught the theory and practice of physic (medicine) in addition to his clinical lectures. He never was officially appointed professor.

[c] Adam Kuhn held only the chair of the theory and practice of physic; Rush held the chair of the institutes of medicine and taught clinical medicine.

[d] The chair of the theory and practice of physic held by Adam Kuhn and the institutes of medicine held by Rush, both since 1892, were combined in 1805 under Rush, who had been lecturing in these two subjects since Kuhn's resignation in 1797.

[e] In 1835 Samuel Jackson took over the chair of the institutes of medicine. Nathanial Chapman continued in the chair of the theory and practice of physic and clinical medicine.

(continued)

Medicine

DATE	NAME
1850–1860	George Bacon Wood
1860–1864	William Pepper, Sr.
1864–1883	Alfred Stillé[f]
1884–1898	William Pepper, Jr.[g]
1899–1910	James Tyson[h]
1910–1911	David Lynn Edsall
1911–1931	Alfred Stengel
1931–1947	O. H. Perry Pepper
1947–1965	Francis C. Wood
1965–1967	James B. Wyngaarden
1968–1977	Arnold S. Relman
1977–	Laurence E. Earley

[f] In 1864 Alfred Stillé held the chair of the theory and practice of physic (it appears medicine and physic were interchangeable at this time).

[g] "In June 1884 he resigned the chair of Clinical Medicine at the University to which he was elected in 1876 and on the same day was elected Professor of the Theory and Practice of Clinical Medicine. By this appointment he succeeded to the chair which his father had vacated at death twenty years before. During the intervening time the chair had been filled by the eminent Dr. Alfred Stillé, who now at Pepper's appointment became Professor Emeritus." (F. N. Thorpe, *William Pepper, M.D., LL.D.* [Philadelphia: Lippincott, 1904], p. 91.)

[h] Title changed to professor of medicine, June 2, 1903.

Microbiology[a]

DATE	NAME
1865–1875	Henry Hartshorn
1875–1876	Horace Binney Hare
1877–1887	Joseph G. Richardson
1887–1891	Samuel G. Dixon
1891–1892	Seneca Egbert
1891–1896	John Shaw Billings
1891–1896	John Shaw Billings
1896–1928	Alexander Crewer Abbott
1929–1932	Seneca Egbert (acting)

Bacteriology/Microbiology		*Hygiene/Public Health*	
1931–1959	Stuart Mudd	1932–1933	David Bergey (acting)
1959–1973	Harold Ginsberg	1933–1939	Henry Field Smith (acting)
1973–1978	Joseph Gots (acting)		
1978–	Neil Nathanson	1939–1944	Arthur Parker Hitchens
		1944–1947	Arthur Parker Hitchens (visiting)
		1950–1963	John P. Hubbard
		1963–1968	Johanes Ipsen
		1968–1971	William Kissick
		1971–1972	Robert Leopold (acting)
		1972–1975	Robert Leopold
		1975	Discontinued

[a] Microbiology at Penn traces its origin to a course on hygiene in the short-lived "auxiliary" school, which started in 1865 and closed in 1898. Hygiene was elevated into a department in 1891 and its name changed to bacteriology and hygiene in 1896. In 1931 the name was split. Bacteriology became microbiology in 1959. Hygiene became public health and preventive medicine in 1939, then community health in 1968; this department was discontinued in 1975.

Neurology[a]

DATE	NAME
1875–1901	Horatio C. Wood
1901–1915	Charles K. Mills
1915–1936	William G. Spiller
1936–1937	William Biddle Cadwalader (acting)
1937–1942	William Biddle Cadwalader
1942–1952	George D. Gammon (acting)
1952–1962	George D. Gammon
1960–1962	A. M. Ornsteen (acting)
1962–1963	Gabriel A. Schwartz (acting)
1963–1967	G. Milton Shy
1967–1973	Lewis Roland
1973–1974	Donald Silberberg (acting)
1974–1982	Arthur K. Asbury
1982–	Donald Silberberg

[a] Neurology was called the Department of Nervous Diseases until 1901.

Neurosurgery[a]

DATE	NAME
1922–1937	Charles Harrison Frazier
1937–1957	Francis C. Grant
1957–1968	Robert Groff
1968–1975	Thomas Langfitt
1975–1986	Thomas Langfitt and Frederick Murtagh
1986–1988	Frederick Murtagh (acting)
1988–	Eugene Flamm

[a] Neurosurgery is a division of surgery, but its head has chairman status.

Obstetrics and Gynecology

DATE	NAME
1765–1808	William Shippen[a]
1810–1834	Thomas Chalkley James[b]
1834–1835	William Potts Dewees
1835–1863	Hugh L. Hodge[c]
1863–1889	R. A. F. Penrose

Obstetrics		*Gynecology*	
1889–1927	Barton Cooke Hirst	1872–1893	William Goodell[d]
		1893–1899	Charles B. Penrose
		1899–1927	John G. Clark

Obstetrics and Gynecology

1927–1941   Charles C. Norris[e]

1927–1935	Edmund B. Piper	1927–1938	Floyd E. Keene
1939–1940	Howard C. Taylor	1941–1950	Franklin Payne
1941–1950	Carl Bachman[f]		

1950–1964	Franklin Payne
1964–1988	Luigi Mastroianni, Jr.
1988–	Michael T. Mennuti

[a] Professor of anatomy, surgery, and midwifery.

[b] Title changed to professor of midwifery.

[c] Title changed to professor of obstetrics and diseases of women and children.

[d] Professor of diseases of women and children in the Summer Medical Association until 1874; thereafter a member of the hospital staff. In 1878 he was made clinical professor of gynecology and, in 1888, professor of gynecology.

[e] Under the combined specialties, Piper and Keene, though holding no professorships, were considered assistants to Norris.

[f] Held the senior chair.

Ophthalmology

DATE	NAME
1870–1874	William F. Norris (clinical lecturer)
1874–1901	William F. Norris[a]
1902–1924	George E. de Schweinitz
1924–1936	Thomas B. Holloway
1936–1937	Alexander G. Fewell (acting)
1936–1960	Francis Heed Adler
1960–1977	Harold G. Scheie
1975–1977	William C. Frayer (acting)
1977–1986	Myron Yanoff
1986–1988	Theodore Krupin (acting)
1988–	William C. Frayer (acting)

[a] The department was called diseases of the eye from its inception in 1874 until 1924.

Orthopaedic Surgery

DATE	NAME
1899–1911	DeForest Willard
1911–1918	Gwilym Davis
1918–1920	Vacant
1920–1942	A. Bruce Gill
1943–1958	Paul C. Colonna
1958–1960	David S. Grice
1960–1961	Edgar L. Ralston (acting)
1961–1977	Edgar L. Ralston
1977–	Carl T. Brighton

Otorhinolaryngology and Human Communication[a]

	DATE	NAME
Diseases of the ear/Otolaryngology		*Laryngology and Rhinology/ Otolaryngology*
1870–1902 George C. Strawbridge	1903–1925	Charles P. Greyson
1902–1925 Burton A. Randall	1925–1933	George Fetterolf

Otolaryngology

1933–1940	George M. Coats
1940–1959	Harry P. Schenk
1959–1973	Philip Marden

*Otorhinolaryngology and
Human Communication*

1972–	James Snow

[a] The department began as diseases of the ear and was renamed otolaryngology when it absorbed the department of laryngology and rhinology in 1925. In 1972 it was given its current name.

Pathology and Laboratory Medicine[a]

DATE	NAME
1875–1889	James Tyson
1889–1899	Juan Guiteras
1899–1903	Simon Flexner
1903–1926	Allen J. Smith
1927–1933	Eugene L. Opie
1933–1948	Edward B. Krumbaar
1948–1954	Balduin Lucké
1954–1967	Dale Coman
1967–1973	Peter Nowell
1973–1978	David T. Rowlands
1980–	Leonard Jarett

[a] Original title was pathological anatomy and histology. Title changed to pathology and laboratory medicine in 1980.

Pediatrics

DATE	NAME
1874–1891	Louis Starr
1890–1891	Hobart A. Hare[a]
1891–1924	Joseph P. C. Griffith
1924–1939	John C. Gittings[b]
1939–1963	Joseph Stokes, Jr.[b]
1963–1972	Alfred M. Bongiovanni
1974–1986	Jean A. Cortner
1986–1990	Richard B. Johnston, Jr.
1990–	Elias Schwartz

[a] Department called the Department of the Diseases of Children. It was changed to pediatrics under Gittings.

[b] Joseph Stokes, Jr., headed the department from 1929 to 1930 while Gittings recovered from an episode of depression.

Pharmacology[a]

DATE	NAME
1768–1789	Adam Kuhn
1782–1789	Adam Kuhn
1789–1791	Samuel Powell Griffiths
1789–1791	James Hutchinson
1789–1796	Samuel Powell Griffiths
1796–1813	Benjamin Smith Barton
1816–1818	John Syng Dorsey
1818–1835	John Redman Coxe
1835–1850	George Bacon Wood
1850–1876	Joseph Carson
1877–1907	Horatio C. Wood, Sr.
1907–1910	David Linn Edsall
1910–1939	Alfred N. Richards
1939–1959	Carl F. Schmidt[b]
1959–1981	George B. Koelle
1981–	Perry B. Molinoff

[a] The department was originally named materia medica and botany, then changed to materia medica in 1784, materia medica, pharmacy, and general therapeutics in 1877, and to its current title in 1910.

[b] A. N. Richards, according to the catalogue, held the chair until 1945. Corner states that Carl F. Schmidt became professor of pharmacology in 1939.

Physical Medicine and Rehabilitation[a]

	DATE	NAME
	1912–1945	Joseph Nylin
	1942–1953	George Morris Piersol
	1953–1983	William J. Erdman
	1983–1987	Emery Stoner
	1987–1988	William J. Erdman (acting)
	1988–	Laurence J. Earley (acting)

[a] R. Tait McKenzie, the first professor of physical education in America, was appointed professor of physical therapy and rehabilitation in 1912. In the late 1920s he phased himself out of this work.

[b] Overlapping dates as Piersol was taught the ropes.

Physiology[a]

	DATE	NAME
	1789–1792	Caspar Wistar
	1792–1805	Benjamin Rush
	1813–1815	Benjamin Smith Barton
	1815–1835	Nathaniel Chapman
	1835–1863	Samuel Jackson
	1863–1878	Francis Gurney Smith
	1878–1885	Harrison Allen
	1886–1920	Edward Tyson Reichert
	1920–1950	H. Cuthbert Bazett
	1950–1952	Carl F. Schmidt (acting)
	1952–1970	John Brobeck
	1970–1990	Robert Forster
	1990–	Paul DeWeer

[a] Originally the institutes of medicine.

Psychiatry[a]

DATE	NAME
1883–1890	John J. Reese
1893–1901	Charles K. Mills
1901–1930	Charles W. Burr
1931–1932	Earl D. Bond (acting)
1932–1953	Edward A. Strecker
1953–1962	Kenneth E. Appel
1962–1973	Albert J. Stunkard
1973–1974	John Paul Brady (acting)
1974–1982	John Paul Brady
1982–1984	George E. Ruff (acting)
1984–	Peter Whybrow

[a] The Department of Psychiatry was established in 1912. Prior to that, it was called the Department of Mental Diseases. Reese, professor of medical jurisprudence and toxicology, and Mills, professor of mental diseases and medical jurisprudence, can be called forerunners because they treated alcoholism and drug addiction. Daniel McCarthy held a new chair of medical jurisprudence from 1904 until he retired in 1939; the subject was dropped until a series of *ad hoc* lectures given by specialists in medicine, neurology, and pathology were given shape by a local lawyer, Laurence H. Eldridge, who became responsible for the course from 1941 until 1967.

Radiation Oncology[a]

DATE	NAME
1977–	Robert L. Goodman

[a] A division of the Department of Radiology until 1977.

Radiology

DATE	NAME
1898–1902	Charles Lester Leonard Instructor in Skiagraphy
1902–1903	Vacant
1904–1939	Henry K. Pancoast
1939–1961	Eugene Pendergrass[a]
1961–1975	Richard H. Chamberlain
1975–	Stanley Baum

[a] Until 1939, radiology was a division of the Department of Surgery.

Research Medicine[a]

	DATE	NAME
	1910–1920	Richard M. Pearce
	1921–1943	J. Harold Austin
	1943–1956	William C. Stadie
	1956–1960	Colin McCloud
	1960–1962	Eugene A. Hildreth (acting)
	1960–	Robert A. Austrian

[a] Once the John Herr Musser Department of Research Medicine.

Surgery

	DATE	NAME
	1765–1805	William Shippen[a]
	1805–1818	Philip Syng Physick
	1819–1855	William Gibson
	1855–1871	Henry Hollingsworth Smith
John Rhea Barton Profes-	1871–1877	D. Hayes Agnew[b]
sors of Surgery	1877–1900	John Ashurst
	1900–1910	J. William White
	1910–1918	Edward B. Martin
	1918–1922	John B. Deaver
	1922–1936	Charles Harrison Frazier
	1936–1945	Eldridge L. Eliason
	1945–1959	I. S. Ravdin
	1959–1972	Jonathan E. Rhoads
	1972–1975	William T. Fitts
	1975–1978	Leonard D. Miller (acting)
	1978–1983	Leonard D. Miller
	1981–1983	Brooke Roberts (acting)[c]
	1983–	Clyde E. Barker

[a] Shippen served as professor of anatomy, surgery, and midwifery.

[b] Title changed to John Rhea Barton Professor of Surgery November 6, 1877. First endowed chair of surgery.

[c] Brooke Roberts was given the title "vice chairman and acting chairman." Miller remained the official chairman and John Rhea Barton Professor of Surgery during this period although he was on leave.

Urology[a]

DATE	NAME
1886–1889	J. William White
1891–1900	Edward B. Martin
1903–1923	Thomas R. Neilson
1923–1945	Alexander Randall
1945–1964	Boland Hughs
1964–1980	John J. Murphy
1980–	Alan Wein

[a] Not a department but a division of surgery, yet, according to David Riesman, "somewhat sanctified . . . by the distinction of the men who taught it." (Corner, *Two Centuries of Medicine*, p. 274.) Originally called genito-urinary surgery, the division became urology under Murphy.

BUILDINGS OF THE SCHOOL OF MEDICINE

BUILDING	DATE	COMMENT
William Shippen's Father's Shed at Fourth above High St.	175?	William Shippen lectured on anat., surg. and midwifery here 1762
The Academy Building and Charity School	1740	John Morgan gave first lectures on the theory and practice of medicine here
Surgeon's Hall	1778?	Not known when this building was built or first used
Medical Hall adjacent to President's House	1807	Benjamin Latrobe, architect
Medical Hall of 1807 renovated	1817	William Strickland, architect
Medical Hall rebuilt in 1829	1829	William Strickland, architect
Medical Hall (now Logan Hall) in West Philadelphia	1874	T. W. Richards, architect
Hare Building	1878	T. W. Richards, architect
Fire in Medical Hall	1888	
Department of Hygiene	1892	Wing added in 1899
Wistar Institute	1894	George W. and D. Hewett, architects
Medical Laboratories (renamed the John Morgan Building in 1987)	1904	Cope and Stewardson, architects
Henry Phipps Institute	1913	Original buildings were houses downtown

(continued)

BUILDING	DATE	COMMENT
Anatomy-Chemistry Building	1929	Stewardson and Page, architects
A. N. Richards Building	1960	Louis Kahn, architect
Robert Wood Johnson Pavilion	1969	Alexander Ewing, architect
Medical Education Building	1980	Geddes, Brecher, Qualls, and Cunningham, architects
Clinical Research Building	1989	Payette Associates (interior) and Venturi, Ranch, and Scott Brown (exterior), architects

APPENDIX III

BUILDINGS OF THE HOSPITAL OF THE UNIVERSITY OF PENNSYLVANIA[a]

BUILDING	DATE	COMMENT
Hospital of the University of Pennsylvania	1874	Building begun 1872, T. W. Richards, architect, drawing instructor, University of Pennsylvania
Peter Hahn Ward	1880	
Henry Gibson Wing	1883	Facilities for chronic diseases; Wilson Brothers, architects
Machine shop for orthopaedics	1883	
Men's clinic moved to Gibson	1886	
Nurses' residence	1886	Gift of Mrs. Richard D. Wood
Mortuary building and chapel	1890	Gift of Mrs. Charles C. Harrison
Nurses' residence addition	1891	
Agnew Wing	1894	Cope and Stewardson, architects
William Pepper, Sr., Laboratory of Cinical Medicine	1895	
D. Hayes Agnew Pavilion	1897	
Addition to nurses' residence	1898	
Student Ward	1899	Two fireplaces included

(continued)

[a] Thanks to Nadine Landis.

BUILDING	DATE	COMMENT
J. Dundas Lippincott operating room	1899	
Eight private rooms adjacent to J. Dundas Lippincott operating room	1899	This must have been constructed when the amphitheater was divided horizontally
New nurses' residence (old renovated)	1899	
Children's surgical ward	1899	
Medical ward for children	1900	J. Crozier Griffiths and Mrs. Longstreth, benefactors
Neurology amphitheater	1900	
Isolation building	1905	
Laundry	1905	
Medical amphitheater removed	1908	
Medical clinic building	1909	Contained clinics, medical lecture room, lab for urine and blood analysis
New maternity building	1916	
Men's dermatology clinic	1922	
J. William White Surgical Pavilion	1912	Begun in 1912
George Secker Pepper Ward	1922	Ward for treatment of metabolic and kidney disorders, diet kitchen, air-conditioned room
First air-conditioned room (adjacent to Pepper Ward)	1922	Built by Simon Leopold and his brother to treat asthma patients
Gynecological Ward (Clark unit) moved to first floor of Dulles	1922	
Laundry enlarged	1923	
Laboratory for occupational therapy	1925	Sabin Colton and Cornelia Sellars, benefactors

(continued)

BUILDING	DATE	COMMENT
Medical Clinic Building moved and Pepper Laboratory demolished	1926	Room made for building the Maloney Building
Martin Maloney Memorial Clinic	1929	
Physical therapy moved to Maloney, fifth floor	1929	
Dental clinic moved to Maloney	1929	
Pharmacy moved to basement of Maloney	1930	
Diet kitchen moved to Dundas Lippincott area	1930	
General and neurosurgery ward	1931	
Dundas Lippincott operating room moved to White Building	1931	
Corner Cupboard Restaurant	1931	
New gymnasium	1932	
George Cox Institute	1932	To study and treat diabetes
Central dressing room first floor Agnew Pavilion	1934	
Orthopaedic Hospital for Nervous and Bone Diseases absorbed	1938	
Agnew Pavilion fire	1939	Agnew private floor and two wards
Eisenlohr private floor	1941	Atop the Agnew-Dulles Building
Agnew-Dulles wing rebuilt	1941	
Neurology moved to neurology building	1942	Old maternity building
Bridge to connect Maloney to neurology	1945	Led from Maloney fourth private floor to Maloney cubicles

(continued)

BUILDING	DATE	COMMENT
Beauty parlor and chapel, third floor Dulles	1948	
Interns' quarters on "long" corridor	1949	
Hospital library	1949	1949 to 1950, library for patients' books on "long" corridor
Medical Alumni Hall, library, admitting room, cafeteria	1952	
Nurses' infirmary moved to orthopaedic ward	1953	
Thomas S. Gates Building	1954	
Chapel moved downstairs under surgical amphitheater	1954	
Diagnostic clinic opened	1954	
Dental clinic opened in Gates	1956	Previously located on second floor, Maloney
"Long" corridor reopened for patients	1957	Ceased to be interns' quarters
Donner radiology building	1958	
Annex for nurses torn down	1958	
Piersol building	1959	
Urology and children's orthopaedic wards demolished	1959	
Nurses' residence moved to English House	1960	
Maloney cubicles renovated to Maloney roomettes	1960	
Clinical research floor	1961	
I. S. Ravdin Pavilion	1962	
Central dispatch established	1964	First patient transport

(continued)

BUILDING	DATE	COMMENT
1st Psychiatric Ward at H.U.P., tenth floor Gates	1965	
Isolation area, fifth floor Maloney	1966	
Maloney Lobby destroyed for Department of Medicine	1966	
Anesthesia Floor added above Eisenlohr	1967	
Eye Ward	1968	
MICU in White Building	1968	
SICU in White Building	1968	
Centrex Building	1969	
Emergency Room renovated	1969	
Cigarette machines removed from H.U.P.	1969	
Children's ward closed	1971	Children's Hospital of Philadelphia moves from downtown to south of H.U.P.
Ravdin Courtyard Building	1973	
Clinical engineering department	1977	
Silverstein Pavilion	1978	
Dental clinic, Silverstein	1978	
Men's and women's medical wards demolished	1983	
Surgical amphitheater became Agnew-Grice Lecture Room	1983	
David Devon MRI Center	1984	
Founders Pavilion	1987	

INDEX

A System of Anatomy (Wistar), 19–20
Abbott, Alexander C. (1860–1935), 124–26
Abbott, William Osler ("Pete") (1902–1943), 216–19
Academy of Natural Sciences, 124, 127
Academy of Philadelphia, 6
Academy of Science meeting to organize the American Medical Association, 40
acetyl CoA, 293
Achilles tendon, repair of, 49
acute contagious diseases, 178
Adams, John (1767–1848), 33
adrenal virilizing hyperplasia, 279
adrenalectomy for high blood pressure, 296–98
Adrian, E. D., 230, 232
Aesculapius, staff of, 3, 205
Agassiz, Louis (1807–1887), 91
Agnew, D. Hayes (1818–1892), 32, 37, 76, 79, 116–18; anatomical school, 39–40; appointed John Rhea Barton Professor, 117; explains blood clotting and bone healing, 117; operation for webbed fingers, 117; surgical instruments developed by, 117; use of eels to clean cadaver bones, 116
The Agnew Clinic (Eakins painting), xv, 117–18, 138
Agnew Pavilion, 146
Allen, Harrison (1841–1897), 68, 83, 91–92; mouth diseases, 92
Allen, Jonathan M., 116
Allen, William M. (1904–   ), 248
Alumni Society (1873), 77
American Argonauts, 60
American Board of Dermatology, 158
American Journal of Medical Sciences, 58, 177
American Journal of Physiology, 23
American Medical Association, 76; committee

on cancer of the uterus, 104; first president, 59; founding of, 40–41; presidents, 77
American Philosophical Society, 32, 98
American Physiological Society, 186
American Tuberculosis Association, 101, 194–95, 198
anaphylactic death (guinea pigs), 132
anatomical amphitheaters, 33
anatomical legislation, 68
anatomical schools, 39–40, 116. *See also* Philadelphia School of Anatomy; Chevat.
Anatomy of the Rat, 130
Anatomy, A System of, 19–20
Anderson, Thomas F. (1911–   ), 237–39, 299; phage studies, 238–39
anesthesiologists (at the University hospital), 267
anesthetics, nonexplosive, 268
animal: care, 148; ligatures, use of, 49; motion, 82
anterior spinal occlusion, 106
antivivisectionist legislation, 148; "Arguments For and Against the Use of Animals for Experimentation," 154; trial, 150
Archer, John (1741–1810), 13
Archiv für Anatomie, 189
Armed Forces Medical Museum, 158
Army Medical Corps, 252
Army-Navy football game, 2, 118
Arsenobenzol (Salvarsan), 180–81
arterial puncture, 155
artery forceps (Agnew) 117
arthritis, 283–84
artificial anus, closure of, 47
artificial respiration, 267
aseptic surgery, 145
Ashton, William, 138

Atlas of Dermatology, 89
Aub, Joseph (1890–1973), 270
Auer, John, 132
Austin, J. Harold (1883–1952), 155
Austrian, Robert (1916–   ), 157
Autumn Course, 70
Auxiliary School of Medicine, 68–70
Avery, Oswald T. (1877–1958), 157
Ayer Clinical Laboratory (Pennsylvania Hospital), 95

bachelor of medicine, 13
Bachman, Carl (1897–   ), 290–91
Baconian science, 11
bacteriology, 125
Ball, Eric G., (1904–1979), 296
ballistocardiograph, 195–96
Banting, Frederick J. (1891–1941), 186
Bard, Samuel (1742–1821), 8, 13
Barnwell, John (1895–   ), 125
Barth, Elizabeth, 220
Barton, Benjamin Smith (1766–1815), 18–19, 59, 115; botanical collector, 18
Barton, John Rhea (1794–1871), 115–16; fracture, 115–16; head bandage, 115; operation for ankylosis, 116; professorship, 78, 100, 115
Barton, Sarah Rittenhouse, 78, 115
Barton, William P. C., 115
Basic Science Correlation Course, 172
Batson, Oscar V. (1894–1979, 244–46; cranial veins, 246; ligation of jugular vein in mastoiditis, 245; vertebral veins, 245
bay chamber to study living tissue, 244
Bayliss, Leonard (1900–1964), 184
Bazett, Henry Cuthbert (1885–1950), 196–98, 230, 264; human temperature regulation, 196–97
Beerman, Herman (1901–   ), 162
Bennett, Mary Alice, 70
Best, Charles, H. (1899–   ), 186
bile, physiology and chemistry of, 254
Billings, John Shaw (1838–1913), 123–25
Birch, William (1755–1834), 32
Black, Joseph, 15
Blakemore, William S. (1920–   ), 297–98
Blockley Hospital, 89
Board of Guardians of the Poor of the City of Philadelphia, 38
Bockus, Henry (1894–1982), 172

Boerhaave, Hermann (1668–1738), 3, 19
Bond, James, 270
Bond, Thomas (1712–1784), 13, 29, 36
Bongiovanni, Alfred M. (1921–1986), 279
botany at Penn, 18
bovine tuberculosis, 212
Bowie, Maurice (1903–   ), 220
Bowman's capsule, puncture of, 183
Boye, Martin, 58
Brady, Ross O. (1923–   ), 292
brain physiology, 272
Brink, Frank, Jr. (1910–   ), 234, 237
Brobeck, John, 221, 268
bromine sensitization of photographic plates, 57–58
Bronk, Detlev W. (1897–1975), 195, 229–32
Brown, Robert B. (1908–1977), 153, 253
Bryan, James, 169
Buchanan, John M. (1917–   ), 292–93
bundle of His, 216
bundle of Kent, 216
Burkett, Dennis, 282; Burkett's lymphoma, 282–83
Bush Hill Hospital, 46
Bush, Vannevar (1890–   ), 231, 261

caduceus, 3, 204–05
Caeserean section, extraperitoneal approach, 49
Caldwell, Charles (1772–1853), 36, 59
cancer, biological properties of cells, 294; mechanism of spread, 294
capillary blood flow, 201
carbon 14 isotopes, 293
carbon dioxide, control of respiration, 266
carbonic anhydrase, 155
Garbutt, John, 99
cardiac clinic, 211
cardiac output (Starr), 194
Carnegie, Andrew, 130; Carnegie Foundation, 167
Carnett, John Berton (1871–1934), 150–51, 153
carotid body, 265
Carson, Joseph (1808–1876), 1, 90
Case, Miss, 220
Castiglione's *History of Medicine,* 177
cells, morphology of living, 243
cerebral circulation, 270

Chambers, Leslie A. (1905–   ), 237, 238, 268

Chambers, Robert (1880–1957), 185, 200

Chambers, Stanley, 159

Chance, Britton (1913–   ), 235, 236–37, 294–96; spectrophotometer, 295–96

Chapman, Nathaniel (1780–1853), 39, 58–60; Swaim's Panacea, 59–60; panel by Mc-Kenzie, 204

Chappel, Charles (1903–1979), 279–281

Charity Hospital (Diagnostic Hospital), 170

cheating scandal, 138

chemical apparatus of Robert Hare, 58

chemical classification of animals (Reichert), 92

chemistry laboratory, Medical Hall, 55

chemotherapy, 2, 177

Chen, K. K., 191–93

Chevat (Chovet), Abraham (1704–1790), anatomical collection of, 39

Chiâri, Hans, 102

childbed fever (puerperal sepsis), management of, 80–82

Children's Hospital of Philadelphia, 277, 284

Chinese drugs, 191–92

cholera studies, 50

Church, John (1774–1806), 36

Churchill, Edward (1895–1977), 251

Clark, Eliot R. (1881–1963), 224, 243–44

Clark, John Goodrich (1867–1927), 46, 102–05; radical cancer operation (Wertheim's operation), 105

Clarkson, Gerardus (1737–1790), 36

climate-controlled room, 186–87

climate chamber to study arthritis pain, 284

clinical clerkships started, 211

Clinical Pharmacology course, 193–94

Cohen, Seymour S. (1917–   ), 279, 299–301

colitis, experimental, 146

College of Physicians of Philadelphia, 46

Collip, James B. (1892–1965), 186

colorimeter, rapid responding for kinetic studies, 295

Coman, Dale Rex (1906–   ), 293–94, 299; Coman report, 301–02

"combination chamber," to study living tissues (E. Clark), 244

committee on medical research, 261

compression chamber, 263

Comroe, Julius (1911–1984), 172–73, 236, 265–66; respiratory research, 265–267

congenital heart disease, 285

containers, individual sealable, 247

convalescent serum for prevention of measles, 246

Cooper, David Alexander (1897–1970), 175

Cooper, David Young III (1924–   ), 267

cordotomy, 108

Corielle, Lewis (1911–   ), 279

Cornelius, Robert, 58

Corner, George W. (1889–1981), 1, 248, 249

corpora albicantia, 102

corpus luteum, 102

Correa de Serra, Abbé José (1750–1823), 20

cortisone, local administration for arthritis, 283–84

Cowell, David (?–1781?), 13

Cox, George S., Institute, 219–21, 249, 278

Coxe, John Redman (1773–1864), 21–22, 23; vaccination, 21; 23

Crick, Francis (1916–   ), 239

Crookes tube, 97–98

Cullen, William (1710–1790), 7, 14

Dale, Henry Hale (1875–1968), 185

Darwin's theory of the origin of species, 92

Davies, Philip W., 234, 237

Davis, J. Stage (1872–1946), 49

Deaver, John Blair (1855–1931), 108–09, 119–21; retractor, 121; aphorisms, 121

Delluva, Adelaide M. (1917–   ), 293

Dercum, Francis X. (1856–1931), 84

dermatology, 157–162; Dermatological Research Laboratory, 158; Duhring's will, 157; Milton Bixby, Hartzell, 157–58, 159; "pest house," 160; John H. Stokes, 159–62; Frederick D. Weidman, 157–59

detoxification of drugs, 183

Diagnostic Hospital, 170

Diasone synthesis, 182

Dick, Elisha Cullen, 59

Discourse (Morgan), 11–12

Dispensary for Skin Diseases, 89

dissolution of lymphatic tissue by mustard gas, 177

divinyl ether, 256

Dixon, Samuel G. (1851–1918), 68, 124

Djerassi, Carl, 249

DNA, 237–38

Dohan, F. C., 220
Donaldson, Henry (1857–1938), 127–29
Dorsey, John Syng (1738–1818), 49, 59–60
Dougherty, T. F., 177
Drinker, Cecil K. (1887–1956), 183
Dripps, Robert D. (1911–1973), 265–68
dual-wave spectrophotometer, 236
ductless glands, 146; and diabetes, 220
duel, last pistol in America, 2
Duffield, Samuel (1732–1814), 13
Duhring, Louis (1845–1913), 89–90, 157, 158, 178; *Atlas of Dermatology*, 89; "Duhring's disease," 89; laboratory, 162; will, 157
Dumke, Paul (1911–   ), 270
dusty lungs, 101

Eakins, Thomas (1844–1916), 117–18, 138
Eck's fistula, 146
Edsall, David Lynn (1869–1945), 138–42, 175, 183
Ehrenstein, Maximilian (1899–   ), 241, 249
Einhorn's tube, 217
Eldridge Reeves Johnson Foundation for Medical Physics. *See* Johnson Foundation for Medical Physics
electromyograph, 230
electron microscope, 238
electron-tube potentiometer, 155
Eliason, Eldridge L. (1879–1950), 252–56
Elmer, Jonathan (1745–1817), 13
Elsom, Katherine O'Shea, 216
Enders, John, 278, 279
endocrine disease, 108
endocrinology, pediatric, 279
entrance examinations, 79
Ephedra vulgaris helviticus, 193
epidermal hyperplasia, 159
Episcopal Hospital, 137
Epstein-Barr virus, 282–83
Erb, William (1907–1987), 107, 253
Erdman, William J. (1921–1989), 205
ether, early use of, 50
Evans, Gerald (1900–   ), 220
evolution, 52
extraocular movement, 106

Farris, Edmund J., 130
Fels, Samuel, 176
Fick principle for measuring blood flow, 270
Fitts, William T. (1915–1980), 297

FitzHugh, Thomas (1894–1963), 175, 212
Flacks, Joel, 293
Fleming, Sir Alexander (1881–1955), 261
Ferguson, L. Kracer, 253
Flexner, Abraham (1866–1959), report on medical education for the Carnegie Foundation, 137, 167
Flexner, Simon (1863–1946), 94–95, 125, 142, 154
Flick, John, 252
Flick, Lawrence (1856–1938), 130–131
flies, transmitters of disease, 54
Florey, Howard (1898–   ), 184
Flosdorf, Earl, 246–47
Forbes, William S. (1831–1905), 68
forceps for arresting hemorrhage (Physick), 46
Forster, Robert E., II. (1919–   ), 268
Fothergill, John (1712–1780), 4–7
Fowler, Ward, 236, 268
Fox Chase Cancer Center, 239
Franklin, Benjamin, 5–6
Frazier, Charles Harrison (1870–1936), 107–10, 139–42, 255; conflict with William Spiller, 107; cordotomy for intractable pain, 107–08; gasserian ganglion, 107; importance of research, 110, 150; thyroid, 108–09
Freeman, Norman, 153
freeze-drying process, 247
Friedman, Maurice, 248
frog tumors (carcinoma), 199
Frost, E. H., 98
fungi that cause disease, catalogue of, 158
Fullerton, Humphrey, 13

G.I. Bill and the Graduate School of Medicine, 171
galvanic generation of electricity, 56
Gambel, Clarence, 281
Garfield, James A., Agnew's patient, 117
Garretson, James Edmund, 40
gas, embolic disease, 265
gasserian ganglion resection, 107
gastric digestion, chemistry of, 22
gastric lavage (Physick), 48
gastric pouches, 146
gastrointestinal intubation, 217
Gates, Thomas S. (1873–1948), 222
Gay-Lussac, Joseph Louis (1778–1850), 21
Gelason, Philip, 267
generation potential, 232–233

geology and minerology, 68

Gerhard, William Wood (1809–1872), 60–61, 77; distinguishes typhoid from typhus, 60

Gerstley, Margaret, 220

Geyer, Samuel, 148

Gibbon, John Heysham (1903–1973), 153, 201, 249–252; heart-lung machine, 251–252

Gibson, Henry, 73

Gibson Pavilion, 73

Gibson, William (1788–1868), 50, 54–55

Gilman, Alfred (1908–   ), 177

Gleason, Philip, 267

Glenn, Elizabeth, 254

glomerula fluid analysis, 185–86

Goddard, David R. (1908–1985), 207

Goddard, John, 58

Goddard, Paul Beck (1811–1866), 57–58; bromine sensitizing method for photography, 57–58

Gohn, Anton, 133; Gohn's complex (tuberculosis), 133

Goldberger, Joseph (1874–1929), 179

Goldschmidt, Samuel, 254

gonadotrophin, purification of, 290

Goodell, William (1829–1894), 76, 80–82; gynecological instruments invented by, 81

Goodman, Louis, 177

Goodspeed, Arthur W. (1860–1943), 97–100, 101

gorget to enter bladder (Physick), 46

Graduate Hospital, 122, 178–79, 247

Graduate School of Medicine, waves of prosperity and disappointment, 171–73

Graham, Clarence, 233

Graham, James D., 247

Granit, Ragnar (1900–   ), 232

Grant, Francis (1891–1967), 107

grave robbing, Shippen accused, 18

gray rat *(Epimys norvegicus)*, 128

Great Windmill Street Anatomical School, 39

Green, Eunice Chase (1895–1975), 130

Greenman, Milton Jay, 127

Griffiths, John Q. (1904–1977), 296

Griffiths, Samuel Powell (1759–1826), 18

Gross Clinic, The (Eakins), 117–18

Gross, Samuel David (1805–1884), 40, 117, 177

Guiteras, Juan (1852–1925), 94, 96, 125

Gurin, Samuel (1905–   ), 290–93

Hafkenshiel, Joseph (1916–   ), 297

Hales, Stephen (1667–1761), 200

Hare Building, 146

Hare, Horace Binney (?–1879), 68

Hare, Robert (1781–1858), 23, 55–58; "deflagrator," 57; oxygen-hydrogen blowpipe, 57; second-class faculty member, 55–56

Harnwell, Gaylord P., 301

Harrison, Charles Custis (1844–1929), 138–39, 141, 167

Harrison, Emily McMichael (?–1902), 153

Harrison, George Leib (1836–1935), will, 150

Harrison Department of Surgical Research, 150–53

Hartline, Haldan Keffer (1903–1983), 232–34

Hartshorn, Henry, 68

Hartzell, Milton Bixby (1854–1927), 140, 157–58; microphotography, 158

Harvey, William (1578–1657), 200

Hatai, Shinkishi (1876–?), 127

Haugaard, Ella (1922–   ) and Neils Haugaard (1920–   ), 156

Hayden, Ferdinand V., 68

Hayes, Isaac, 41

Heacock, Edward, 205

heart-lung machine, 251

heart sounds, study of mechanism of production, 214–15

Heilbrunn, Lewis V. (1892–1959), 207

hemoglobin crystals, 92

hemopholus influenza, 198

Henderson, Yandell (1873–1944), 195

Henle, Gertrude (1912–1987) and Werner Henle (1920–1987), 278, 281–83; "interference phenomenon," 281

Henry, Joseph (1797–1878), 56, 58

hepatitis, investigation of, 200

Hershey-Chase experiment, 239

Heymans, Joseph, 193, 250

high-altitude chamber, 263

Hill, A. V. (1903–1941), 219–20, 230

His, Wilhelm (1831–1904), 103

"history rounds," 1, 2

Hittorf tube, 97

Hodge, Hugh Lenox (1796–1873), 70

Hodgkin's disease, 101

Hoeber, Rudolph O. A. (1873–?), 207, 269

Hollander, Joseph L. (1910–   ), 283–84; climate chamber to study arthritis, 284

Holmes, Oliver Wendell (1809–1894), 60, 81

hookworm, 54

Hopkinson, Mary (1905–1986), 249–52; heart-lung machine, 250

Horner, William E. (1793–1853), 33, 49–51, 58, 61, 127; anatomical discoveries, 51; extraperitioneal approach for a Caesarean section, 49; pathology discoveries, 50; tensor tarsi muscle, 49; Z-plasty, 50

horse, foot position while running, 82–83

horseshoe crab, 233

Horvath, Steven, 283

Horwitz, Orville (1909–   ), 195, 235

Hospital of the University of Pennsylvania, 70–76, 84, 88, 119, 145, 148, 205, 225; first wave of additions, 73–76; medical faculty vs. clinical faculty, 76; Pepper proposes, 71–73

Houssay, Bernard (1887–1971), 221

Huger, Francis Kenlock (1773–1855), 204

Hunter, John (1728–1793), 7, 14, 46

Hunter, William (1729–1777), 7, 14, 39

Hutchinson, James H. (1834–1889), 23

Hygiene, School of, 123–27; Abbott and, 124–26; Billings, John Shaw, 123–26; fund-raising for, 123–24; wavering support from trustees, 126–27

Hyoscyamus Niger, 18

IBM, 252

industrial hazards, 101

infectious diseases, 123

infectious mononucleosis, 283

influenza pandemic, 198

influenza vaccine (Austrian), 281

instantaneous photographs, 58

Institute for Environmental Medicine, 263

Institute for the Study of Venereal Diseases, 160

insulin action, 156–57

isolette, development of, 279–80

Itzkowitz, Harold, 297

Ives Herbert, 205

Ivey, Robert (1881–1974), 205

Jackson, David (? –1801), 13

Jackson, James (1777–1868), 60

Jackson, Samuel (1787–1872), 58; panel by McKenzie, 204

Jacobs, Merkel (1884–1970), 200, 205–07, 255

James, Thomas Chalkley (1766–1835), 22, 36, 39, 59

Jeffers, William, 296

Jefferson, Thomas, 21

Jefferson Medical College, 37, 89; near-merger, 168

Jenner, Edward (1749–1823), 178

Jennings, William N. (1860–1945), 97–99

John Morgan Building, 119, 145

John Morgan Society, 138

John Rhea Barton Professor of Surgery. *See* Barton, John Rhea

Johns Hopkins Hospital, 103, 123, 137

Johns, Richard J. (1925–   ), 267

Johnson Foundation for Medical Physics, 229–39, 268–69, 294–96

Johnson, Eldridge Reeves, 229

Johnson, Julian (1906–1987), 109, 153, 253, 255

Joyner, Claude (1925–   ), 270

Keen, William Williams (1837–1932), 40 67

Kelley, Howard A. (1858–1943), 102

Kent, A. F. Stanley (1863–?), 216

Kern, Richard (1891–1982), 212

Kety, Seymour (1915–   ), 172, 270–72

King, Helen Dean (1869–1955), 127

Kinnersly, Ebenezer, 13

Kirby, Charles K., 269

Kirby, E. R. (1865–1935), 138

Kitasato Institute of Infectious Diseases, 95

Kite, Anna S., 205

Klaer, Fred H. (1878–1915), 212

Koch, Robert (1843–1910), 132, 133

Kolmer, John (1896–1962), 179

Koop, C. Everett (1916–   ), 279

Koprowsky, Hilary (1916–   ), 130

Krumbhaar, Edward Bell (1882–1966), 176–78, 195, 212; precursor discovery to chemotherapeutic agents, 177; invents names, 177

Kuhn, Adam (1741–1817), 13–14, 28, 29, 36, 39, 45

labor, artificial induction of, 22

Laboratory for Dermatological Research, 162

Laboratory of Hygiene, 146

Lackman, David (1911–   ), 238

lactic acid formation, 219

Lambertsen, Christian J. (1917–   ), 263–

65; Institute for Environmental Medicine, 265

Landis, Eugene M. (1901–1987), 200–02, 251; physiology of blood circulation, 200–01

Lankanau Surgical Clinic, 121

Larrey, Dominique Jean (1766–1842), 51

Latrobe, Benjamin Henry (1764–1820), 33

Lavoisier, Antoine Laurent, 21

Lawrence, James Valentine O'Brion, 39

Lawrence, John, 13

Lea, Henry C. (1825–1909), 123–24, 126

Lehr, Herndon B. (1923–1979), 198

Leidy, Joseph (1823–1891), 51–54, 67, 91, 117; discovers *Trichina spiralis*, 54; speculates on origin of life, 52–53; medallium by McKenzie, 204

Leonard, Charles Lester (1861–1913), 100–01

Leopold, Charles, and Simon S. Leopold (1892–1957), first air-conditioned room in a hospital, 186–87

Levis, Richard J. (1827–1890), 40

Lewis, Paul A. (1879–1929), 132

Lewis, Sir Thomas (1881–1945), 213

light sensitivity, color vision, 232

Lilly, John C., 235–37

Lindauer, August (1906–1972), 296–97, 298

Linneaus, Carolus (1707–1778), 14

lithotomy, 46

Livingood, Clarence (1911–   ), 161

Livingston, A. E. (1883–?), 184

Lombard (of Geneva), 60

Long, Crawford, 204

Long, Cyril Norman Hugh (1901–1970), 219–21

Long, Esmond R., 133–34

Lucké, Balduin (1889–1954), 198–200, 254; Lucké carcinoma, 199

Ludlow, John Livingston (1819–1888), 38

Ludwig, George D., 268–69

Lukens, Francis D. W. (1899–1978), 219, 221, 278, 297

Luria, Salvatore (1912–   ), 238

Lusk, Graham, 97

lyophilizer, 247

Ma huang, 192

Mackenzie, Colin, 7

MacLeod, Colin M., 157

Makepeace, A. W., 248

Maloney, Martin, 212

Maloney Clinic, 154, 211–13, 229

malonyl CoA, 293

Malphigi, Marcello (1628–1694), 200

manikin for practice of intravenous injections, 162

Maragliano, Edoardo (1849–1940), 132

Marshall, John (1755–1835), Chief Justice of the United States, 46, 138

Marshall, John (1855–1925), dean of the medical school, 78, 139

Martin, Edward B. (1859–1938), 108, 119; inkstand with bullet hole, 119

mask for artificial respiration, 267

materia medica, 2, 13

maternity ward, 73

Maury, Francis Fontaine (1840–1879), 89

Maxwell, James Clerk (1831–1879), 45

McAllister, Robert M. (1922–   ), 279

McCarthy, Daniel J. (1874–1958), 137

McClintock, James (1809–1881), 39

McCollum, Robert, 283

McKenzie, R. Tait (1867–1938), 202–05; sculpture, 204–05; caduceus, 204

McMichael, Morton (1807–1879), 71

Medical Hall, of various dates, 33, 138

Medical Inquiries and Observations upon Diseases of the Mind (Rush), 17

medical jurisprudence, 65

Medico-Chirurgical College, 198

Meldrum, Andrew N. (1876–1934), 155

Mendel, Lafayette (1872–1935), 97

Merck Chemical Company, 254

Mercurochrome, 187

Mercury, staff of, 3, 204–05

menopause, cause of early, 103

Meyer, Adolf (1866–1950), 128

microchemical techniques, 186

microchemistry, 93; of poisons, 93

micromanipulator, 200

microscope observation chambers to study living cells, 244

Miller, T. Grier (1886–1981), 171, 193, 212, 216–19; relief of intestinal obstructions, 217–19

Miller, William, 285

Miller-Abbott tube, 218–19

Millikan, Glenn, 236–37

Mills, Charles K. (1881–1931), 105

Mitchell, John McKay, 172

Mitchell, S. Weir (1829–1914), 67, 79, 93, 96, 141; specialized hospitals, 67
Monod, Jacques (1910–1976), 299
Monroe, Alexander (secundus) (1717–1813), 7, 48
Montgomery, Hugh (1904–   ), 201, 235, 251
morbid anatomy, 70
Morehouse, George R. (1829–1908), 67
Morgan, John (1735–1789), 6–9, 11–15; *Discourse*, 11–12, 222
Morris, Benjamin, 6, 12
Morton, Harry (1906–1988), 238
mouth-to-mouth artificial respiration, 267
"Mrs. O'Flaherty," 80
Mudd, Stuart (1893–1975), 238, 246–47, 281; freeze-drying process, 246–47
mumps vaccine, 278
Musser, John Herr (1883–1947), 153, 155
mustard gas, 177
Muybridge, Eadweard (1830–1904), 82–84, 92; medical faculty join him, 84
mycological preparations, 158

Neefe, John R., 216
Neil, John, 76
neurology, 105; clinics, 84
neuropathology laboratory, 109
neurotropic viruses, 281
New York State Medical Society, 40
Nicholson, Jessie (1903–1987), 284
Niederman, James, 283
nitrous oxide to measure cerebral blood flow, 270–72
Noguchi, Hideyo (1876–1928), 95–96
norprogesterone (10-norprogesterone), 249
Norris, Charles C. (1878–1961), 104
Norris, George W. (1808–1875), 60
Norris, William F., 76
North American (newspaper), 71
Nuttall, Thomas, 20
Nylin, Josef B. (1874–1945), 205

O'Brien, Helen, 155
obstetrical forceps, 187; leg holders, 187
obstetricians, 80–82
Ogden, Bertha and Henrietta, 148–50
Opie, Eugene L. (1873–1971), 95, 132–33
orchectomy for prostatic hypertrophy, 118
origin of life, 52

orthopaedic surgery, 145
Osborne, William, 46
Osler, Georgiana, 217
Osler, William (1849–1919), 60, 87–89, 94, 103, 175
osmotic pressure experiments, 239
otologist, 245
outpatient department, Hospital of the University of Pennsylvania, 211
Owen, Richard (1804–1892), 54
oxygen, chamber for treating pneumonia, 155; high partial pressures, 263; tension in tissues, 234; toxicity, 156; oxygen-hydrogen blowpipe (Hare), 2
oxygenator (heart-lung machine), 252

pH measurements, 155
Paget, Sir James (1814–1899), 54
Pancoast, Henry K. (1875–1939), 101; tumors, 101
Pancoast, Joseph, 50
Pasteur Institute (Paris), 299
patent ductus arteriosus, 286
Pathological Museum (Pennsylvania Hospital), 9
pathology, 94–97, 140; Pepper Laboratory, 80
Pearce, Richard M. (1874–1930), 154–55, 176
pediatric surgery, 279
Pemberton, James (1723–1809), 7
Pendergrass, Eugene (1895–1980), 101
penicillin: treatment of syphilis, 160; in oil, 182; production of, 261–262
Penniman, Josiah, 222
Pennock, Caspar Wistar (1801–1886), 60, 77
Pennsylvania Dental College, 40
Pennsylvania Gazette (Franklin), 5, 12
Pennsylvania Hospital, 5–6, 13, 60, 95
Penrose, R. A. F. (1827–1908), 76, 80
Pepper Laboratory, 80, 100, 105, 141, 153
Pepper, Oliver Hazzard Perry (1884–1962), 11
Pepper, William, Sr., 80, 171
Pepper, William, Jr. (1843–1898), 77–79, 126–27, 133, 139; founding of University hospital, 70–73
Pepper, William III (1874–1947), 159, 264
Perry, Robert (of Glasgow), 60
"pest house" (dermatology), 160
Peter Bent Brigham Hospital, 185
phage, biochemistry of, 299–300; connection to host, 239; separation of DNA from, 239

pharmacology, 2
Pharmacy, Philadelphia College of, 21
Philadelphia Almshouse, 36, 60, 70; residents resign, 37
Philadelphia Dispensary, 18
Philadelphia Dissecting Rooms, 39
Philadelphia General Hospital, 89, 106, 116–18, 172, 175
Philadelphia School of Anatomy, 39, 116, 170
Philadelphia School of Operative Surgery, 116
Philosophical Hall, 32
Phipps Institute, 130–34; first sites unsavory, 131–32; Lawrence Flick, 130–32; Paul Lewis, 132; Esmond Long, 133–34; Eugene Opie, 132–33; Henry Phipps, 130; Mazyck Ravenel, 132
physical medicine and rehabilitation, 205
physical therapy (department), 212
Physick, Philip Syng (1768–1837), 45–49; absorbable sutures, 48; closed an artifical anus, 47; new bougies, 46
physiology: chair, 19, general course, 207
Piersol, George Arthur (1856–1924), 243
Piersol, George Morris (1880–1966), 205
Pillsbury, Donald M. (1902–1980), 162
Pincus, Gregory (1903–1967), 247
Piper, Edmund B. (1881–1931), 187–88
Plant, Oscar (1875–1939), 184
plastic surgery, 198
pneumoconiosis, 101
poisons, microchemistry of, 93
poliomyelitis, research on, 95
Polyclinic College for Graduates in Medicine, 179
Polyclinic Hospital, 105
potassium, isolation of, 21
Potts, Jonathan, 13
Potts, Sir Percival (1714–1788), 7
precordial electrocardiogram, 215
"preliminary course," 70
Preston Retreat, 80–81, 82
Prevost, Harriet C. (18?–1912), 153–54
Priestley, Joseph (1833–1904), 20
Pritchett, Henry (1857–1939), 167–168
"Problems of the Professional Guinea Pig," 217
prostatic obstruction, treatment of, 46
public health, 68, 123
pulmonary artery studies (Gibbon), 250
pulmonary diffusion capacity, 268
pulmonary embolism, 251

Pupin, Michael (1858–1935), 98
purified protein derivative (PPD), 133
purine molecule (origin of atoms), 292

Quinn, Dorothy, 220

Radio Corporation of America, 238
radioisotopes as metabolic tracers, 291
radiology, 101
radium to treat uterine carcinoma, 104
Raiziss, George (1884–1945), 179, 182
Rashkind, William J. (1922–   ), 284–286
rat: albino, 128; breeding (Wistar Institute), 127
Ravdin, Isidore S. (1894–1972), 80, 108, 150–53, 252, 254–257, 267; expert on the liver, 254; 20th General Hospital, 255–56
Ravenel, Mazyck Porcher (1861–1946), 132
Rawson, A. R., 195
reaction kinetics, 295
Read, Charles, 191
Red Cross Base Hospital No. 20, 150
Redman, John (1722–1808), 6, 14
Reese, John J., 68
Reichert, Edward Tyson (1855–1931), 84, 92–93, 196; chemical proof of Darwin's theory of evolution, 92–93; snake venom, 93
Reid, John, 270
Reis, Emil (1865–?), 104
Reivich, Martin, 272
research medicine, 153–57
respiratory pigments, oxidation reduction, 236
respiratory control, hydrogen ion concentration, 265
Retrospectroscope (Comroe), 267
Review of Scientific Instruments, 237
Reyes syndrome, 281
Rhoads, Jonathan E. (1907–   ), 153, 257, 279
Rhodes, Edward, 70
Richards, Alfred Newton (1876–1966), 140, 191, 199, 249, 261; how the kidney makes urine, 183–86; microtechniques developed, 186; World War II effort, 261–63
Richards, T. W., 73
Richards-Miller report, 170–71, 222–24
Richardson, Joseph G., 68
Ricketts, Howard Taylor (1871–1910), 140
rickettsia, structure of, 238
Riesman, David (1867–1940), 175–76

Robbins, Frederick C., 278
Roberts, John B., 170
Robinette, Edward B., 214
Robinette Foundation, 214
Robinson, George (1878–19?), 138
Rock, John (1890–19?), 247
Rockefeller Foundation, 126
Rockefeller Institute, 182
rocket motors, precursor, 57
Roentgen, Wilhelm Konrad (1845–1923), 99
roentgenology, 101
Rogers, Robert E. (1813–1884), 67, 78
Rose, Edward (1898–1987), 212
Rosemond, George, 297
Rosenthal, Otto (1898–1980), 137, 252–53
Roughton, F. J. W. (1899–1972), 155
Rush, Benjamin (1745–1813), 14–18, 29, 36,
    39, 46; improves an insane ward, 17; psy-
    chology of the mind, 17; bloodletting, 18
Rush, William, 19

Saint George's Hospital, 46
Saint Joseph's Hospital, 38, 51, 71
Sakami, Warwick (1916–   ), 292
Salvarsan, 180; litigation, 178
Saubourad, Raymond, 158
Sayen, John (1914–   ), 235
Schamberg, Jay Frank (1870–1934), 178–82;
    Arsenobenzol, synthesis of Salvarsan, 179–
    82; Dermatological Research Laboratories,
    179–182; Schamberg's disease (progressive
    pigmentary dermatosis), 178
Schlumberger, Hans, 200
Schmidt, Carl F. (1893–1988), 184, 191–93,
    265–66, 270; ephedrine brought to the
    United States, 193
Schnabel, Truman G., Jr., 195
School of Medicine, appropriate education for
    teachers in, 23; basic sciences vs. practical
    medicine, 68–70; buildings early in the 20th
    century, 145–46; cheating scandal, 138–39;
    clinical teaching, 35–38; curricular reform,
    76–78; division during the Revolution, 29–
    32; early buildings, 32–35; David Edsall,
    139–42; entrance examinations, 79; exami-
    nations behind a screen, 35; first courses,
    12; first degrees, 13; first plan, 7; four-year
    course, 78–79; Frazier's contentious reforms,
    139–42; medical faculty vs. clinical faculty,
    76; mergers with local medical schools and
    hospitals, 167–70; reorganized administra-
    tion, 222; Richards-Miller report, 222–25
Schwann, Herman (1915–   ), 269–70
Scientific Research, United States Office of,
    231, 261
Seibert, Florence, 133
Semmelweiss, Ignaz (1818–1865), 82
serum, preservation of, 246
seton, for treating fractures, 48–49
Shattuck, George C. (1845–1923), 60
Shattuck, Lemuel, 60
Shigella flexneri, 94
Shippen, William (1736–1808), 6–9, 12, 14,
    15
Silliman, Benjamin (1779–1864), 55
single-fiber nerve impulses, measurement of,
    230
smallpox vaccine, 21
Smith, Allen John (1863–1926), 96–97, 140,
    142, 158
Smith, Edgar Fahs (1854–1928), 21, 58, 141,
    mergers proposed and made, 167–170
Smith, Henry Hollingsworth (1815–1890), 38,
    61–62; treatments for nonunited fractures,
    61
Smith, William (1727–1803), 13
snake venom studies, 93
Sokoloff, Louis (1921–   ), 272
Sonne, John, 293
Spaltzholz, Werner, 103
spectrophotometer, dual wavelength, 295
Spiller, William G. (1863–1940), 105–08; con-
    flict with C. H. Frazier, 107; cordotomy for
    intractable pain, 107–08; vascular occlusion
    of the brain stem, 106
spinal anesthesia, 268
spinal cord, location of pain tracts in, 117
spinal headaches, 268
spinal trauma, 150
spontaneous generation, 52
"spring course," 70
Stadie, William C., 155–57; buffering capacity
    of hemoglobin, 155; insulin action, 157; ox-
    ygen toxicity, 156; potentiometer, 155; Sta-
    die-Riggs tissue slicer, 156
Stanley, Wendel M. (1904–1971), 236
starch crystals, 92
Starr, Isaac (1895–1989), 193–96; ballistocar-
    diograph, 194–96
Stelwagen, Henry, 158

Stengel, Alfred (1868–1939), 140–41, 175, 210, 222, 229; Maloney Clinic, 211–212
Stevens, Lloyd, 253
Stillé, Alfred (1813–1900), 60, 76, 77, 87
Stokes, John Hinchman (1885–1961), 159–61; circus, 161
Stokes, Joseph (1896–1972), 216, 277–79
Stokes, T. Lane, 252
Stokes–McCloud gauges, 247
Strawbridge, George, 76
streptomycin (tuberculosis), 133
Strickland, William, 33, 55
Struthers, Francis, 269
sulfa drugs, synthesis, 182; sulfapyrazene, 178; sulfathiozolaline, 178
Summer Medical Association, 70
superior sulcus tumors (Pancoast) 101
Surgeon's Hall, 20, 32; "elaboratory," 19
surgical research, 146–53
Sutnick, A. (1928–), 297, 298
Swaim's Panacea, 59–60
Sweet, J. Edwin (1876–1957), 118, 146–150; research contributions, 146–48; vivisectionist attack and trial, 148–50
syphilis, experimental, 182

Target, John D. (1868–?), 138
Taylor, Alonzo, E. (1871–1975), 140
Taylor, Ivan B., 267
telegraph, 21
temperature control studies, 196–97
tensor tarsi muscle (Horner), 49
Thénard, Louis Jacques (1777–1857), 21
Theorell, Hugo (1903–1982), 295
thymine formation, cell death from inhibition of, 300
thyroid service, 108
tuberculosis, studies to prevent, 130
tic douloureux, 107
Tilton, James (1745–1822), 13
Topping, Norman (1908–), 172
toxicology, 93
Treatise on Pathological Anatomy, 50, 51
Treatise on Special and General Anatomy, 51
Trichina spiralis, discovery in breakfast ham, 54
Trichophyton interdigitale, 159
trustees, 12, 22
tuberculin, purification of, 133

tuberculosis drugs (ethambutolil, isoniazid, rifampiin, streptomycin), 133
20th General Hospital, 255, 267
typhoid, 60, 77
typhus, 60
Tyson, James (1841–1919), 70, 87, 125, 140

ultrasound, 269
Undergraduate Medical Association, 104–05
urethral obstruction and catheters, 46
urology, 2
uterine cancer, 103

vaccination, 21
vaccines, development of, 130
vacuum systems, 247
van Leeuwenhoek, Antony (1632–1723), 200
Vandam, Leroy (1914–), 268
Vars, Harry M. (1903–1983), 97, 254
venereal disease (syphilis), 160
vertebral veins, 244–46
Victor Talking Machine Company, 229
viral-produced carcinoma, 199
Virchow, Rudolf (1821–1902), 108
virology, 281
vision, mechanism of, 233; physiology, 232
vocal membrane, 51
von Bergman, Ernst (1836–1907), 108
von Furth, Otto, 97
von Hebra, Ferdinand Hans (1816–1880), 89
von Humboldt, Friedrich Heinrich Alexander (1769–1859), 20

Walker, Arthur (1896–1955), 184
Warburg respirometry, 252
Ward K, 105
Waterhouse, Benjamin, 21
Watson, James (1928–), 239
Watson, Thomas J., 252
Way, Nicholas (??–1793 or 1797), 13
Wearn, Joseph (1893–), 185
weather and arthritis, 287
Weidman, Frederick D. (1881–1956), 157; studies or xanthoma, 159
Weidner, P. A. B., 179
Weinstein, George L. (1908–1988), 247–48
Welch, William Henry (1850–1934), 94, 124–26
welding, gas and electric origin, 57

Wertheim, Ernst, operation for uterine cancer, 104

Whipple, Allen O., 256

Whipple, George H. (1878–1976), 140

Whitaker, W. C., 220

white blood cells, pathology of, 177

White Haven Sanitorium, 130, 131

White, C. Y., 137

White, J. William (1850–1916), 79, 100, 118–119, 138–39, 202, 253; last pistol duel in America, 118; orchectomy, 118–19; use of X-rays, 118

Williams, Horace, 216

Wilson, David Wright (1889–1965), 289–93

Winegrad, Albert, 219

Wistar Institute 127–30; albino rat, 127–30; collection, 127; Henry Donaldson, 127–29; Hilary Koprowsky, 130

Wistar, Caspar (1761–1818), 19–20; first American textbook on anatomy, 19–20; Wistar parties, 20

Wistar, Isaac J., 127

wisteria, 20

Wolff-Parkinson-White syndrome, 216

Wolferth, Charles C. (1887–1965), 212–16, 295–98

Women's Medical College, 40, 167

Wood, Francis Clark (1901–   ), 215–16

Wood, General Leonard (1860–1927), 222

Wood, George B. (1797–1879), 68, 76

Wood, Horatio C (1841–1920), 68, 79, 88, 90–91; *A Treatise on Therapeutics*, 91

Wood, Mrs. Richard D., 73

Woodhouse, James (1770–1809), 20–21, 23, 55; experimental chemist, 20–21

Wormley, Theodore G. (1826–1897), 93–94; early toxicologist, 93; microanalytical techniques, 93; wife did plates for his textbook, 94

Wyatt, George R., 299

X-rays, 97–101; burns, 100; first, 98; to treat Hodgkin's disease, 101; to see anatomy, 100, 245

yellow fever, 17, 23, 96

Young, John Richardson (1782–1804), 22; food digestion, 22

Z-plasty, 49

Zenker, Albert, 54

Zirkle, Raymond E., 237

Zintel, Harold, 298